PRODUCTIVE AGING

AN OCCUPATIONAL PERSPECTIVE

T0343268

PRODUCTIVE AGING

AN OCCUPATIONAL PERSPECTIVE

Marilyn B. Cole, MS, OTR/L, FAOTA

Professor Emerita of Occupational Therapy

Quinnipiac University

Hamden, Connecticut

Karen C. Macdonald, PhD, OTR/L

Adjunct Professor of Occupational Therapy

Sacred Heart University

Fairfield, Connecticut

Housatonic Community College

Bridgeport, Connecticut

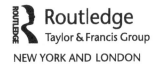

Routledge
Taylor & Francis Group

NEW YORK AND LONDON

Marilyn B. Cole and Karen C. Macdonald have no financial or proprietary interest in the materials presented herein.

First published in 2015 by SLACK Incorporated

Published 2024 by Routledge
605 Third Avenue, New York, NY 10158

and by Routledge
4 Park Square, Milton Park, Abingdon, Oxon OX14 4RN

Routledge is an imprint of the Taylor & Francis Group, an informa business

© 2015 Taylor & Francis Group.

Library of Congress Cataloging-in-Publication Data

Cole, Marilyn B., 1945- , author.
  Productive aging : an occupational perspective / Marilyn B. Cole, Karen C. Macdonald.
    p. ; cm.
  Includes bibliographical references and index.
  ISBN 978-1-61711-077-1 (alk. paper)
  I. Macdonald, Karen C. (Karen Crane), author. II. Title.
  [DNLM: 1. Aging. 2. Occupational Therapy. 3. Aged. 4. Quality of Life. 5. Retirement. WB 555]
  RA776.75
  613--dc23
                    2015003428

ISBN: 9781617110771 (hbk)
ISBN: 9781003525981 (ebk)

DOI: 10.4324/9781003525981

DEDICATION

This book is dedicated to four of our participants who have passed away during the course of this 3-year project. All of them died in Laslett's Third Age, meaning in the midst of living a full and productive life. Isn't that what we all want for ourselves and those we love?

Patricia (Figure 1) died suddenly of a stroke in December 2012. At age 91, it was not her first, but she had recovered most of her functioning from the previous one. She still functioned independently, attending activities and classes at the retirement community where she lived, staying in touch with her family, and volunteering regularly. She had just completed writing a memoir of her time living in India, which her family is having published as a tribute to her life.

Ken (Figure 2) came home from a train trip to visit his daughter in Philadelphia one weekend in 2013, ate a late supper with his wife, and died suddenly of a massive heart attack. He'd had heart disease for over 10 years, and took measures to minimize the risk, not only with surgery and medication, but also by running, exercising at a gym, and eating a healthier diet. The university where he taught had to find someone to take over his classes. His wife had to hire workers to complete his home repair projects; she took over the care of his tropical fish. Ken died in the midst of living a full and productive life.

Johanna (Figure 3) practiced law from her hospital bed. She was still signing papers, editing documents, and talking with clients on the phone 2 days before her death. At age 73, she lost her 2-year battle with ovarian cancer in December 2013. Much of her time was also donated to community organizations. She was a devoted mother and grandmother. All of her grandchildren spoke at her wake of the hours she had spent caring for them, teaching and inspiring them. At her funeral service, the church was packed with hundreds of people she had helped and befriended.

Suzy (Figure 4) died peacefully in her own home at age 98. She lived alone, took good care of her house and yard, and drove a car. She continued to enjoy cooking, baking and craft activities, and she participated in many social organizations until the week before her death. With the help of friends and family, Suzy was able to successfully age in place.

The authors thank these four who died, and all of the 36 living participants in our Productive Aging Study, for their generosity in sharing valued life lessons, their courage in taking charge of their own aging, and their many recommendations and examples. Their skills in self-management, sustaining social connections, and engaging in self-fulfilling activities gave us the inspiration to write this book.

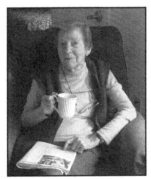

Figure 1. Patricia.

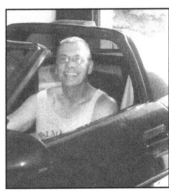

Figure 2. Kenneth McGeary, June 5, 1944-March 2, 2013.

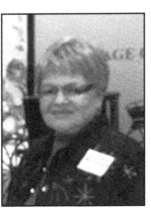

Figure 3. Johanna.

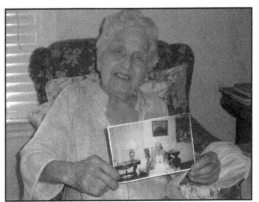

Figure 4. Suzy.

Contents

ACKNOWLEDGMENTS

I would like to thank my OT colleagues, many of whom contributed to the Productive Aging Study as both advisors and participants. My colleagues at Quinnipiac University continue to inspire me, and enable me to continue doing research through an interdisciplinary grant. Recognition also goes to my OT masters students over the years, who always taught me as much as I taught them. A special thanks to Quinnipiac University professor Martha Sanders for contributing some original writing from her own research and teaching materials to the chapter on the older worker. My connections with Baldwin Senior Center in Stratford afforded me a place to introduce fieldwork students to the joys of geriatric practice with well-elderly, who impressed them with their fitness and active lifestyles, and the upbeat setting of the CARES adult day program. My thanks to Diane Puterski, director at Baldwin, and Erin McLeod, director at CARES, for their interview information. The American Occupational Therapy Association has also offered encouragement for authors, like Karen and I, to explore uncharted waters of wellness and community practice, and given us documents such as the Centennial Vision (AOTA, 2007) that support and validate the emerging practice area of productive aging.

Finally, a big thank you to Karen, my co-author, who expertly led me through the complexities of qualitative research and collaborated with me so enthusiastically throughout the long process of writing this book.

Marilyn B. Cole

I would like to express my appreciation to my family and friends who have offered inspiration and support through all my years enjoying a career in occupational therapy. At Quinnipiac University, the University of Bridgeport, and New York University, professors offered guidance and support for learning and professional growth. Working at the Jewish Home for the Elderly introduced me to my love for geriatric occupational therapy, and I am indebted to them for their willingness to encourage creative avenues for occupational therapist roles. I wish to thank Laurie Wallace, OTR/L, who saved my functional life. My students at Housatonic Community College and Sacred Heart University, through their excitement to learn, promote my own ongoing growth. I thank Marli Cole for inviting me to join in this opportunity to explore exciting possibilities for roles of OTs related to productive aging. I am grateful to the participants who embraced the importance of this topic, and contributed their time and thoughts so generously. I thank my husband, Geno Piacentini, who listens, offers feedback on yet another project, and joins with me in sharing so many occupations that define our fully-lived life.

For contributions to this book, I would like to thank the following occupational therapy colleagues who generously offered their expertise and opinions: Dr. Jody Bortone, Dr. Estelle Breines, Janice Conway, Dr. Liz Lannigan, Dr. Mary Ellen Johnson, Dr. Rosalie Miller, Ellen Rabinowitz, Mickey Reed, Dr. Pam Story, and Laurie Wallace. I would also like to thank Louise Norrell, Carol Fox, and Dorothy Crofut for sharing insights regarding their personal experiences with caring for older adults. Appreciation is extended to Betsy Bowen and her assistant for their highly skilled work with word processing.

Karen C. Macdonald

REFERENCE

American Occupational Therapy Association. (2007). AOTA's Centennial Vision and executive summary. *American Journal of Occupational Therapy, 61,* 613-614.

ABOUT THE AUTHORS

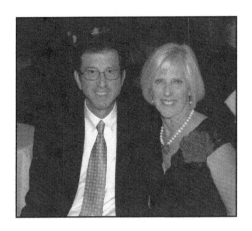

Marilyn B. Cole, MS, OTR/L, FAOTA began her occupational therapy career in mental health, creating programs for inpatient psychiatry at Eastern Pennsylvania Psychiatric Institute in Harrisburg, Pennsylvania and Middlesex Hospital in Middletown, CT, and mental health day treatment at Lawrence and Memorial Hospitals in New London, CT. Throughout her part-time and full-time teaching at Quinnipiac University, beginning in 1982, she continued to practice and also train students at the West Haven VA Hospital, and consulted at Fairfield Hills Hospital in Newtown, CT.

To expand her knowledge, she became certified in Sensory Integration, and for 3 years, practiced in pediatrics at the Newington Children's Hospital and worked with children in surrounding public school systems. Her education includes a bachelor of arts in English from the University of Connecticut, a year of art education at Rhode Island School of Design, a graduate certificate in Occupational Therapy from the University of Pennsylvania, and a master's in Clinical Psychology from the University of Bridgeport. Beginning in the 1990s, Marli consulted and also trained students at St. Joseph's Manor, a long-term care facility in Trumbull, CT.

After retiring from full-time teaching at Quinnipiac for 25 years, and practicing OT in mental health, pediatrics, and geriatrics, Marli has written four textbooks: *Applied Theories in OT: A Practical Approach* (with Roseanna Tufano, 2008), *Social Participation in Occupational Contexts* (with Mary Donohue, 2010), *Group Dynamics in OT*, 4th Edition (2012), and the current one, *Productive Aging: An Occupational Perspective*.

Throughout her professional career, Marli has regularly presented at local, national, and international conferences (Melbourne, London, Montreal, Stockholm, Sydney) and has supervised student experiences in England, Costa Rica, and Australia. She has completed research studies in sensory integration, mental health assessment, time management, therapeutic relationships, group size and cohesiveness, and with students, created training videos for Donohue's Social Profile. She currently holds an interdisciplinary grant from Quinnipiac University with physical therapist Professor Russell Woodman, DPT, for which she educates patients with lower back pain with a self-management program entitled "Protecting Your Back." Some of the photos from that program appear in the chapter on self-management.

Marli and husband, Marty Schiraldi, enjoy sailing, cruising, and visiting with their five children and eight grandchildren. They are at home in Stratford, CT and Freeport, Bahamas.

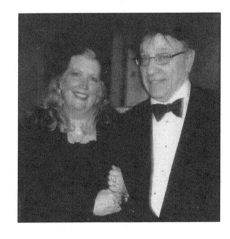

Karen C. Macdonald, PhD, OTR/L has specialized in geriatric occupational therapy for 35 years. Her undergraduate degree in occupational therapy was from Quinnipiac University. She received her master's degree in Counseling the Aging from the University of Bridgeport. At New York University, she earned a PhD in occupational therapy.

Roles in adult day care and long-term care as a clinician included program design and intervention for individuals and groups with acute and chronic conditions. Eventually specializing in dementia management, she was the Coordinator of the Special Care Unit at the Jewish Home for the Elderly in Fairfield, CT.

Over the years, she has participated in public speaking, research, and consulting roles. Currently, she teaches at Sacred Heart University and Housatonic Community College. She is listed in Marquis' *Who's Who in America* and *Who's Who in the World*.

Personal interests include travels and social organizations with her husband, Geno Piacentini, as well as quilting, gardening, and visiting nearby seashores.

INTRODUCTION

We are excited to offer a very different style of publication related to geriatric occupational therapy. It combines original research with evidence-based reviews and in-depth exploration of the productive occupations of older adulthood. This book is directed toward occupational therapy (OT) students (assistants, masters, and doctoral), and OT practitioners (both OTs and OT assistants). It explores the needs of current and future older adults who represent a new client culture and population. For OT practitioners and students, the lessons serve to inform the new geriatric practice. Future clients who wish to be productive agers will, in addition to traditional OT services, also seek new avenues for self-management, prevention, and wellness. As health services rapidly change and evolve, OTs need to update their knowledge to prepare for their new and significant roles in promoting ability and independence for current and future senior clients.

As OT authors, we wanted to write a timely book about productive aging for students and practitioners that would add to existing texts that skillfully address geriatrics conditions, assessments, and intervention principles and practices. Recently, the American Occupational Therapy Association identified productive aging as an emerging practice area in conjunction with their Centennial Vision for 2017 (AOTA, 2007). AOTA's Centennial Vision also encourages original research to promote evidence-based and occupation-based practice, and urges anticipation of OTs' emerging roles in new health care systems to address the needs of the rapidly expanding population of older adults. Throughout the text, key terms are identified in italics.

Responding to these needs, and to ensure that our information was current, we designed a qualitative research project to explore the topic of productive aging. We sought the perspectives of 40 individuals whom we defined as successful seniors, based on their current engagement in productive occupations. What led to their high level of sustained skills? What was important to their health and wellness? What were facilitators and barriers to their performance of preferred occupations? Based on findings, and in comparison with published literature, we hoped to propose new opportunities for OT practitioners to promote active engagement and participation for individuals, groups, and populations. The content reflects several objectives that we had as researchers and authors:

- Understanding the current generations and diverse cultures of older adults
- Appreciating the changing role of OTs in both medical model and community-based services, especially their potential contributions in primary care
- Identifying and analyzing key themes that contributed to sustaining independence and function for today's productive older adults from wellness to end-of-life care
- Offering real life examples and current evidence through an original qualitative research project (the Productive Aging Study [PAS]), including the final proposal of a grounded theory of Conditional Independence to promote productive aging in OT practice
- Providing a user-friendly format to encourage personal thought or group discussion through related learning activities
- Assisting the reader in consideration of expanded possibilities for OTs having roles as group facilitator, educator, consultant, and advocate
- Expanding awareness of the importance of groups as a means of intervention to promote health, wellness, and quality of life
- Considering future trends and potential areas of practice for OT, and pathways toward developing emerging areas of practice

Because we wished to invite the reader to join in our process of discovery, we have interspersed personal journal entries, case studies, and results of interviews or submissions called "Expert's Experience" within the chapters. A detailed description of the methodology is included in Appendix I. A list of participants with thumbnail biographies appears in Appendix II. Throughout the text, interdisciplinary and OT roles are reviewed.

Knowledge about productive aging holds importance for both traditional medical settings and emerging areas of practice, such as wellness programs for community groups and populations. Who are OT's future clients, with a shared experience of decades of vast change and adaptation? How may OTs expand their roles for client-centered and holistic services, anticipating needs and designing new types of intervention programs? Through focused reviews of literature and completion of the PAS, we synthesized findings to reveal multiple secrets of successful and productive aging. These may serve as guidelines for designing effective OT interventions for this emerging area of practice. In doing the PAS, we also reasoned that participants would become examples and case studies in the book, and that photographs of participants would illustrate the productive occupations being described.

Because this book is designed for entry level OT/OTA students and OT practitioners, learning activities accompany each chapter in a workbook format. These activities encourage readers to personalize the information presented, examine their own previous experience and attitudes, or further explore areas specific to their own areas of current or emerging OT practice. The term *OT practitioner* refers to either occupational therapists or occupational therapy assistants, because titles are designated in different ways according to the state in which practice occurs. We consistently used the title OT or OTA.

Section I: The New Geriatric Practice (Chapters 1 through 5) sets the stage for understanding the way that productive occupations of older adulthood will guide future OT practice. As defined in this text, productive aging goes beyond healthy lifestyles and prevention of health conditions, in promoting self-management, social connections, and self-fulfilling occupations.

- *Who* are the upcoming generations and cultural subgroups that help define our future clients?

- *When* will they need help with some predictable yet challenging life tasks and transitions?

- *Where* will future geriatric OT practitioners work?

- *How* will the roles of OT practitioners (OTs and OT assistants) change with the evolving health care climate and reimbursement sources outside the medical model?

- *Why?* The wealth of evidence presented, including new and emerging theories of aging that define the Third Age of retired yet healthy and active seniors, and a new appreciation for the importance of social relationships and connections embedded (Laslett, 1989) in productive occupations, overwhelmingly support *why* OTs need to embrace productive aging in the new millennium.

Section II: Productive Occupations in Older Adulthood as Defined Through Productive Aging Study (PAS) (Chapters 6 through 15) presents the findings of the PAS, broken into themes representative of occupational roles defined as significant by the participants in contributing to productive aging. The first theme, Self-Management, was so all-encompassing that it was divided into several chapters as separate categories: Home Manager, Caregiver, Volunteer, Older Worker, and Lifelong Learner. Final chapters in this section describe the remaining two themes of Social Connections and Self-Fulfilling Activities.

Chapters 14 and 15 address future OT geriatric practice. Chapter 14 proposes an original grounded theory for OT. It synthesizes the themes of analyzed data into several hypotheses toward generating a grounded theory, identified as Conditional Independence. A model is presented in which OT practitioners design interventions toward client-directed skills required for structured function through application of adaptive strategies. These include Situational Adaptation, Structured Performance, and Intentional Abilities. In the final chapter, future possibilities for OT programs and services are identified. The need for ongoing research and program development is promoted to support the continued advancement of OT as a profession.

We have used the original research of the PAS to supplement literature reviews, as well as our extensive professional and personal experiences with elders. The PAS participants sincerely wished to share their "secrets to successful aging" so that people would establish these life roles and habits at a younger age, in order to arrive at retirement years with established routines for wellness. Older adults themselves might read portions of this text to discover valuable lessons about how to age productively. The reader is encouraged to follow their recommendations, not only for OT intervention strategies with older clients, but also to apply to their own eventual years of productive aging. Hopefully, the material found in this book will promote a deeper understanding of the breadth of possibilities for OT roles in gerontology in the coming years.

REFERENCES

American Occupational Therapy Association. (2007). AOTA's Centennial Vision and executive summary. *American Journal of Occupational Therapy, 61*, 613-614. Retrieved from http://dx.doi.org/10.5014/ajot.61.613.

Laslett, P. (1989). *A fresh map of life: The emergence of the Third Age.* Cambridge, MA: Harvard University Press.

Section I

The New Geriatric Practice

This section sets the stage for the new occupational therapy (OT) gerontology practice from the viewpoint of productive aging. Older clients are increasing in both numbers and diversity, with health care needs beginning with prevention; establishing healthy lifestyles; nurturing self-management, independence, and autonomy; and focusing on engagement in valued occupations throughout the continuum of care. The following chapters broadly define productive occupations, and provide evidence for their importance for health and wellness. They further explore the diverse generations, cultures, and adult life stages and describe the processes of some predictable life transitions. They address OT practitioners' (both occupational therapists and assistants) roles across the continuum of care, under both medical and community models, applying the new *Occupational Therapy Practice Framework: Domain and Process, 3rd Edition* (AOTA, 2014) for the area of productive aging.

Chapter 1: What Is Productive Aging? defines productive aging from both an interdisciplinary and an occupational perspective. It introduces a condensed summary of the Productive Aging Study methodology as a foundation for understanding the context of our inquiry and introduces the three themes derived from it:

1. Self-Management
2. Social Connections
3. Self-Fulfilling Activities

It also includes a review of OT services across the continuum of health care, describing how occupational therapists can enable productive occupations, both in the community, and within the traditional health care settings, such as home care, rehabilitation centers, and long-term care.

Chapter 2: Generations and Diversity in Older Adulthood explores some of the diverse ways older adults might categorize themselves, including theoretical life stages, generations, and multicultural groups. It includes a rich description of the generations comprising new millennium senior citizens, ranging from Baby Boomers to traditionalists. Multidisciplinary theories of aging are presented, along with projected demographics related to the "greying of America." Cultural groups based on urban or rural dwelling, ethnicity, and sexual orientation make cultural sensitivity and competency essential features for OT professionals. The chapter also highlights the importance of the expression of empathy for new graduates and practitioners to best relate to older clients with diverse backgrounds.

In **Chapter 3: Transitions in Older Adulthood**, life transitions of older adulthood are explored. Typical developmental or circumstantial changes may lead to altered abilities, roles, and function. Retirement, health changes, relocating (moving), changes in social relationships, widowhood, and end of life topics represent possible periods of vulnerability for which OT practitioners may provide valuable interventions.

Cole MB, Macdonald KC.
Productive Aging: An Occupational Perspective (pp 1-2).
© 2015 Taylor & Francis Group.

Chapter 4: Continuums of Care reviews continuums of care, including medical, community, and nontraditional models; settings that offer minimal to total care; and wellness to acute or chronic illnesses or disabilities. Settings for OT practice are described with examples of roles and functions for the OT practitioner in various setting throughout these continuums.

Chapter 5: Occupational Therapist's Roles in Productive Aging enlarges the spectrum of OT roles in geriatric practice, including applying the *Practice Framework* *3rd Edition* (AOTA, 2014), and addressing productive occupations with individuals, groups, and populations.

REFERENCE

American Occupational Therapy Association. (2014). The occupational therapy practice framework: Domain and process, 3rd edition. *American Journal of Occupational Therapy, 68,* S1-S48.

1

What Is Productive Aging?

Marilyn B. Cole, MS, OTR/L, FAOTA and Karen C. Macdonald, PhD, OTR/L

"Every day you accomplish something positive is a good day…whether for your personal needs or for the needs of others."
(Participant, Geno)

Productive aging is an emerging practice area in OT. Because its focus is wellness and not illness, OT has not yet been integrated into the current medically funded geriatric practice. Yet, its importance for the health and well-being of older adults is critical, highly supported with evidence, and central to the future of geriatric OT practice in the 21st century. Once understood by OT practitioners, productive aging will become highly relevant not only for well elderly, but also for those at all levels of health challenges across the continuum of care. The need to be productive, useful, needed, valued, and loved does not end with a stroke, heart attack, fractured hip, or diagnosis of terminal cancer. Productive occupations give older adults a reason to look forward to each day.

This chapter provides the reader with an overview of the rest of this book. First, we review the various definitions of productive aging and how this topic changes geriatric practice for occupational therapists as well as for other health care providers. Second, we review the history and the interdisciplinary literature on the general topic, providing evidence for the importance of continued productive roles to the health and well-being of older adults. Third, we place productive aging in the context of occupation, citing the American Occupational Therapy Association's (AOTA's) Centennial Vision (2007), the AOTA's *Occupation Therapy Practice Frame, 3rd Edition* (OTPF III) (2014), and the

contributions of occupational science. Finally, we provide an overview of our original qualitative productive aging study (PAS), with suggested implications for changes in OT practice to better serve our future clients who wish to continue or develop their own productive occupations, making their older adulthood the most healthy, self-fulfilling, and meaningful stage of life possible.

PRODUCTIVE VERSUS SUCCESSFUL AGING

The term *productive aging* was first introduced by Robert Butler, founding director of the National Institute on Aging and 1976 Pulitzer prize-winning author (Butler, 2003; Butler & Gleason, 1985; Gilleard, Higgs, Hyde, Wiggins, & Blane, 2005). He used the term broadly, referring to the many ways in which older adults continue to contribute to their own health, to their families and communities, and to society (Leland, Elliott, & Johnson, 2012). As a gerontologist and psychiatrist, Butler knew that neither dementia nor disability were inevitable outcomes in normal aging. He wanted to change the way society viewed older adults. Perceptions of older people as frail, senile, and dependent often made them victims of

Cole MB, Macdonald KC.
Productive Aging: An Occupational Perspective (pp 3-16).
© 2015 Taylor & Francis Group.

age discrimination, or ageism, another term he coined in 1968. With the current explosion in the American aging population (20% by 2030) (United States Census Bureau, 2009) and an ever-increasing life expectancy among older Americans (20 to 30 years post-retirement), there is growing concern among policy makers about their cost to the health care system. When we refer to aging as "productive," we must change our perceptions from negative to positive and appreciate the potential for older adults to balance out their costs in Medicare dollars by continuing to contribute and serve society through their many and varied productive occupations.

A self-awareness exercise may be helpful in understanding your personal feelings and beliefs about old age and older adults. Some biases and stereotypes have led to ageism, where individuals have a range of negative connotations about the elderly. Common among these negative views are beliefs that senior citizens are slow, unable to learn or try new things, chronically ill, dependent, and needy. Please take a few minutes to explore your own preconceived ideas about older adults by filling out the worksheet below:

Learning Activity 1: Exploring Beliefs About Older Adults

Briefly describe the following:

1. What have been your personal experiences with older adults? Describe one specifically.

2. What are your general impressions of the issues and needs of older adults?

3. What is your opinion about current health services for seniors?

4. What does it mean to be an older adult in America today?

5. In the table below, list some positive and negative stereotypes of "an old person" that you have heard. Include "politically incorrect" labels such as "slow" or "old geezer."

NEGATIVE STEREOTYPES	POSITIVE STEREOTYPES

6. Considering the list of stereotypes, briefly discuss the following:
   - Where do these views come from?
   - Which are realistic?
   - How do they vary culturally or internationally?
   - What is the role of TV, movies, and other media?
   - How do you think they should be changed?

BEYOND SUCCESSFUL AGING

As a positive approach to aging, productive aging represents the next step beyond successful aging. Rowe and Kahn (1998) are credited with introducing the term *successful aging* as a (then) revolutionary outcome of their analysis of the MacArthur Foundation Study of Successful Aging. They defined successful aging as "growing old with good health, strength, and vitality" (Rowe & Kahn, 1998, p. 33), with three defining characteristics:

1. Low risk of disease and disease-related disability: Achievable by taking steps to lower one's risk through adopting a healthy lifestyle.

2. High mental and physical function: Maintained through continued applications in everyday occupations and personal projects.

3. Active engagement with life: Individually defined through continued social roles, group memberships, and frequent interactions with other people.

Successful aging, as defined above, is achievable for almost everyone through increased attention to environment and lifestyle factors.

Occupational scientists Carlson, Clark, and Young (1998) have further defined the art of successful aging with the following three areas of pursuit:

1. Achieving a sense of control over one's life: Planning and structuring one's own life by selecting areas of occupational focus and exerting control over one's environment.

2. Practicing healthy habits: For example, exercising regularly, stopping smoking, maintaining a nutritious diet, seeking preventive medical treatment, participating in social networks with family and friends, continuing in productive activity whether paid or unpaid, and engaging in activities that make one happy.

3. Achieving continuity with one's past: Older adults choose to continue with activities they have engaged in throughout their lives, with a goal to "preserve and maintain internal and external structures…using strategies tied to their past experiences of themselves and their social world" (Atchley, 1989, p. 183). These ideas have been more recently conceptualized as preserving "social identity, a strong predictor of health and well-being, even for people who live with chronic illness" (Tarrant, Haggar, & Farrow, 2012).

The areas of pursuit outlined above have been applied within OT well-elderly studies and their replications (Clark et al., 1997, 2011; Mountain & Craig, 2011) and can serve as a road map for the occupational therapist's role in promoting productive aging with healthy or at-risk older adults. However, with the help of OT, even elders who are chronically ill, disabled, or bedridden, can achieve a measure of satisfaction and well-being through engagement with others and with meaningful occupations that support their social and personal identities (Carlson et al., 1998).

Learning Activity 2: Exploring Successful and Productive Aging

1. Thinking of your own aging, how would you apply Rowe and Kahn's (1989) guidelines for successful aging to maintain your health and prevent disability? Describe three ways.

    a.

    b.

    c.

2. How is successful aging different from productive aging?

3. Projecting yourself into the future, what do you envision doing at age 65?

    a. Describe your lifestyle.

    b. Describe the environment in which you would be living (home, family, community).

    c. In what productive occupations would you regularly participate? List three.

4. Write one sentence defining productive aging in your own words.

WHAT IS AN OCCUPATIONAL PERSPECTIVE?

An occupational perspective is defined as a focus on the activities that make up one's life roles. Occupational therapists have already acknowledged the link between occupations and productivity. *Productivity* refers to occupations, both paid and unpaid, that contribute to "the maintenance or advancement of society as well as to the individual's own survival or development" (Creek, 2014, p. 40). Productive occupations are closely connected to the social roles often identified as meaningful by older adults themselves. An occupational science study identified five productive occupations reported by older adults in the United Kingdom (Knight et al., 2007). Their rates of participation were the following: (1) 30% volunteer, (2) 89% home-maker, (3) 27% caregiver, (4) 23% paid employee, and (5) 10%

student. This study cited enjoyment and altruism as the main reasons for engaging in productive occupations (Knight et al., 2007). A U.S. study reported that 85% of Americans older than age 60 years participated in one or more productive activities over a 9-month period, including paid work, volunteering, caregiving, and providing informal assistance to others (Hinterlong, 2008). Because older people, in continuing their productive roles, also contribute to their own health and well-being, we added the role of "self-manager" to the above list of productive occupations.

ROLES OR OCCUPATIONS?

While OTs understand that paid work, volunteering, and education or lifelong learning are areas of occupation, as stated in the OTPF III (AOTA, 2014), older adults themselves often think of these as roles. The OTPF III defines roles as "sets of behaviors expected by society, shaped by culture and context that may be further conceptualized and defined by the client" (AOTA, 2014, p. S27). Working and volunteering are productive roles that are recognized and defined by society, but they are also occupations because they have specific sets of activities or tasks that define them. *Occupations* are defined by the AOTA (2014) as "daily life activities in which people engage. Occupations occur in context and are influenced by the interplay among client factors, performance skills, and performance patterns. Occupations occur over time, have purpose, meaning, and perceived utility to the client…" (p. S43).

Learning Activity 3: Defining Productive Roles and Occupations

1. Write a list of your own current productive occupations. Describe each briefly.

    a.

    b.

    c.

    d.

    e.

2. How do you think these might change within the next 5 years?

3. Write a list of social groups you belong to. What is the role you play in each?

    a.

    b.

    c.

    d.

4. What are the activities or tasks associated with the productive *occupation* of a student?

5. Explain the *role* of a teacher. How is this similar/different from teaching as an *occupation*?

Evidence for Productive Aging

Gerontology research itself has undergone a transformation over the past several decades, largely fueled by what some have called the "era of the Third Age," which refers to a larger, healthier older population (Carr & Manning, 2010). Laslett (1989, 1997) originated the concept of the Third Age with his developmental theory in which he acknowledges four basic ages. The Third Age, by definition, begins at retirement, and brings with it the new life tasks of pursuing creativity and self-fulfillment and serving the unmet needs of society. Qualitative research methods have been critically important in changing the focus of aging studies away from decline and disengagement and toward the positive aspects of aging. Rowles and Schoenberg (2002) describe three major trends in Third Age inquiry: (1) capturing the experience of aging from the perspective of older adults themselves; (2) recognizing the importance of context, including both physical and social environments; and (3) understanding the roles of reactivity and reflexivity in qualitative gerontology (i.e., the researchers' consideration of their own experiences when interpreting the personal narratives of study participants).

In recent years, the relatively early retirement of skilled and knowledgeable older workers without equivalent younger replacements in the work force has prompted a redefinition of retirement as "a period of productivity, not just a period of leisure" (Carr & Manning, 2010, p. 24). Three areas of gerontology research address productivity: "work in later life, lifelong learning, and volunteerism or unpaid work" (Carr & Manning, 2010, p. 24). For example, Rocco, Stein, and Lee (2003) found that patterns of work participation shaped the extent to which leisure is defined in a productive way. For example, watching Jeopardy on TV provides mental stimulation as viewers try to answer the difficult questions, whereas playing golf or tennis promotes physical fitness goals for participants.

Some researchers have found a strong connection between engagement in meaningful activities and improved well-being (Rossen, Knafl, & Flood, 2008), while others found that social participation in an organized group contributed positively to an older person's ability to manage stress, deal with loss, and promote improved quality of life (Hutchenson, Yarnal, Staffordson, & Kerstetter, 2008).

Much of this interdisciplinary geriatric research, while not specifically OT, supports the value of occupational engagement and social participation as part of what might be called the "Third Age lifestyle," or "the activities and roles associated with being in the Third Age" (Gilleard et al., 2005; Carr & Manning, 2010, p. 27). Chapter

2 provides a fuller description of Laslett's and other contemporary theories of aging.

The evidence for productive aging to date was reviewed extensively by Leland et al. (2012), noting ample research to support the health benefits of productive activities in older adulthood. The AOTA (2010) has identified some of the activities included in their definition: "Productive aging involves care of self and others, management of home, engagement in leisure and physical activities, civic engagement, and social interactions which can involve travel, entertaining, and visiting with friends" (AOTA, 2010), giving a broad and holistic perspective for OT practitioners to follow (Leland et al., 2012, p. 8).

Productive Aging and Occupational Therapy

The AOTA's Centennial Vision has identified productive aging as a key societal need in the 21st century. "Our society's rapidly aging population, increased longevity, the changing world of work, and Baby Boomers' focus on quality of life issues are some of the factors that will increase the need for services in this area" (AOTA, 2012).

Furthermore, the AOTA's evidence-based practice initiative has generated summaries of existing research on the relationship between productive occupations and health for community-dwelling older adults (Stav, Hallenen, Lane, & Arbesman, 2012). They found a "multidisciplinary appreciation for occupational engagement and associated well-being" as well as highlighted "the health effects of engagement in a wide variety of occupations and activities" (Stav et al., p. 301). Good health, well-being, and lower mortality risk are strongly associated with physical activities (occupations) like gardening, walking, dancing, swimming, shopping, and home maintenance; active paid work or volunteering; and social participation. In evidence reviews, occupations involving social interaction are shown to reduce physical and cognitive decline in older adults, even in the presence of chronic health conditions (Stav et al., 2012).

Theorists have observed that the OT professional paradigm, which provides the general approach across the span of practice, has changed over the past several decades from one that is mechanistic, narrowly defined, and medically based to one that is community-based—holistic, client-centered, and systems oriented (Cole & Tufano, 2008). Yet in today's geriatric OT practice, many positions are still defined by the medical model. That will hopefully change when current students become advocates for the role transformation that has already occurred on the professional level. Occupational therapists can demonstrate a wider role in the area of productive aging by pursuing some of the goals outlined in this book: supporting self-management, focusing on wellness and prevention early in the process of chronic health conditions, and taking advantage of the benefits of social interaction by providing many more interventions in a group format.

A meta-analysis of the types of geriatric research found recurrent themes in falls, pain, and functional difficulty, and driving abilities for older adults (Murphy, 2011). Their recommendation for future research suggested exploring topics related to higher functioning and productive aging. Murphy (2011) highlighted topics of need for research, paid work, and volunteering coincided precisely with the themes presented in the our PAS.

PRODUCTIVE AGING STUDY: AN OVERVIEW

Because productive aging represents a new perspective for OT gerontology practice, we decided to do our own qualitative study using a purposive sample of 40 successful agers, defined by their current engagement in at least three of six productive occupations described in the occupational science literature (self-manager, paid worker, volunteer, caregiver, home maintainer, and lifelong learner). Our goals were to increase our own understanding of how productivity fit into the everyday lives of (mostly) retired participants and to learn some of their strategies, techniques, and motivations for continuing to be actively engaged in productive occupations, despite some considerable health challenges and advancing ages (age range: 52 to 98 years). A detailed description of the methodology and results of the study appears in Appendix I. The following is a summary.

Research Design

To research the topic of productive aging, we investigated the self-described qualities and skills of older adults whom we defined as successful seniors. This meant those who were retired and leading active lives while residing independently in the community. The need for the study was justified because, although productive aging was a blossoming area of interest in gerontology, as well as an important emerging area of practice in OT, little research had been completed. Some of our research questions to explore productive aging included the following:

- How do they do it?
- What contributed to and sustained their productive aging?
- How would they define productive aging and its elements?
- How could their answers be analyzed and translated into principles for future OT practice?

Because we wanted in-depth subjective data from the participants, we chose a qualitative method. A semi-structured interview format included background information and ten semi-structured interview questions; and a shorter form was adapted for use by a few individuals (see Appendix I). All participants received a cover letter and signed a consent form giving authors permission to publish both information and photographs in our resulting textbook.

Part of the research design included establishing an anticipated process and schedule for data collection and related review of literature. Immersion into the topic included ongoing brainstorming, journal writing, and the collection of any community or published materials related to the topic.

Data Collection

A preliminary fieldwork study was completed with one participant, which led to some minor changes on the interview form. We created lists of potential participants and began interviewing. During the interviews, principles of active engagement and prompts for additional clarification were utilized. As data collection continued, we were using the following inclusion criteria:

1. Retired (including working part-time by choice)
2. Community dwelling (including retirement communities)
3. Participating in at least three of six productive roles/ occupations:
   a. Self-manager
   b. Home manager
   c. Caregiver
   d. Volunteer
   e. Paid worker (reduced hours from full-time)
   f. Student/lifelong learner

Health conditions were not addressed as a part of the study. Instead, the focus was on active occupations and participation, regardless of possible existing conditions. A snowball effect occurred, as individuals heard about the research and eagerly volunteered to participate. We realized that the participants were rather homogeneous in socioeconomic status and ethnicity and, therefore, applied purposive sampling to promote cultural diversity.

Most interviews took place in the individual's home, with a single face-to-face interview. The authors took notes by hand. Interviews usually took 45 to 50 minutes. When we reached a total of 40 participants, we had established a sense of saturation, with recurring themes and findings. We also needed to set a boundary with data collection, which would usually be only four to eight participants for a qualitative study. We knew we were gathering valuable information to

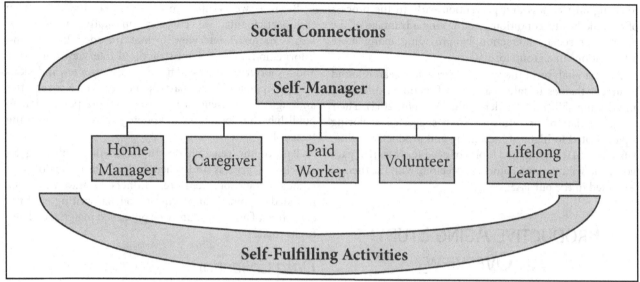

Figure 1-1. Components of Self-Management. In retirement, the self-manager controls choices of engagement in other productive occupations and structures and schedules these roles to match skills, motivations, strengths, and limitations within cultural, social, temporal, and other environmental demands and expectations. Social connections and self-fulfilling occupations occur both within and outside these defined productive roles. (From Productive Aging Study by M. Cole and K. Macdonald, 2015.)

aid in understanding issues for evolving practice areas for OT and approaching answers to the age-old human question, "How can I live a long, healthy, and happy life?" Data collection lasted 8 months. Some interviews were adapted to be conducted by phone, hard copy, or e-mail responses. Photographs were taken depicting participants engaged in a typical productive occupation of their choice.

Data Analysis

Data analysis began as soon as data were gathered, and then was built on by findings of subsequent interviews. We would read results aloud to each other, taking notes on emerging themes. Initial coding began for apparent clusters and categories, which led to the identification of three main themes: *ability*, *activity*, and *attitude*.

The participants consistently described examples of varied activities within the context of self-care and self-motivation, along with concurrent issues such as interpersonal relations and managing their structural space and place. These were consistent with a classic Person-Environment-Occupation (PEO) model associated with occupational performance literature (Law & Dunbar, 2007).

Using concept map techniques, we expanded these themes further to identify additional elements and relationships between topics. We created posters to note issues that were frequently repeated and themes that were apparent by their absence. We used the OTPF II (AOTA, 2008) as an additional organizing structure for topics. The process continued using principles of constant comparative analysis. This included ongoing reflection on prior results as "making meaning" progressed. As data analysis

was evolving, results were mentioned to participants who were interviewed later during the data collection phase. Their feedback consistently concurred with our findings and interpretations.

Their quotes were transcribed into thematic categories. At this point, inductive reasoning was used to consolidate assorted themes through a process known as *funneling*. The data were grouped into larger general themes to serve as a foundation for final extensive analysis. These categories included the following:

1. Self-management

2. Social connections

3. Self-fulfilling activities

Self-management was an enormous theme on which other productive roles depend (Figure 1-1). Therefore, it was divided into several subthemes depicting five additional productive occupations: home manager, caregiver, volunteer, older worker, and lifelong learner/student. These six categories became the basis for further research through extensive literature review.

Issues of trustworthiness and confirmability were considered throughout the project. The authors critiqued each other's work and engaged in some peer review when discussing proposed findings with colleagues.

As we neared completion of the research, we designed a formal "exiting the field" in which we included a system for member checking. A final letter containing a summary of the interview findings was sent to all participants 6 months after the final interview. On a separate sheet, we requested written feedback for what they agreed or disagreed with or to suggest changes. The majority replied very quickly, with confirmation of our findings and suggestions for further or clarified descriptions.

Data Synthesis

The results of an interdisciplinary literature search, both classic and current, served as a final step of "triangulation." The data had been analyzed from the perspective of the two researchers and some peers, the feedback from participants, and comparison with related literature.

Findings were organized into content for separate chapters in Section II. Each chapter includes sections of definition of a topic, participant perspectives, relationship to practice settings, and occupational therapy role.

A final level of synthesis occurred in the development of a grounded theory—conditional independence. Chapter 14 describes the process of generating hypotheses and developing a proposed new theory and its related components. After completion of the PAS, a manuscript was sent to our publisher, SLACK Incorporated. Three reviewers offered helpful objective commentary for the format and content, with constructive feedback for the presentation and promotion of the PAS findings in a textbook format.

RESULTING THEMES OF PRODUCTIVE OCCUPATIONS

Analysis of the interview content generated three main themes: (1) self-management, (2) social connections, and (3) self-fulfilling activities. These themes form the basis of Section II of this book, where they are explored more deeply, along with their own literature reviews, applications to the continuums of care, and OT practice guidelines. Placed together, we propose a grounded theory of productive aging—conditional independence—which is more fully described in Chapter 14.

In the remainder of this introductory chapter, we will highlight how these themes change the focus of OT practice in meeting the needs of older clients who wish to continue to live their lives as productive agers.

Theme 1: The Prominence of Self-Management

The standout feature from our study was the central role of self-management in successful and productive aging. People who take charge of their own aging process can prevent much of the anticipated physical and mental decline and can prolong their own healthy lives. Here is where OT can make a significant difference. Armed with this new evidence, we can inspire clients to develop and strengthen good self-management skills, and empower them to direct their energy toward the occupations most important to

them. Good self-managers make wise and informed choices about the occupations they will continue or enter in older adulthood. They will gather with intention the support and resources they need through social relationships, networks, and connections. They will safeguard their health by building healthy routines and staying informed about how to best cope with chronic health conditions and generally taking good care of themselves. They will not hesitate to advocate for themselves or their loved ones, and they will make good decisions about when to take calculated risks and when to ask for help. They will come to understand their own strengths and limitations and will balance their lives between social obligations and taking time for self-renewal. These are the tasks within the productive occupation of self-management, about which OT students and professionals must learn, to truly meet the needs of 21st century older adults.

The grounded theory of conditional independence, derived from our qualitative study, is all about self-management. Its importance spans the developmental stages of older adulthood, applying equally to independent seniors aging in place and across the continuum of wellness and disability to dependency and palliative care.

We define *self-management* for older adults as the self-directed ability to control and manage their own aging process, to set realistic and meaningful occupational goals, and to structure their lives and daily self-fulfilling activities in ways that continue and reinforce important social and occupational identities, and create and maintain social roles and connections that they find satisfying. Self-management requires good higher-level cognitive functioning, including abstract thinking directed toward self-reflection and insight, reasoning and problem solving, future planning, judgment, mental flexibility, and the ability to prioritize and adapt, especially when dealing with changing or unexpected situations.

Characteristics of self-management include the following: self-direction and self-discipline, health consciousness and staying informed about health-related issues, maintaining a positive attitude, and attention to a planned lifestyle. The ability to manage oneself will determine the other productive occupations one chooses and the extent and contexts of participation, including engaging in paid work, volunteering, caregiving, maintaining one's home, and/or pursuing creative endeavors and lifelong learning. In other words, the choice to pursue productive roles or occupations in older adulthood depends on whether the person, as self-manager, decides that these occupations are important to continue or pursue in the current stage of life.

Designing Occupational Therapy Interventions to Support Self-Management

If an OT were to design an individual or group intervention to support the role of self-manager, topics might include the following:

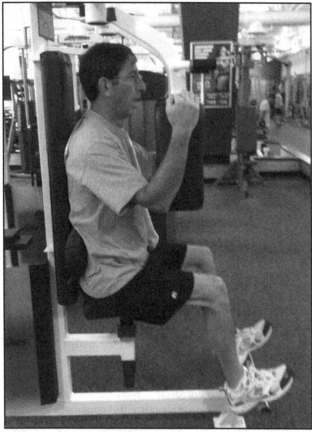

Figure 1-2. Marty stays fit by going to the gym, despite lower back pain. He uses a lumbar support pillow to protect his back while exercising.

- Lifestyle factors that include daily physical exercise, good nutrition, and a balance of productive and enjoyable activities and relaxation (Figure 1-2).
- Self-care routines (activities of daily living [ADL]) that accommodate one's daily activities.
- Health maintenance issues, such as getting annual medical and dental check-ups, checking vision and hearing, and following up with specialists.
- Building health maintenance into daily routines and activities, such as joint protection, energy conservation, and medication compliance.
- Time management: How daily, weekly, monthly, and yearly activities are structured, incorporating both occupational goals and priorities and balancing personal needs and social connections.
- Identifying social networks and groups, and intentionally reaching out to maintain social connections.
- Planning social events with others as a way to continue valued social relationships.
- Challenging oneself mentally through lifelong learning, problem solving, or work and volunteering as a way to maintain higher mental abilities and to prevent cognitive decline.

- Mobility and safety: Both functional and community mobility, including safe driving, walking, and neighborhood safety and maintaining a risk-free home.
- Care of home and belongings: Looking at expenses and value received, standards of organization and cleanliness, and balancing priorities for home maintenance and productive pursuits.
- Choosing to continue or to change productive roles in conjunction with life circumstances, such as needing to care for a sick relative, continuing paid work to supplement finances, or retiring to accommodate the desire to travel while still healthy enough to enjoy it.
- Exploring and practicing the role of self-advocacy with respect to ageism, health, or social issues affecting one's choices and quality of life.

These are some of many areas of intervention to support the self-manager role. A more detailed discussion of self-management can be found in Chapter 6.

Learning Activity 4: Managing Self-Care and Balance

- What daily routines of self-care do you have?
- What do you do to maintain your health and energy?
- How would you change your routine to accommodate an illness such as a cold?
- How do you manage time so that your obligations are fulfilled?
- What signs do you recognize if you are pushing yourself too hard? Not hard enough?
- How well do you manage your various roles and activities? Give some examples.
- What are your top three goals? (awareness of priorities)

Theme 2: Using the Power of Social Connections

The PAS supports social connections, the occupations within self-management, and self-fulfilling activities as important components of productive aging. However, our participants conveyed something that is often overlooked in OT literature—that their productive occupations are usually deeply embedded within, interrelated with, and inseparable from their social networks. For example, work, leisure, volunteer, and learning activities all have important social features, are often shared with or performed in the company of others, and require social interaction as a part of occupational performance. Family members share household duties. Workers interact with coworkers, customers, and supervisors. Volunteers and caregivers interact in various capacities with those they serve. Even when parts of these occupations are performed alone, people have internalized social standards and usually consider the expectations of others.

The health-related literature taught us much about social connections in productive aging. First, we learned that social connections, networks, and support can actually prevent illness, disability, and even premature death (Holt-Lunstad, Smith, & Layton, 2010). Social identity, that part of self-identity that comes from group membership and interaction with others, plays an important role in this process. We know that older adults with strong social identities are generally healthier and have a greater sense of well-being (Tarrant et al., 2012). The interdisciplinary research suggests that it is largely the social aspects of occupations that provide older adults with the protection they need against morbidity and mortality and promote vitality and life satisfaction in aging.

Occupational Therapy Interventions for Social Participation

Social participation may be foremost in the minds of older clients who wish to continue their meaningful social roles and relationships, despite emerging health conditions. Social participation is one of the eight occupations included in the OTPF III's domain, but it does not easily translate into separate "activities" as some of the other occupations do, making it necessary for OT practitioners to be creative with designing social participation interventions. As mentioned earlier, there are complex transactional relationships between social participation and the productive occupations of worker, caregiver, volunteer, home maintainer, and lifelong learner. In their self-manager role, clients must navigate these complex relationships, manage functional challenges, overcome internal and external barriers, and adapt the tasks and strategies that will allow them to continue to engage in the occupations and social roles they choose.

To address social participation, occupational therapists first need to understand how clients view the social connections embedded within their productive occupations. Are the most valued social relationships found within a work role, a volunteer role, or a caregiving role? How important is it to share home management with a spouse, partner, or other family members? What do clients need to be able to do in order to maintain their social connections within these occupations? Which self-fulfilling activities are shared with family, peers, and friends?

Some examples of areas of focus for OT in social participation might include the following:

- Going out to lunch with friends.
- Volunteering to help with simple crafts at an adult day care center.
- Hosting a book discussion group for six couples on a Saturday evening.
- Shopping for groceries and cooking dinner each day with spouse.
- Resuming caregiving for 3-year-old grandson 3 days per week.
- Participating in a church fair committee meeting, taking on one aspect to lead.
- Attending a yoga class at a senior center with friends.
- Driving 2 hours to spend Thanksgiving with extended family.
- Returning to work part-time as a greeter for a home improvement store.

For each of these examples, there are social components and activity components. The OT will address client factors, health conditions, and contexts or environments as well as occupational and social aspects. The main point to keep in mind is to address the situation holistically and with continued client collaboration, sometimes also including spouses or significant others when designing an effective OT intervention.

Learning Activity 5: Social Connections in Occupational Therapy Interventions

Choose one example from the below list as a goal for a 75-year-old home care client who is recovering from a left knee replacement.

1. Find prognosis for knee replacements and precautions on a reliable website or in textbooks or other resources. List and describe briefly.

2. Relative to your chosen goal, discuss the physical and mental requirements for doing this activity, including preparation, transportation, and physical and social environments.

3. What problems or barriers do you foresee? List three potential barriers for client collaboration and problem solving. For each, what might be some potential ways to remediate, adapt, or compensate?

4. To what extent would assistance from others help this client to achieve his goal? How might the contexts or environments be adapted without taking away the benefits for the client?

Occupational Therapy Groups Use the Power of Social Connections to Facilitate Client Goals

Considering the overwhelming evidence supporting the importance of social connections for the health and well-being of older adults, OTs increase their awareness of the need to provide interventions within a group format. While OT alone can certainly improve occupational performance, that same intervention introduced within a

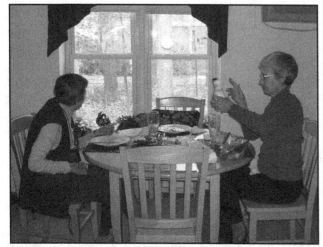

Figure 1-3. Valnere checks ingredients for a healthy meal for herself and her mother, Patricia.

carefully selected group of clients with similar health challenges adds the essential ingredient of social support and identity. Occupational therapists have the skills to design and facilitate groups using a client-centered approach (Cole, 2012). Sometimes, older adults who live independently would be better served by having occupational therapists organize groups to address the common issues of aging, such as fall prevention, fitness and flexibility, driver safety, and overcoming sensory issues such as poor hearing or low vision. The researchers in a widely recognized well-elderly study (Clark et al., 1997, 2011) provided occupation-centered group interventions. Their outcomes unequivocally support the value of OT groups in maintaining wellness, increasing life satisfaction and well-being, and reducing health costs. These weekly groups, which met consistently in the same place and time, and with the same leader and participants over a 9-month period, focused on the concept of occupation and topics relevant to the lives of the individual participants. Some of these group modules are described briefly below.

- Occupation, health, and aging: Focused on defining occupation and illuminating its relationship to health using a range of self-analysis and reflective activities, such as answering the questions "How do you experience ageism?" or "What has retirement meant to you?" or asking members to present their current hobbies and projects.

- Transportation and occupation: Including educational presentations, outings, exploration, and special events.

- Finances and occupation: Looking at how finances affect occupations, gathering local resources for inexpensive social and leisure activities, and learning how to prevent financial abuse and scams (e.g., the group game The Price Is Right).

- Physical and mental activity: Includes managing stress, identifying occupations that promote physical fitness,

and participating in mentally challenging activities or ways to improve memory.

- Dining as an occupation: Includes nutritional information for healthy aging (Figure 1-3), ways to manage chronic conditions through diet, exploring the evidence on nutritional supplements, medication and food interactions, and reading and understanding food labels (e.g., group adventure finding low-fat items in a grocery store).

- Time and occupation: How occupations provide continuity past-present-future, occupational rhythms and routines, how familiar occupations provide a sense of well-being and normalcy, how historical events affect occupations, and special activities for specific seasons and holidays.

- Home and community safety: How home and community affect occupations, what adaptations have been (or could be) made to facilitate occupation, what are community safety concerns, gathering and posting a list of emergency phone numbers and instructions, or exploring one another's homes as a group to screen for safety, putting together a neighborhood watch plan.

- Relationships and occupation: Explores issues of friendships, loneliness, companionship, dealing with grief and loss, group problem solving for troubled relationships, dealing with bothersome neighbor issues, exploring the influence of culture, discussing how occupations are shared, and promoting connectedness with others and avoiding social isolation (Mandel, Jackson, Zemke, Nelson, & Clark, 1999).

Please refer to the book entitled *Lifestyle Redesign: Implementing the Well Elderly Program* (Mandel, Jackson, Zemke, Nelson, & Clark, 1999) for a more complete description of these excellent group-based OT interventions. A replication of the U.S. study in the United Kingdom produced similar positive evidence for OT group intervention (Mountain & Craig, 2011). The Well Elderly studies provide some of the best evidence to date for the effectiveness of OT group interventions with community dwelling older adults (Clark et al., 1997, 2011; Mountain & Craig, 2011).

Many more examples of OT group interventions and programs are appearing in the recent literature. These group programs focus on individuals with physical disabilities just as often as mental health issues. For example, a social group for men with Parkinson's disease focused on "community life, meaningful pursuits, and valued roles of members, helping them to live life to the fullest" (Porter, Mazonson, & Tickle-Degnen, 2011, p. 18). Dale (2008) describes an "Up to Date Club" in Danville, IN, comprising women ages 65 to 93, for whom she offers OT educational sessions related to healthy aging. A "Matter of Balance" is a multicomponent group intervention explicitly aimed at reducing excessive concerns about falling and activity avoidance, a program that has been evaluated through two

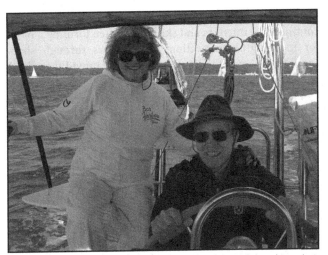

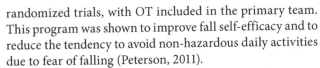

Figure 1-4. Mary and Malcolm belong to a sailing club, taking their turns as "crew."

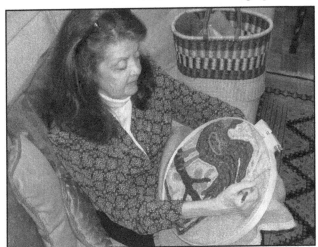

Figure 1-5. June's advice to retirees: "Learn something new." She takes classes in rug-hooking and often designs her own patterns.

randomized trials, with OT included in the primary team. This program was shown to improve fall self-efficacy and to reduce the tendency to avoid non-hazardous daily activities due to fear of falling (Peterson, 2011).

OT groups can harness the power of social connections by facilitating positive interactions among members, reinforcing and strengthening important social identities, and linking past, present, and future productive occupations through sharing and processing group activities (Figure 1-4).

Please see Chapter 12 for a fuller description of Social Connections.

Theme 3: Developing Self-Fulfilling Activities

People in retirement look for meaningful ways to spend their time. We know from the interdisciplinary literature that people can prevent cognitive decline, even that due to Alzheimer's disease, through engaging in mentally challenging activities and pursuing lifelong learning (Landau et al., 2012). The occupations people engage in throughout their lives offer many mental challenges, as well as opportunities for creative problem solving, adaptation, and the necessity of learning new skills. People are also motivated by their own values and beliefs to pursue occupations that are meaningful for them, and this process continues after retirement. The OT and occupational science literature tells us that people adapt best to the inevitable transitions of older adulthood through continued pursuit of occupations that give their lives meaning. Jonsson (2011) and Jonsson, Josephsson, and Kielhofner (2001) called these engaging occupations—meaningful projects that helped older adults in Sweden to successfully transition to retirement.

However, there is also a more basic reason that older adults seek self-fulfillment in older adulthood, and that is to continue their own personal growth, an important developmental task of older adulthood (Baltes & Baltes, 1990; Laslett, 1989). A New Zealand occupational science study questions prior research setting parameters of physical activity for successful aging, finding social and spiritual aspects of occupational engagement just as significant to the preservation of health and longevity (Wright-St. Clair, 2012). In this study, participants spoke of "doing what matters," referring to having one occupation that was of "primary importance to them" (Wright-St. Clair, 2012, p. 44). Some self-fulfilling occupations cited in this study by participants well into their 80s and 90s were playing the piano, growing tomatoes, writing poems, doing tapestry, grooming a dog, and building a model boat. This suggests that OT practitioners and researchers look beyond the spectrum of everyday activities to help older clients to continue their participation in the subjectively compelling occupations that matter most to them (Figure 1-5).

A Canadian study deepened the focus on meaningful occupations by looking at participation levels over time (Menac, 2003). Results of this study showed that greater happiness was associated with three activity categories: (1) solitary leisure activities, such as handiwork hobbies, reading, writing, music or art; (2) productive activities, such as light housework and gardening; and (3) spending time in social groups. Higher levels of engagement did predict survival over 6 years; however, even when participation levels decreased over time, continued engagement in chosen occupations showed no decline in happiness. This finding stresses the importance of continuity and the role of self-fulfilling occupations in connecting past, present, and future with enduring occupational (and social) identities.

Occupational Therapy Interventions for Self-Fulfilling Activities

Some of the activities included here might fall under the occupations of "play" or "leisure" in the OTPF III (AOTA, 2014). However, the self-fulfilling aspect adds another dimension—that of continued growth and development and life satisfaction. Today's older clients tend to see even leisure activities as productive, promoting physical or mental fitness, encouraging relaxation, or overcoming stress. Aspects of self-fulfilling activities often include social participation (e.g., playing Bocce ball, bridge, or poker; designing and making quilts to commemorate an event or to raise money for a cause; or planting flowers to be admired by neighbors and visitors). Solitary activities might include walking and exercising, reading, needlecraft, writing poems, playing computer games, or repairing lawnmowers. Their meaning for the individual depends on many factors, including past accomplishments, skill level, personal interest or motivation, time, equipment and materials, and access to assistance or mentoring when desired. However, the social context within which activities are performed, or the internalized social expectations for them, cannot be ignored. OT practitioners collaborate with older clients to overcome barriers to performing self-fulfilling occupations, either individually or through group interventions.

Learning Activity 6: Identifying Self-Fulfilling Activities

As an occupational therapist, you are asked to design a program for an assisted living facility, with a goal of encouraging creative self-expression for a group of residents with arthritis.

1. Explain how you might evaluate the interests of this population.

2. Explore and explain the health benefits of doing creative activities for persons with arthritis.

3. Choose two specific activities and use task analysis to outline the requirements or demands for the activity itself. What equipment and supplies are required? What are the physical, emotional, social, and financial considerations?

4. Discuss how these two activities encourage creativity. How will residents be able to express their individuality through them?

5. Using these examples, explain how self-fulfilling occupations enhance health, well-being, and life satisfaction in older adulthood.

To summarize, engaging in self-fulfilling occupations fosters continued personal growth and development in older adulthood by supporting lifelong personal and social identities, encouraging creative self-expression, providing continuity of interests and skills, and often forming a basis for meaningful connections with others through sharing interests, mentoring or teaching, or providing valued contributions to society.

Please see Chapter 13 for a fuller description of self-fulfilling activities.

PRODUCTIVE AGING ACROSS THE CONTINUUM OF CARE

The "Occupational Therapy Guidelines for Productive Aging for Community-Dwelling Older Adults" outlines the application of OT domains and the process of evaluation, intervention, and outcomes for serving productive agers in a variety of community settings (Leland et al., 2012). The process begins with screening—using interview, observation, or informal testing to determine whether older adults are experiencing difficulty with desired occupations. The screening provides an opportunity for the occupational therapist to educate potential clients and their significant others about the importance of productive occupations for maintaining health and well-being. Excellent examples of evaluations, interventions, and outcomes in both medical- and community-based settings are outlined in this text.

This textbook extends the role of OT productive aging beyond community dwellers, and across the continuum of care. Older adults in assisted living, subacute rehabilitation, or long-term care facilities can also continue to lead productive lives. Within such facilities, residents continue self-management by choosing what they will continue to do for themselves and how much help they want to accept from others. They still find ways to follow their lifelong interests, hopefully with the help of an OT professional who understands its importance for their health and well-being. They can still interact with friends and family and take intentional steps to connect with others through social activities, whether eating meals together, playing card or board games, doing line dancing, celebrating birthdays and holidays, or participating in book discussions. Occupational therapists could take a leading role in establishing such group activities within care-based facilities. As we have also learned from the interdisciplinary research, even people with moderate to severe dementia can re-establish social connections and achieve a much-needed sense of belonging through participation in group activities that evoke shared memories with others of their own generation (Haslam, Jetten, Haslam, & Knight, 2012).

See Chapter 4 for further considerations related to the continuum of care. See Chapter 5 for a more extensive discussion of the role of OT in productive aging.

JOURNAL ENTRY (M. C.)

Occupational therapists have historically seen patients and clients more holistically than the medical model advocates. They must, after all, look at occupation as the standard and not some measurement of strength, range of motion, or cognitive calculation. Medicine, in embracing the scientific method, has often ignored the client's emotions, motivations, social positions and roles, and cultures and environments in the service of precision. But OT, even in embracing the medical profession in the mid-20th century, never really abandoned the person. That is why Mattingly and Fleming (1994) unveiled the OT reasoning process as having multiple tracks, only one of which embraces scientific precision (procedural reasoning), and the others recognizing the whole person as more than the sum of his or her parts.

For OT, joining the health care system was a double-edged sword. It brought the profession needed recognition and status and served as the basis for often generous reimbursement over the years. It gave our scholars the scientific tools to build a knowledge base and develop evidence to support its theories. But for at least the past three decades, the medical payment system has tied our hands, holding OT to standards of accountability that often seemed irrelevant to the real occupational needs of the client.

Of course, this phenomenon has occurred in other disciplines as well. The World Health Organization (2001) took the lead in boldly redefining health as greater than the absence of disease, considering the effects of physical and social environments and giving priority to the outcomes of engagement in activities and participation in life. Medical systems generally have recognized the depersonalizing effects of focusing too narrowly on diseases, symptoms, and prescriptions and moved slowly in the direction of patient, client, and family centeredness. Health care professionals across the board have felt the constrictions of an antiquated medical reimbursement system that is too much grounded in politics, bureaucratic policies, and the actuarial tables of insurance corporations. Clearly change is needed. But whether the U.S. Affordable Care Act (2010) brings these changes remains to be seen.

Where does that leave the OT professional who just wants to enable clients to participate in the occupations that give their lives meaning? Yes, we have the necessary background in anatomy, physiology, and traditional medical knowledge and still need to use these tools. But for occupational therapists the answer also lies in both creativity and advocacy. For at least a decade, the leaders of our profession have advocated community-based interventions that include not only individuals, but also organizations and populations, and focus not only on remediation, adaptation, and compensation, but also on wellness and prevention. Isn't it time to come out from under these medical constraints of reimbursement? More of us need to take nontraditional jobs in communities, apply for grants to develop innovative community programs, and develop services with such strong appeal that people are willing to pay for them directly without relying on insurance or Medicare reimbursement to sustain them.

SUMMARY

People are living longer. Research has already shown that if we choose healthy lifestyles, keep fit, eat right, challenge ourselves mentally, and remain engaged with others in the community, we increase our chances of staying healthy well into our 80s or longer. This is within our control, if we make the right choices. Rowe and Kahn (1998) called this successful aging. We are occupational therapists, interested in the everyday activities people do and how we can help them to prevent disability or overcome barriers such as injuries or chronic health conditions, or social attitudes so that they can keep on doing what they want to do. Current research (Carr & Manning, 2010) shows that older adults who choose to remain active in their communities and to continue their productive roles are more likely to live longer, healthier lives while using up fewer health care dollars. Remaining productive is better for elderly citizens and cost-effective for our national budget.

We asked productive agers to share with us some of their secrets of success, and their answers fell into three categories: (1) self-management, (2) social connections, and (3) self-fulfilling activities. These themes, along with the productive occupations already identified by occupational scientists of paid worker, home maintainer, volunteer, caregiver, and lifelong learner, form the basis of a holistic OT approach. We also note that productive occupations and social roles have a complex transactional relationship that makes it difficult to address them separately. This leads to our strong recommendation that OT interventions be delivered, whenever possible, within a group format.

REFERENCES

American Occupational Therapy Association. (2007). AOTA's Centennial Vision and executive summary. *American Journal of Occupational Therapy, 61,* 613-614.

American Occupational Therapy Association. (2008). The occupational therapy practice framework: Domain and process, 2nd Edition. *American Journal of Occupational Therapy, 62,* 625-683.

American Occupational Therapy Association. (2010). *Nearly recession-proof profession celebrates national awareness month* (Press Release). Retrieved from http://aota.org/News/Media/PR/2010-Press-Releases/2010OTMonth.aspx?FT=pdf.

American Occupational Therapy Association. (2012). *Productive aging.* Retrieved from http://www.aota.org/practice/productiveaging.

American Occupational Therapy Association. (2014). The occupational therapy practice framework: Domain and process, 3rd Edition. *American Journal of Occupational Therapy, 68*, S1-S48.

Atchley, R. C. (1989). A continuity theory of normal aging. *The Gerontologist, 26*, 183-190.

Baltes, P. B., & Baltes, M. M. (Eds.). (1990). *Successful aging: Perspectives from the behavioral sciences.* New York: Cambridge University Press.

Butler, R., & Gleason, H. P. (1985). *Productive aging: Enhancing vitality in later life.* New York: Springer.

Butler, R. N. (2002). The study of productive aging. *Journals of Gerontology, 57*, S323.

Carlson, M., Clark, F., & Young, B. (1998). Practical contributions of occupational science to the art of successful ageing: How to sculpt a meaningful life in older adulthood. *Journal of Occupational Science, 5*, 107-118.

Carr, D., & Manning, L. (2010). A new paradigm for qualitative research in the United States: The era of the Third Age. *Qualitative Sociology Review, VI* (April), 16-33.

Clark, F., Azen, S., Carlson, M., Mandel, D., Zemke, R., Hay, J., ... Lipson, L. (1997). Occupational therapy for independent living older adults: A randomized controlled trial. *Journal of the American Medical Association, 278*, 1321-1326.

Clark, F., Jackson, J., Carlson, M., Chou, C., Cherry, B., Jordan-Marsh, M., & Azen, S. (2011). Effectiveness of a lifestyle intervention in promoting the well-being of independently living older people: Results of the Well Elderly 2 randomized controlled trial. *Journal of Epidemiology and Community Health.* Retrieved from http://jech.bmj.com/content/early/2011/06/01/jech.2009.099754.abstract.

Cole, M. (2012). *Group dynamics in occupational therapy: The theoretical basis and practice application of group treatment* (4th ed.). Thorofare, NJ: SLACK Incorporated.

Cole, M., & Tufano, R. (2008). *Applied theories in occupational therapy.* Thorofare, NJ: SLACK Incorporated.

Creek, J. (2014). The knowledge base of occupational therapy. In W. Bryant, J. Fieldhouse, & K. Bannigan (Eds.), *Creek's occupational therapy and mental health* (5th ed., pp. 27-47). London, UK: Churchill Livingstone Elsevier.

Dale, L. (2008). Healthy aging through social participation. *OT Practice,* December, 24-26.

Gilleard, C., Higgs, P., Hyde, M., Wiggins, R., & Blane, D. (2005). Class, cohort, and consumption: The British experience of the Third Age. *Journal of Gerontology: Social Sciences, 60B*, 305-310.

Haslam, C., Jetten, S., Haslam, A., & Knight, C. (2012). The importance of remembering and deciding together: Enhancing the health and well-being of older adults in care. In C. Haslam, & A. Haslam (Eds.), *The social cure* (pp. 297-316). New York: Psychology Press.

Hinterlong, J. E. (2008). Productive engagement among older Americans: Prevalence, patterns, and implications for public policy. *Journal of Aging and Social Policy, 20*, 141-164.

Holt-Lunstad, J., Smith, T. B., & Layton, B. (2010). Social relationships and mortality risk: A meta-analytic review. *PLOS Medicine, 7*(7), e1000316. Doi:10.1371/journal.pmed.1000316.

Hutchenson, S., Yarnal, C., Staffordson, J., & Kerstetter, D. (2008). Beyond fun and friendship: The red hat society as a coping resource for older women. *Ageing & Society, 28*, 979-999.

Jonsson, H. (2011). The first steps into the Third Age: The retirement process from a Swedish perspective. *Occupational Therapy International, 18*, 32-38.

Jonsson, H., Josephsson, S., & Kielhofner, G. (2001). Narratives and experience in an occupational transition: A longitudinal study of the retirement process. *American Journal of Occupational Therapy, 55*, 424-432.

Knight, J., Ball, V., Corr, S., Turner, A., Lowis, M., & Ekberg, M. (2007). An empirical study to identify older adults' engagement in productivity occupations. *Journal of Occupational Science, 14*, 145-153.

Landau, S., Mintun, M., Joshi, A., Koeppe, R., Peterson, R., Aisen, P., ... Jagust, W. (2012). Amyloid deposition, hypometabolism, and longitudinal cognitive decline. *Annals of Neurology, 72*, 578-586.

Laslett, P. (1989). *A fresh map of life: The emergence of the Third Age.* Cambridge, MA: Harvard University Press.

Laslett, P. (1997). Interpreting the demographic changes. *Philosophical Transactions of the Royal Society B: Biological Sciences, 352*, 1805-1809.

Law, M., & Dunbar, S. (2007). Person-environment-occupation model. In S. Dunbar (Ed.), *Occupational therapy models for intervention with children and families* (pp. 27-50). Thorofare, NJ: SLACK Incorporated.

Leland, N., Elliott, S., & Johnson, K. (2012). *Occupational therapy practice guidelines for productive aging for community-dwelling older adults.* Bethesda, MD: AOTA Press.

Mandel, D., Jackson, J., Zemke, R., Nelson, L., & Clark, F. (1999). *Lifestyle redesign: Implementing the well elderly program.* Bethesda, MD: AOTA Press.

Mattingly, C., & Fleming, M. (1994). *Clinical reasoning: Forms of inquiry in a therapeutic practice.* Philadelphia, PA: FA Davis.

Menac, V. (2003). The relation between everyday activities and successful aging: A 6-year longitudinal study. *Journal of Gerontology: Social Sciences, 58B*, S74-S82.

Mountain, G., & Craig, C. (2011). The lived experience of redesigning lifestyle post-retirement in the UK. *Occupational Therapy International, 18*, 48-58.

Murphy, S. L. (2011). Update on geriatric research in productive aging. *American Journal of Occupational Therapy, 65*, 197-205.

Peterson, E. (2011). Reducing fall risk: A guide to community-based programs. *OT Practice,* September, 15-19.

Porter, S., Mazonson, N., & Tickle-Degnen, L. (2011). Supporting social participation in individuals with Parkinson's disease: A story of the Parkinson's men's group. *OT Practice,* August, 17-18.

Rocco, T., Stein, D., & Lee, C. (2003). An exploratory examination of the literature on age and HRD policy development. *Human Resource Development Review, 2*, 155-180.

Rossen, E., Knafl, K., & Flood, M. (2008). Older women's perceptions of successful aging. *Activities, Adaptation, & Aging, 32*, 73-88.

Rowe, J., & Kahn, R. (1998). *Successful aging.* New York: Dell Publishing.

Rowles, G., & Schoenberg, N. (2002). *Qualitative gerontology: A contemporary perspective.* New York: Springer Publishing.

Stav, W., Hallenen, T., Lane, J., & Arbesman, M. (2012). Systematic review of occupational engagement and health outcomes among community-dwelling older adults. *American Journal of Occupational Therapy, 66*, 301-310.

Tarrant, M., Haggar, M., & Farrow, C. (2012). Promoting positive orientation towards health through social identity. In J. Jetten, C. Haslam, & A. Haslam (Eds.), *The social cure: Identity, health and well-being* (pp. 39-54). New York: Psychology Press.

United States Census Bureau. (2009). United States Population Projections. Retrieved February 23, 2011, from http://www.census.gov/population/www/projections/summarytables.html.

World Health Organization. (2001). *International Classification of Functioning, Disability, and Health.* Geneva: Author.

Wright-St. Clair, V. (2012). Being occupied with what matters in advanced age. *Journal of Occupational Science, 19*, 44-53.

Generations and Diversity in Older Adulthood

Marilyn B. Cole, MS, OTR/L, FAOTA

Just as the percentage of older adults in the population is rapidly increasing, their attributes are also becoming more diverse, making many preconceived ideas outdated. This chapter explores some different ways older adults have been categorized, both in scholarly literature and in the media: developmental stages, historical generations, and cultural backgrounds. While these categories increase our general understanding of future older adult clients, they are not intended to describe every individual, and their use does not replace therapeutic use of self in understanding each person as unique.

First, we look at developmental stages as a way to understand the physical, psychological, and social attributes within the aging process. Several contemporary theories of aging are well researched and highly compatible with OT models. Aging research provides ample evidence that physical and cognitive decline are *not* an inevitable result of growing older. Theories of aging give occupational therapists a framework for understanding aspects of normal development in older adulthood, so that it is easier to identify the impact of health conditions, occupational contexts, and individual life circumstances.

A second way to categorize older adults is by their generation. This gives us a sense of the historical events they have experienced and how these have affected their beliefs, values, attitudes, and personalities. These generations have been defined by social science research, as well as longitudinal population studies. The identified characteristics of traditionalists (who experienced the Great Depression and World War II) vary substantially from the characteristics of

their children, dubbed Baby Boomers, who grew up in relative prosperity and participated in the enactment of sweeping social changes such as civil rights, anti-war protests, feminism, and sexual freedom. These two generations, who will soon make up equal parts of occupational therapists' older clients, have very diverse values and beliefs about occupations and health care in older adulthood.

Third, we will look at cultural differences as subcategories of older adults, such as urban vs. rural settings and different ethnic or other minority groups. Multicultural understanding also gives occupational therapists important insight into how to best communicate with older clients who may not have the same expectations for occupational performance as those of mainstream America.

Learning Activity 7: Exploring Your Own Experiences With Older Adults

1. Describe some of your personal experiences with older adults.

2. What is your general impression of their issues and needs?

3. What do you already know about health services for seniors?

4. Would you hope to work in a geriatric setting as an OT practitioner? Why or why not?

5. What does it mean to be an older adult in America today?

Cole MB, Macdonald KC.
Productive Aging: An Occupational Perspective (pp 17-32).
© 2015 Taylor & Francis Group.

TABLE 2-1
LASLETT'S FOUR AGES
First Age: Preparing for life and work
Second Age: Working to support self and family life
Third Age: Retirement, self-fulfillment, and service to society
Fourth Age: Dependence in one or more activities of daily living
Adapted from Laslett, P. (1989). *A fresh map of life: The emergence of the Third Age.* Cambridge, MA: Harvard University Press.

6. How do you think the goals of an individual older than 75 years might differ from your own goals? Explain.

CONTEMPORARY THEORIES OF OLDER ADULTHOOD

Currently, a new graduate could easily find a choice of geriatric OT positions in skilled nursing facilities, adult day cares, or home health agencies. These positions serve Fourth Age (Laslett, 1989) populations who already have functional limitations, regardless of their chronological age. Third Agers, according to Laslett (1989), have retired from obligatory work roles but remain healthy and engaged in a wide variety of productive occupations. These potential clients most likely live independently, although some may have opted to live in retirement, assisted living, or senior housing communities. Occupational therapy roles with these older adults focus on wellness, prevention of disease or disability, and adaptations when dealing with chronic health conditions. Their OT goals might be overcoming obstacles and adapting tasks and environments that allow them to continue active participation in the social and occupational roles of their choosing.

Development and maturation, once thought to end at age 18 years, are now understood to continue throughout the lifespan. However, within the second half of life, developmental stages become less likely to occur at any specific age. The contemporary theories summarized here tend to be defined by changes in focus and selection of different types of activities (occupations) that represent changes in one's self and social identity, changing roles in society, and altered views of the world.

Laslett's Four Ages

Laslett (1989, 1997) bases his theory on current demographics, accounting for extended life spans, improvements in health care, increased percentages of elders in the population, and trends in work and retirement. Roles in society, rather than chronological age, define the four ages listed in Table 2-1. Clients in geriatric OT practice would likely fall into either the Third or Fourth Age categories.

The newly defined Third Age begins at retirement, meaning the necessity of working to support oneself has ended. It emerged because of the growing distance between retirement and the onset of functional disability seen in world demographics, leaving 15 to 30 years of healthful living in retirement. Laslett's theory allows for gainful employment well into the Third Age, but working thereafter is by choice because children have grown and left home and other sources of income (pensions, social security benefits) are usually available (Laslett, 1989). The demographics show that while the legal retirement age remains between ages 60 and 65 years, today's older adults remain healthy and energetic well beyond that age. In 2011, the average life expectancy was 78 years for men, and 81 years for women, (U.S. Department of Health & Human Services-Centers for Disease Control and Prevention, 2011). Furthermore, retirement no longer signifies an endless vacation, but comes with two additional life tasks: self-fulfillment and service to society. In other words, without the responsibilities of working to support a family, Third Agers are free to pursue their lifelong dreams, to express their creative talents, or to start a second career. But according to Laslett's theory, they also have an obligation to direct some of their efforts to solving the problems of society.

Beginning in Europe in the 1980s, Universities of the Third Age (U3As) now have thousands of campuses across the globe (Formosa, 2010). Their purpose is twofold: to offer education to older adults in retirement, and to engage in research on the aging process itself, with the goal of maintaining wellness and increasing longevity. One of the critiques of current U3As has been their focus on liberal arts, "when nowadays retirees are embracing the philosophies of active and productive ageing by engaging in consumer lifestyles, and some, even seeking to re-enter the labor market" (Formosa, 2010, p. 8). However, the very existence of U3As confirms the notion that "very old people in their 80s and 90s can still 'do', 'grow', and 'become' even if they have experienced loss of some physical and mental functions. Simply by living and continuing to grow in a spiritual sense, these elderly people are demonstrating a creativity that can help all of us to become more human" (Withnall, 2002, p. 97). Lifelong learning, therefore, holds a central place in both the Third and Fourth Ages of older adulthood.

The emergence of Third Age theory offers occupational therapists a unique opportunity—that of creating group and individual interventions that focus on prevention, wellness, and promotion of health and well-being. The Third Age is a stage of life in which people remain engaged with others and continue to play important roles in society. When health challenges arise, their goal may likely be to remediate, adapt, or compensate for some lost capacities, so that they can continue their chosen occupational roles. Some examples of new practice areas with this age group are home adaptation, work site adaptation, compensation for vision or hearing loss, fall prevention, adapted mental and physical fitness programs, and finding, defining, and/or adapting meaningful volunteer positions for older adults.

Laslett's Fourth Age is defined in occupational terms, making the distinction easy to identify: dependence in one or more activities of daily living (Laslett, 1989). Logically, most OT clients would fall into this category. However, there are more complex differences between Third and Fourth Ages involving differing patterns of social participation, interest in activities, and emotional and spiritual dimensions. A growing body of evidence supports the notion that entering the Fourth Age denotes a significant change in self and social identity, spirituality or meaning in life, and views of time, space, and the state of humanity.

Socioemotional Selectivity Theory

Socioemotional Selectivity Theory (SST) further defines the changes that occur within Laslett's Fourth Age. When Carstensen (1992) first defined SST, some reasoned that the tendency of elders to narrow their social connections to only their more emotionally significant relationships resonated closely with Cumming and Henry's (1961) mid-century discovery of disengagement theory. However, upon further investigation, SST represents a much more positive view of social and emotional choices with advancing age. The primary assumption in this theory is that people make choices about their social and emotional life based on their future time perspective (Carstensen, Isaacowitz, & Charles, 1999; Lockenhoff & Carstensen, 2004). For example, in a study of friendships over middle and late adulthood, Wright and Patterson (2006) found that younger adults tend to expand their social networks based on common interests and activities and a need for novel and diverse experiences, using a future time perspective. Older adults, perceiving a shorter time left to live, preferred smaller social circles made up of familiar, deeper, and emotionally meaningful relationships. SST also guides people's selection of goals. Younger adults seek goals that expand their horizons, while older adults choose goals that increase their emotional experience and meaning in life (Penningroth & Scott, 2012). Some examples of older adult goals in this study are helping others, staying close to family, and enjoying planned events in the near future. Meaning in life is typically defined as a strong sense of purpose (Krause, 2009). In a group of four studies involving meaning in life, Hicks, Trent, Davis, and King (2012) found a strong correlation between the perception of limited future time in older adults and their experience of positive affect and meaning.

Occupational therapists can apply SST in their selection of activities and goals with older clients whose time left to live is growing short. Some researchers have attempted to draw a parallel between the Third and Fourth Ages by observing their changing interest in specific activities. Adams (2004) defined three categories of activities in her Change in Activity and Interest Index-Revised (CAII-R): active instrumental, active social, and passive social spiritual, based in part on the SST theory. She found that Third Agers more often chose active social activities such as attending concerts and lectures, meeting and getting to know new people, and going to new restaurants or places. Third Agers also chose active instrumental activities, such as entertaining others at home, making and creating things, or shopping and buying things. In contrast, Fourth Agers tended to withdraw from these types of activities, opting instead for passive social spiritual interests such as visiting/hearing from family, taking pleasure in small things, or spiritual life (prayer, meditation, religious services). In an updated study, the CAII-R was used to differentiate older adults normally transitioning to the Fourth Age from those with depression (Adams, Roberts, & Cole, 2011). Third Agers who prematurely withdrew from active social activities were more often struggling with poor health and increased depressive symptoms (Adams et al., 2011). For occupational therapists, this important distinction can only be made by determining the true life stage and supporting the client in determining which goals and activities are truly meaningful within that context.

Developmental Life Stages of Older Adulthood

Jung and Erikson pioneered the extension of adult development theory into later life. Jung (1933) observed the tendency for introversion in later years, focusing on more philosophical and spiritual issues. Out of Erikson's eight stages of psychosocial development, only the final two apply to older adulthood: generativity vs. self-absorption and ego integrity vs. despair (Erikson, 1963; Westermeyer, 2004). Although Erikson (1963) envisioned his eight stages as epigenetic, requiring resolution of conflicts in a defined hierarchy, the tasks are potentially reversible and do not necessarily follow a rigid sequence or specific timing (Vaillant, 1993). The primary focus of generativity is "the culmination of adulthood when the individual becomes a responsible guide or mentor for the next generation" (Westermeyer, 2004, p. 30). More recently, two aspects of generativity have been identified by McAdams, Hart, and Maruna (1998): (1) a desire to play an active role in the next generation, and (2) empathy or compassion for others. The extension of generativity into old age was demonstrated by Shmotkin, Blumstein, and Modan (2003), who found that volunteer roles resulted in more positive psychological functioning and reduced mortality risk for the 75 to 94 age group. The primary focus of Erikson's (1963) integrity phase is the personal satisfaction with one's accomplishments and contributions, giving importance to the tasks of reminiscence and life review, the late life resolution of unfinished issues, and reconciliation of rifts with significant others in the past. Joan Erikson, Erik's wife and frequent collaborator, wrote at age 93 about the need for solitude as a possible Erikson's Ninth Stage, a "deliberate retreat from the usual engagements of daily activity...a paradoxical state that does seem to exhibit a transcendent quality" (Erikson & Erikson, 1997, p. 25).

Gerotranscendence Theory

Gerotranscendence, echoing Joan Erikson's (Erikson & Erikson, 1997) observations, focuses on the positive potential of cognitive changes that occur as the aging individual constructs a new reality, one that shifts from pragmatic and materialistic, to a more cosmic and transcendent world view. This internal, contemplative way of life, which trades in meaningless socialization for solitude, appears to be accompanied by an increase in life satisfaction (Tornstam, 1997, 2000, 2011). The cosmic dimension, which conceptually unites the past and present, may symbolize true wisdom for the older individual. In this state, the individual feels free to select only activities that are meaningful and to ignore the necessity for social reciprocation or convention.

Continuity Theory

Continuity theory proposes that throughout the lifespan, adults make adaptive choices that tend to maintain their self-identity and existing perceptions of self and the world (Atchley, 1989; Atchley & Barusch, 2004). Social identity theory (Jettan, Haslam, & Haslam, 2012) and other theories of social support provide much evidence that this is true. Social convoys, for example, are social groups or networks that continue to interact as one ages (Rowe & Kahn, 1998). For example, groups of friends from school tend to keep in touch as they grow up and age together. This metaphor applies to families and extended families, who move along the road of life together (convoy), sharing each others' joys and sorrows, and assisting each other as needed. Because the absence of social support has been associated with significantly higher mortality for older adults (Lyyra & Heikkinen, 2006), the formal and informal social networks of elderly have been studied extensively. Social support for older adults may provide emotional comfort, guidance, companionship, information, and physical assistance.

Baltes' Theory of Selection, Optimization, and Compensation

This theory applies to the entire lifespan but has particular relevance for the transitions of older adulthood, where life goals and priorities change with both retirement (Laslett's Third Age) and the onset of dependency (Laslett's Fourth Age) (Baltes & Smith, 2001). The rebalancing of life priorities may be best accomplished with careful planning, as one plans for retirement by saving and investing money, but may also be accomplished by establishing and maintaining social networks, civic engagement, and leisure activities apart from paid work throughout the adult years. Baltes' theory suggests that as older adults experience declining energy levels, physical capacities, and other limitations, they will choose top priority occupations (select) and focus remaining resources (optimize) more narrowly on the most important activities. Social and community resources will then be called upon to compensate for those necessary occupations that the older person either cannot do (such as driving or managing finances) or elects not to do (such as cleaning house, grocery shopping, and other instrumental activities of daily living). SOC provides useful guidelines for intervention with older adults who need assistance with the transitions of older adulthood, described in the next chapter.

GENERATIONS DEFINED

While developmental stages offer needed guidance in designing OT interventions, it is also necessary to understand a client's life history from a generation's perspective. This is important because life experience shapes the clients' view of health care, and influences their expectations of OT services. Keeping in mind that each individual is different, we can categorize older adults currently over 60 into one of two generations: traditionalists or Baby Boomers. Strauss and Howe (1991) first introduced generational theory in the 1980s, when they noticed that in market research, people who fought in World War II differed dramatically from people who grew up afterward. Sociologists have defined traditionalists as having birth dates approximately between 1901 and 1945, while Baby Boomers were born approximately between 1946 and 1964 (Xenakis, 2010).

Traditionalists—The Greatest Generation

Dubbed "The Greatest Generation" by Tom Brokaw (2000), traditionalists include primarily those who fought in World War II or engaged in home-front, war-related activities. Some of their historical experiences most likely included poverty and survival during the Great Depression in the 1930s, patriotism and sacrifice during the 1940s war years, and industrial rebuilding, trust in government, and dedication to family and community during the prosperous years that followed. Traditionalists believed in hard work, saving for the future, adherence to rules, and loyalty and respect for authority (many having worked for the same company for most of their careers). In later years, they expect recognition for their experience and to be treated with respect. In their view, others should adhere to good grammar and manners, use self-discipline, behave responsibly, and honor their commitments. As the title implies, traditions are very important to members of this generation, who especially celebrate holidays geared toward patriotism and reinforce family and religious values.

Older traditionalists also learned many lessons from living through the Great Depression in the 1930s. Remembering what it was like to go without, they hesitate to throw away anything that might be needed at a later time. They squirrel away bits of string, empty containers, stray buttons, and wrapping paper. They are members of the "clean plate club," always finishing the food they have served themselves so as not to waste it. They mend their socks and sew patches on their clothing. Some still compost their trash, save seeds to plant next spring, and hang out clothes to dry in the sun, so as not to waste energy because it costs money. Their habits of saving and watching their dollars have served them well in the past and given them survival skills to apply in the future. They cannot understand how younger generations can be so wasteful; they may have been the original conservationists who recycle everything.

The youngest members of this generation would now be in their late 60s, making the majority of older adults traditionalists. However, within this generation is wide variation, not only in the historical events they have experienced, but also in their own roles within that context. Women, for example, may have played a supportive role to their husbands as homemakers and mothers or they may have developed their own careers, fulfilling their parents' dreams for a better future. Some men played active military roles, while others, being too old or too young to serve, worked in agricultural, commercial, or war-related industries on the home front.

Learning Activity 8: Understanding a Traditionalist

Today's college students may be lucky enough to have known their own grandparents and great-grandparents, who were members of The Greatest Generation.

1. As a learning activity, try writing a few paragraphs about a person in your family who was a traditionalist.

2. What life experiences did this person encounter, and what lessons did he or she learn from these experiences?

3. How did traditional values and characteristics help this person deal with occupational challenges later in life?

Case Example: George

George was born in 1902, the youngest of six children in rural Massachusetts. His ancestors came from England and fought in the Revolutionary War. He was the first in his family to get a college degree in 1929, and he worked for an engineering company through the depression years. The company was contracted to create a signal system for the U.S. military during World War II. George spearheaded the project, and later went on to develop communication systems to tally airline reservations, national election results, banking information, and trades on the New York Stock Exchange—systems that paved the way for the modern computers. He worked for the same company for 41 years, valuing loyalty and devotion to the good of the corporation over personal recognition. As a traditionalist, George needed the support of a wife at home looking after the house, the children, the meals, and general home maintenance.

When George had a stroke in 1975, his eyesight declined significantly. For an occupational therapist, he was an ideal client—eager to follow instructions and highly motivated to meet or exceed occupational goals. After just 6 weeks at a rehabilitation hospital, his strong work ethic helped him to recover nearly normal function (other than eyesight), and he continued to work as a consultant for the same company even after his official retirement. His wife provided transportation to and from work. As the years went on, George became hard of hearing and his eyesight diminished to near blindness. A home health occupational therapist adapted his home for maximum independence in daily functioning, including a talking clock, tactile cues for the home's thermostat, tape placed on the TV remote and the controls for the microwave, and an adapted telephone. His wife became his eyes and ears, but he continued to keep the balance for his checkbook in his head and signed all his own checks with the help of an adapted writing board. Despite physical limitations, George held onto his most important life roles—working as an engineer and remaining head of his household. With his adapted telephone and through writing letters on his writing board, he kept in touch with family and lifelong friends. Coworkers continued to call him for advice or to advise him of the latest work news. Through his adapted TV remote and a set of adapted headphones, he kept up with local and national current events. Although he never owned a computer, he was very much aware of its development and felt an integral part of the communication tool it had become. George died at age 97, still in the role of head of household, with the assistance of his wife and daily home health workers (Figure 2-1).

Case Example: Jeanne

Jeanne, a homemaker, had a very different experience. Born in 1914 in New York City, she married right after high school, and spent her young adulthood caring for her home and raising three children. As the oldest daughter in an Italian American family, she became the matriarch, the keeper of family traditions, holding large family dinners each Sunday and planning many social events, including birthday and anniversary celebrations, baptisms and first communions, family vacations and reunions, and later weddings and wakes. Jeanne's forte was cooking: she had

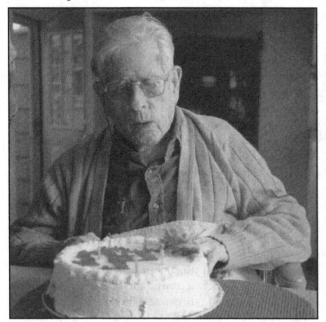

Figure 2-1. George celebrates his 94th birthday.

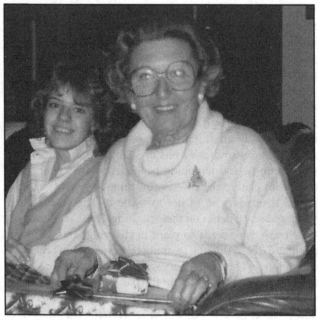

Figure 2-2. Jeanne prepares to unwrap her Christmas gifts at a family gathering (with granddaughter Charlot).

all the old family recipes memorized and taught most of the women in her family to cook. Members of her large and growing family called on her frequently for advice, which she gave out abundantly with discretion and without judgment. In difficult times, she acted as the thread that held the family together. For example, when her son and his wife were going through a difficult divorce, she moved in to take care of her three grandchildren, often mediating arguments and guiding with a firm but gentle voice. She championed traditional values, but also understood the need for compromise.

Later, when her husband died suddenly from cancer at age 59, Jeanne had to cope with life alone for the first time. She had to learn how to drive so she could shop and do errands from her suburban Connecticut home. She found a job as a secretary, where she worked for 10 years to help pay for her children's education. In time, she retired and sold her home, opting for two condominiums, one in Connecticut and the other in Florida. With children grown, Jeanne's social life became more central, although family always came first.

As an older adult, arthritis and stenosis caused Jeanne nearly constant pain, which she stoically endured. An occupational therapist helped her adapt her kitchen in Florida so that she could continue her favorite pastime—cooking and entertaining. Walking became difficult because of arthritis in her hip, and she never fully recovered from a total hip replacement. At age 75, Jeanne required assistance with driving and shopping, which she mostly received from friends and neighbors while in Florida. Her stenosis often caused dizziness, and she experienced two serious falls during the next few years. In one instance, she gashed her scalp and received over 50 stitches at the emergency clinic.

Finally, she had to move in with her daughter, whom she depended upon for most home management activities. She signed over the deeds for both condos to her daughter and oldest son. Because of her failing mobility issues, she could not be left alone, and attended an adult day care program until she died at age 84 (Figure 2-2).

Learning Activity 9: Understanding Characteristics of Traditionalists

1. What are some of the expectations for male vs. female roles and occupations for traditionalists?

   a. Male

   b. Female

2. How did George fulfill the traditional male role expectations?

   a. What social roles did he value most?

   b. List and briefly describe three occupations he most identified with throughout his life.

3. How did Jeanne fulfill the traditional female role expectations?

   a. What social roles did she value most?

   b. List and briefly describe three occupations she most identified with in her life.

4. Choose either Jeanne or George to answer these questions:

   a. Give three examples of how his or her life reflected traditionalist characteristics.

b. Give three examples of how being traditionalists may have caused conflict with people they encountered from later generations.

The values of traditionalists contrast dramatically with the next generation, who may have been their rebellious and socially active children.

Baby Boomers

Baby Boomers (born between 1946 and 1964), defined officially by the increase in birth rate immediately following the end of World War II, have further identified themselves by the mission of righting the wrongs they saw in society through rebellion against prevailing social norms. Baby Boomers are credited with staging peaceful demonstrations that promoted the Civil Rights Act and brought an end to the Vietnam War. They advocated for sexual equality and racial integration in community organizations and in the workplace. Early Baby Boomers were dubbed "hippies" in the 1970s (antiestablishment, sexual freedom, personal growth/gratification) and "yuppies" in the 1980s (spend now, pay later). The historical events they experienced include the Civil Rights and Women's Movements, the Vietnam War, the sexual revolution, the Cold War with Russia, the birth of Rock & Roll, the advent of space travel, and rapid advances in technology.

Because the American dream was promised to them as children, Baby Boomers have been described as entitled, greedy, materialistic, and ambitious. From their experience with social activism in the 1960s and 1970s, Baby Boomers have learned to question traditions, distrust government, and believe strongly in their own ability to create change. They feel quite comfortable challenging authority, demanding their own rights or the rights of others, and organizing and working in teams to raise awareness and enact needed changes in public policy.

On the downside, sociologists have accused Baby Boomers of being spendthrifts, living beyond their means and racking up mountains of debt. They also have been dubbed workaholics who invented terms like *24/7*, meaning they take phone calls and communicate via e-mail even when home, on weekends, and while vacationing. In fact, they never stop working and may have difficulty knowing how to relax and socialize outside of work after they retire.

Baby Boomers are just beginning to enter their retirement years and are anticipating ways to promote their own healthy aging. Current life roles often include being members of the "sandwich" generation, meaning having simultaneous caregiving roles for both underage children and aging parents. Not surprisingly, their attitudes about caregiving responsibility might differ significantly from that of their traditionalist parents. Occupational therapists may need to address Baby Boomers' perceptions of caregiving and how that might be different from their parents' view of family caregiving responsibility (Table 2-2).

Case Example: Pam

Pam always wanted to be a nurse. She attended a bachelor's degree nursing program at a large state university in the 1960s, a time of considerable campus unrest and social turmoil. As soon as Pam settled into her freshman classes, the campus erupted with demonstrations following the assassination of President Kennedy in the fall of 1964. She remembers marching through the campus quadrangles to the tune of Ray Charles' "Hit the Road, Jack," while on weekends classmates taught her do the "Peppermint Twist" at local fraternity houses. Campus organizers recruited the impressionable Pam to write and sign letters to senators and congressmen, and participate in peaceful demonstrations calling for civil rights reforms and an end to the war in Vietnam. Although Pam remembers watching the Beatles' Ed Sullivan debut on the dorm TV, she preferred to listen to the deeper lyrics of Joan Baez, Bob Dylan, and Marianne Faithful. In spite of the lessons from anatomy and physiology professors, she did "inhale" the joints passed to her at parties and rock concerts at nearby jazz festivals.

After college, Pam worked for 2 years in a general hospital before marrying and staying home with her children. However, she remained active in local and professional organizations and soon found herself organizing fundraising activities for the parent-teacher association and advocating for more services for returning war veterans. As a graduate nurse without a full-time job, Pam became involved in an interdisciplinary committee advocating for the recognition of post-traumatic stress disorder (PTSD), a signature mental illness of returning Vietnam veterans who had seen combat close-up. In the 1970s, PTSD was not yet recognized as an official diagnosis, so the Veterans Administration (VA) hospitals did not provide or pay for any type of treatment. Pam claims that the eventual inclusion of PTSD in the *Diagnostic and Statistical Manual of Mental Disorders* revision of 1980 is one of her personal accomplishments.

After both her children were grown, Pam divorced, remarried, and moved across the country, racking up years of working as head nurse for the VA's psychiatric units in several major cities. While she never smoked, Pam often struggled with weight gain and loss, and at age 60 was diagnosed with type II diabetes mellitus, for which she alternately takes insulin or goes on strict crash diets. Now, with a good government pension, Pam has retired at age 62. She does miss working, especially interacting with people and the physical exercise her position provided.

Naturally extraverted, Pam has maintained many social contacts through her profession, her blended families, and her weight loss support groups. Through her second husband, Pam has inherited a large extended family, although none of her own relatives or grown children live nearby. Still, she has a difficult time with self-discipline regarding her diet, lack of exercise, and the scheduling of

		TABLE 2-2	
		FOUR GENERATIONS IN MAINSTREAM AMERICA SUMMARIZED	
	BIRTH YEARS	**HISTORICAL EVENTS**	**POSITIVE & NEGATIVE TRAITS**
Traditionalists: "The Greatest Generation" (Brokaw, 2000)	1902 to 1945	World Wars I and II, the Great Depression, Medicare and Social Security began, air travel, super-highways, Big Band era, movies, TV	Trust in government; respect for authority; loyalty to country, employer, community organizations, organized religions, expect others to take responsibility and keep their promises
Baby Boomers: "Me" Generation "Aging Boom"	1946 to 1964	Economic prosperity, Civil Rights Movement, Vietnam War, sexual revolution, space program, Cold War, rock and roll music, color movies, and TV	Hard working, workaholics; idealistic; committed to harmony, sense of entitlement, self-centered, belief in social activism, spend now, save later, long-term commitments to employers, careers
Generation X: Slackers, X-ers	1965 to 1980	Both parents working, latchkey kids, widespread use of personal computers, economic uncertainty, rise in divorce rate, country music, rap music	Entrepreneurial, flexible and creative, comfortable with technology, skeptical and cynical, lazy, pampered by parents, question authority figures, prefer flexibility in workplace
Millennials: Generation Next	1981+	E-mail, Internet, cell phones, immediate access to information, globalization, violence and terrorism in the United States	Tech-savvy, attuned to and appreciate diversity, skilled multitaskers, lacking basic literary fundamentals, very short attention spans, distracted and distractible, not loyal to job

Adapted from Ethics Resource Center, 2010.

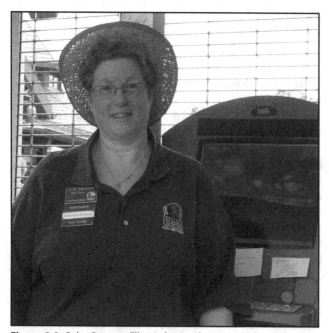

Figure 2-3. Baby Boomer Ellen is busier than ever in her retirement. Here, she is volunteering at a local zoo.

her time. Currently, she's considering going back to school or volunteering in a foreign country where her nursing skills are needed. But first, she needs to get her diabetes mellitus and her weight under control. It has never occurred to Pam that she is getting old, and she looks forward to better things in her future.

Learning Activity 10: Identifying Features of Baby Boomers

1. What characteristics of the Baby Boomers does Pam carry with her from the above description?

2. How did the historical events she experienced influence her life?

3. If Pam were referred to you for OT, what might be some appropriate OT goals?

4. How might you treat Pam differently from a traditionalist with similar medical concerns (Figure 2-3)?

MULTICULTURAL DIVERSITY: SUBGROUPS OF OLDER ADULTHOOD

Culture means more than just race, ethnicity, or where our ancestors came from. Culture affects almost every aspect of everyday life, from the language we use, to the food we eat, to the nature of our relationships with others, what life roles we play, to the goals we set for ourselves, and our expectations of others. Even our self-identity and our view of the world around us is deeply embedded in our culture. Many people are unaware of their own culture until they find themselves immersed in a different one, such as when they travel to another country or move to a different geographic locale.

Urban Versus Suburban and Rural Cultures

When interviewing productive older adults, we noticed very different attitudes and expectations for community services between New York City dwellers and those living in suburban Connecticut. Some people who have lived all their lives in a city have never needed to learn how to drive a car. For them, driving cessation would be a nonissue because most can catch a bus or a subway a few yards outside their front door. In a large city, a wide variety of health services might be found within a few blocks from home, with the nearest drug store just across the street. On the other hand, in the suburbs and rural areas, being unable to drive renders an older adult dependent on others for even basic necessities like grocery shopping.

In a study of mental health attitudes among rural and urban older adults, researchers found that city dwelling elders placed a higher value on mental health services and were more likely to seek help there than their rural dwelling counterparts (Hayslip, Maiden, Thomison, & Temple, 2010). Averill (2012) found that rural older adults in the southwestern United States had less access to health services and needed assistance with prescription renewal, transportation, in-home caregiving, and overcoming cultural and language barriers. Interestingly, a study of the incidence and severity of depression did not show significant differences between urban- and rural-dwelling seniors (Zimmerman, 2012).

Effects of Urbanization for Older Adults

Urbanization refers to growing concentrations of populations in cities. This represents the global tendency for younger people to move from rural areas where their parents may have lived their entire lives to the cities where they can obtain higher education and training and can more easily find higher paying jobs. In developing countries such as China, India, or Brazil, three-generational households used to be the norm, within which elder family members were respected and cared for by their children and grandchildren. However, urbanization has often left elders in these societies behind, in isolated rural areas where access to health and caregiving is difficult or nonexistent. In some countries, such as sub-Saharan Africa, adult children not only move to cities to find work, but also leave their young children behind to be cared for by their grandparents, a phenomenon that is only heightened by the HIV-AIDS epidemic (Hooyman & Kiyak, 2011).

In the United States and other industrialized nations such as the United Kingdom, Western Europe, Japan, and Scandinavia, urbanization occurred much earlier, probably in the late 19th and early 20th centuries, and these nations have instituted government programs that provide pension and health care benefits for their older citizens. Urbanization has the effect of splitting up families or separating them by generations in different areas of the country and weakening strong ties and/or family caregiving obligations. From a social perspective, urbanization takes away some of the power and status elders once held in their families and their communities because in cities, and in the media, "youth is glorified as the embodiment of progress and achievement" (Hooyman & Kiyak, 2011, p. 52). This trend is compounded by the rapid development in technology and the Internet, leaving older adults with the label of "digital immigrants" positioned clearly on the wrong side of the hypothetical digital divide (Prensky, 2001).

Occupational therapists need to consider the pros and cons of urban living for older clients. Some positive aspects include a wide range of living quarters, products and services, public transportation, and diversity of social connections. Cons included traffic congestion, crime, and higher costs. In suburban or rural settings, older adults must depend on driving to meet basic needs and socialization and may have less access to services and fewer choices. Suburban settings often necessitates shopping at megamalls and "big box" stores.

Filial Piety and the Status of Elderly

In Asian countries, including Japan, China, Taiwan, Korea, Thailand, and the Philippines, filial piety, defined as a "sense of reverence and deference toward elders" and a "lifelong indebtedness to one's parents" (Hooyman & Kiyek, 2011, pp. 54-55), is a deeply embedded cultural tradition. Perhaps it began with the Hindu belief in ancestor worship. However, in modern times, the greatest impact is in families, where the younger members feel a strong obligation to care for their parents and grandparents, to seek their guidance, and to honor their wishes. Urbanization in these countries has compromised this tradition, often leaving elderly relatives dependent on strangers or governments to sustain them. In China, because of its long-standing one child per family rule, there are not enough younger relatives to care for older Chinese citizens, placing an increasing burden on the government to create public programs to fill the void. According to He, Sengupta, Zhang, and Guo (2007), 77% of China's older adults live in isolated rural areas, while their adult children have migrated to cities to work, a pattern repeated in surrounding nations also experiencing rapid economic growth. Some rural living elders live in "skipped generation" households, where they are left to care for grandchildren and sometimes still receive financial support from children, which eases the burden. However, Asian women, to whom family caregiving responsibilities traditionally fell, no longer want to leave their jobs to fulfill this obligation.

Latin American countries, including South and Central America and the Caribbean, which are primarily Christian, also have a strong tradition of caring for their older relatives within families. Hispanic immigrants do not readily accept the notion of moving grandparents to long-term care facilities, which they view as a denial of filial obligation. They usually opt to mobilize extended family members as caregivers in home and community settings (Gelfand, 2003). Adult day care in Hispanic immigrant neighborhoods has become a more acceptable option, (e.g., the El Portal Latino Alzheimer's Project in Los Angeles) (Aranda, Villa, Trejo, Ramirez, & Ranney, 2003).

Conversely, many American nursing homes, assisted living residences, and home health agencies hire predominantly female Latin American immigrants to fill low paying jobs, including both housekeeping/maintenance and direct health care (Leutz, 2007). While these workers may possess the necessary skills and work ethic, they often do not speak English well enough to adequately communicate with the predominantly non-Hispanic elderly residents.

Hispanics make up about 15% of the United States population, and this is projected to become 25% by 2050. About half of these are Mexican Americans. Statistics tell us that mortality rates are generally lower for Hispanics than for non-Hispanic Whites, despite their lower income, education, and access to health care. Researchers attribute this phenomenon to the Hispanic elder's greater connectedness with family, faith, culture, and community (Falcon, 2005). This may be a key ingredient for the health and longevity of all older Americans.

Despite urbanization, in most cultures, families continue to play a pivotal role in the care of elderly parents and relatives. However, this trend will be challenged as the percentage of older adults in the population increases, especially if the economy continues to decline.

Lesbian, Gay, Bisexual, and Transgender Issues in Aging

According to the American Psychological Association (2014), the growing population of lesbian, gay, bisexual, and transgender (LGBT) older adults experience unique economic and health disparities and are at higher risk for some specific conditions in their older years. Because of a lifetime of facing stigma and abuse, as well as lack of legal protection, many LGBT older adults are reluctant to disclose their sexual preferences in health care settings for fear of discrimination and rejection. Many fear that caregivers will not be open-minded, affirming, and supportive. Social isolation is a major concern because members of this disadvantaged group often lack the support of adult children or extended families whom their heterosexual counterparts generally rely on for caregiving as they age (American Psychological Association, 2014).

The Centers for Disease Control and Prevention (CDC) (2012) identifies a pronounced gap in research on health disparities with LGBTs in terms of health and aging. Several subsequent studies funded by the CDC are summarized by Fredriksen-Goldsen (2012). There are an estimated 2% of adults over age 50 years who self-disclose as lesbian, gay, bisexual, or transgender living in the United States. As an at-risk population, LGBTs experience significant health disparities, even when controlling for differences in age distribution, income, and education. They have a higher incidence of disability (41% of those over age 50 years) and mental distress and depression (31%), and they are more likely to smoke and engage in heavy drinking than their heterosexual counterparts. Female members have a heightened risk for cardiovascular disease and obesity and are less likely to have a mammogram. Older gay men are more likely to experience poor physical health, perhaps because many are now living into old age with HIV. Within the LGBT group, diabetes mellitus is significantly more common among older bisexual men than among older gay men. Another national study funded by the CDC (2012) confirms the higher disability and depression rates and additionally reports that 53% experience loneliness and 27% have experienced the death of a partner. Historically, older LGBT members have spent most of their lives masking their sexual orientation or identity, with "their stories largely silenced" (Fredriksen-Goldsen, 2012, p. 5). There is good reason for this because most have experienced serious victimization: 82% were victimized at least once, 64% reported 3 or more times, 68% experienced verbal insults, 42% were threatened with physical violence, 27% were hassled by police, 27% were rejected for housing, 22% were not hired for a job, and 20% had their property damaged. However, a lack of disclosure prevents discussions about sexual health, hepatitis, hormone therapy, breast cancer, or HIV risks. With disclosure, some (13%) have already been denied admission to a medical or care facility. They expect to rely on partners or friends from their LGBT communities to care for them as they age; of those receiving care, 54% comes from a partner or spouse, and 27% from a friend.

Baby Boomers, because of the tremendous cultural shifts in attitude toward LGBT that have occurred in their lifetimes, are more likely to disclose their sexual orientation. According to a MetLife (2006) survey, a surprisingly high percentage of this group take on caregiving roles (one in four), with caregiving shared equally among men and women: 36% were caring for aging parents, 18% for partners, 14% for friends, and 12% for other nonrelatives. The majority (three-quarters) of LGBTs from the Baby Boomer generation also reported important connections with what they have called "families of choice" (i.e., a group of close friends who either share or are respectful of their sexual lifestyle). The MetLife (2006) Baby Boomer study also reports some major concerns or fears of aging LGBTs about their older years. Women mostly feared outliving their income, while men feared becoming, sick, disabled, and dependent. Only half of those surveyed expected that health care professionals would treat them with dignity and respect. Additionally, less than half had completed written wills or living wills, which spelled out their end-of-life wishes, yet "such documents are particularly important for LGBT older adults given the current lack of legal protection" (MetLife, 2006, p. 5). granted to heterosexual couples and families regarding health care decisions, visitation privileges, insurance coverage, and qualification for publicly funded financial or health programs

In summary, the culturally competent OT practitioner needs to be sensitive to and respectful of the many types of diversity in older adults. Types might include ethnicity, sexual orientation, political viewpoints, and spiritual beliefs and practices. While awareness of cultural characteristics and differences is helpful to our overall understanding of diverse groups of older adults, occupational therapists need to avoid falling into the trap of stereotyping people in any of these categories and remain sensitive to individual values and lifestyles.

Learning Activity 11: Exploring Cultural Bias in Aging

Mildred, at age 86, has moved to a cluster housing facility to be closer to her daughter's family. She still drives but restricts herself to daytime and short distances and avoids heavy traffic and questionable weather conditions. It is now possible for her to drive 30 minutes to visit her daughter, son-in-law, and grandson without going out of her driving comfort zone. However, she now finds herself the only Jewish person amidst a retirement community of Christians. Additionally, she has some digestive difficulties and religious restrictions on the foods she can eat, and these prevent her from enjoying pizza parties or sharing birthday cakes, the only social events to which she has been invited by other residents. Mildred is normally quite sociable, has had a long and rewarding career in health care, and has kept up with many former coworkers, most of whom live too far away for her to visit easily. She wonders if she made the wrong decision to move to such a place, where she obviously feels like an outsider.

1. Fill in the blanks on the empathy statement below to best express your understanding of Mildred's emotional responses to her situation. You seem to feel _____ because

   _____.

2. Write three follow-up questions you might ask to further understand Mildred's dilemma.

   a.

   b.

   c.

3. How do you think this situation might affect Mildred's health and well-being as she ages?

4. As an OT practitioner, which areas of occupational performance would you identify as important, and what interventions would you suggest for Mildred? Explain your reasoning.

THE GLOBAL AGING BOOM

The "aging boom" is a worldwide phenomenon caused by lower fertility rates, advances in health care, and increased longevity. Currently, 60% of the world's older adults live in developing countries, which may increase to 75% by 2020. Of developed countries, Japan has the highest percentage of those older than age 65 years (22%) followed by Italy (20%), Germany, and Greece (19%) (Population Reference Bureau, 2008). As the proportion of older adults rises and urbanization continues as predicted, governments will need to put policies in place to provide for them. They generally do so with programs such as Social Security and Medicare in the United States, with younger workers paying into the programs that support retirees. In this country as well as abroad, medical and pension plans are threatened with insolvency when the proportion of elders receiving benefits exceeds the proportion of workers paying into entitlement programs. Governments have the choice of importing immigrant workers or encouraging older adults to continue working longer to fill the void, but these efforts are confounded by the current economic recession. The global aging boom is likely to affect broad aspects of life, including distribution of wealth and financial resources, structure of markets, employment conditions, and immigration and taxation policies, as well as the cost and structure of global medical care, among many others.

The status of older adults in traditional societies has been sustained by the balance between their contributions to society and the costs of supporting them. Some older adults' ability to contribute stems from their sources of power, such as material possessions (wealth, real estate holdings), knowledge (history, traditions, expertise, wisdom of life experience), and social authority (public reputation, interpersonal connections). Older adults who still hold some power in the form of money or social influence prefer to use it in exchange for needed services and to remain in control of their own lives as they age, rather than becoming dependent on others, especially their families (Hooyman & Kiyak, 2011). The new challenge for health care and public policy makers is to intervene earlier in the aging process, and design programs that preserve wellness, and encourage and enable older adults to continue making contributions to society that allow them to maintain their social identity. This both preserves their health and well-being, and prevents them from becoming a premature burden on either their families or society (Jettan et al., 2012).

COMMUNICATING RESPECT AND EMPATHY FOR DIVERSE OLDER ADULTS

Cultural competence requires health care workers, including occupational therapists, to cultivate an attitude of nonjudgmental acceptance and collaboration when working with older adults. This might begin with an understanding of the client's stage of development, the generation into which they were born, and the traditions of their country of origin. However, the true test of cultural competence lies in our therapeutic use of self and the ways in which we communicate with each individual. Therapeutic use of self is utilized throughout the therapeutic process, which "allows OT practitioners to develop and manage their therapeutic relationship with clients by using narrative and clinical reasoning, empathy, and a client-centered, collaborative approach to service delivery" (AOTA, 2014, p. S12).

The OT process begins by establishing a rapport through asking thoughtful questions about the older adult's life, the activities or occupations that give his or her life meaning, the roles and social identities that person maintains, and the social networks with whom he or she interacts. Showing a genuine interest in the ways in which a person participates in life communicates an attitude of *respect* and acceptance, regardless of the problems the client may be facing. This represents an important first step in developing a therapeutic relationship.

The next phase of the OT evaluation entails a discussion of the current challenges or situations the client faces, including health issues, symptoms, disabilities, lost roles, troubled relationships, and external barriers to a desired level of engagement with others and in meaningful occupations. To fully understand the perspective of the client, the occupational therapist expresses empathy for the feelings and situations the client describes. This is the best way to establish trust and to encourage the client to more fully describe the problem areas that will form the focus of therapeutic intervention.

Empathy may be defined as an understanding and appreciation of the emotions, beliefs, and views of another person, even when those emotions, beliefs, and views are not the same as our own. We first communicate empathy nonverbally through our facial expression and gestures, our universal language when dealing with other cultures. When using words, occupational therapists must choose words that accurately describe the type and degree of the intensity of emotion the client is expressing. For example, if the client uses an angry voice when explaining how his boss unfairly terminated his employment, the occupational therapist might express empathy by saying, "You sound furious with your boss for not recognizing how hard you have worked." This comment shows that you understand his feeling and the reasons for it, so that he can then move on and get closer to problem solving how he will deal with his current life situation.

Learning Activity 12: Communicating Empathy

Your client, Oliver's wife, Emma, is having trouble coping with the care needs of her very demanding husband, who has just come home from the hospital following rehabilitation for a hip replacement. She complains of feeling tired from being frequently awakened with her husband's complaints.

1. What are some emotions she might be feeling? Name three.

2. Fill in the sentence below. Be sure to include an accurate word for Emma's feelings, and a summary of the reason for her feeling from her perspective. "You seem to feel _____ because _____." If you are unsure the words you chose are correct, you can check back with "Is that right?"

3. Name three emotions Oliver might be feeling.

4. Fill in the sentence below for Oliver. Be sure to include an accurate word for his feelings, and a summary of the reason for it from his perspective. "You seem to feel _____ because _____." Likewise you can check back with "Is that right?"

By expressing empathy, the OT establishes trust in the therapeutic relationship, which encourages further self-disclosure on the part of clients. As OT practitioners continue an initial interview, they more quickly learn who their clients are and what occupations are important and meaningful to them. This not only establishes rapport, but also supports their roles as equal partners in the therapeutic process, whose wishes will be respected. It answers the following questions: "What do they want to be able to do" and "Why can't they do it?"

NEW GENERATIONS OF OCCUPATIONAL THERAPY PRACTITIONERS

Earlier we described some of the generations from which our older adult clients might come. Two additional generations (see Table 2-2) are Generation X and Generation Next (Millennials), as defined by the Ethics Resource Center (2010). These generations, along with the Baby Boomers, represent the current workforce, including graduating OT students and professionals who provide services to the older generations. By understanding the different attributes of each, communication may be facilitated, making it easier to reach a common understanding regarding the goals and health care needs of older clients around which to design effective interventions.

Sociologists create descriptions of the different generations for many reasons, the most common of which is market research (likes, dislikes, interests, buying behaviors). However, the generations themselves have been separated by trends such as birthrate, as well as political views, social behaviors, attitudes, and general personality characteristics. Strauss and Howe (1997) studied the impact of various generations throughout American history and discovered a repeating pattern following crisis wars such as World War II, which they named the "Fourth Turning." Each generation plays a different social role leading up to the next crisis war:

1. Hero generation (fighters who resolve crisis, and become subsequent civic leaders; e.g., GI generation)

2. Artist generation (grow up during crisis period; e.g., Silent generation)

3. Prophet generation (grow up in the glow of success, make social changes that lead to the next crisis; e.g., Baby Boomers)

4. Nomad generation (grow up in shadow of prophets, feeling alienated and cynical but able to lead others in a crisis period).

While the validity of this social generations theory is unclear, it does predict the trends of the upcoming generations—Generation X being the cynical Nomads and Generation Next about to become a new generation of Heroes.

Generation X (X-ers)

This generation immediately following the Baby Boomers has been defined primarily by a reversal in the birth rate both in the United States and abroad. The children of Baby Boomers, many X-ers grew up as latchkey kids whose parents both worked or they were supported by single parents. Their chief complaint usually has to do with being left to fend for themselves, without the presence or guidance of responsible adults. On the positive side, their parents showered them with material gifts and encouraged their creative talents with lessons and group memberships. As workers, they have become self-starters, determined learners, and creative and flexible in their work roles. They often prefer to figure things out for themselves or to invent better ways of doing their jobs. Members of this generation are currently in middle adulthood and may have worked in a variety of organizations or settings while establishing their careers.

Generation Next (Millennials)

Teens and young adults in this generation are currently younger than age 30 years, about the age of the majority of new graduates in OT starting or continuing in their first jobs. The defining characteristic for them is having grown up with computers and technology, making them the first "digital natives" (Prensky, 2001). They are also called Millennials, and they experienced terrorism and violence in the world (e.g., September 11, 2001) at an early age. The Pew Research Center (2007) reports that Millennials' most important goals are getting rich and being famous. Their heroes tend to be entertainers rather than world leaders, and they learn most of what they know about the world through the Internet and social networks. Having grown up with political correctness, they readily accept other races, nationalities, and religions, as well as lesbian, gay, bisexual, and transgendered lifestyles. When dealing with older adults, ageism is not an issue.

Interestingly, most Millennials have maintained close relationships with their parents and grandparents, reporting frequent contact, either daily or weekly. They seem to have a natural respect for older adults generally and communicate effectively with them. In spite of their own greater skill and knowledge of technology, Millennials admire their elders and often find their role models among their family members rather than public figures. Politically, they are less cynical than their predecessors in Generation X about governments and corporations and are somewhat better informed about local, national, and world events. About 75% of Millennials say their parents have helped them financially (Pew Research Center, 2007).

Baby Boomers as Occupational Therapy Practitioners

Although new graduates are likely to come from newer generations, OT practitioners who are themselves Baby Boomers are likely to remain in the workforce for some time. Baby Boomers in 2014 would range in age from 50 to 68 years of age, and most would have upward of 25 years of work experience, placing them as senior therapists, managers, or possibly educators. When encountering clients from their own generation, there would be an expectation of greater understanding and empathy, given their shared history and characteristics, but this may not always be true. Baby Boomer occupational therapists may also be in a unique position to mentor younger generations of therapists, but because they have practiced mainly within the medical model of health care, they may have difficulty moving to an emerging practice area that does not have an established system of reimbursement. Alternatively, as they near retirement, they may welcome broader OT roles within the community that are more compatible with the changing health care trends and professional mandates such as the OT Centennial Vision. Because Baby Boomers have a history of participating in social change, OT practitioners from this generation may have the skills and confidence to lead the profession to new forms of reimbursement outside the medical model. See Chapter 4 for a more in-depth discussion of health care reimbursement systems.

INTERGENERATIONAL/ MULTICULTURAL CHALLENGES AND OPPORTUNITIES

With such diversity among older adults, gaining a true understanding of who they are as people can become very complex. It is hoped that reviewing the many possible ways older people might define themselves will make it easier for OT practitioners to appreciate their older clients as individuals with unique histories, lifestyles, attitudes, and priorities that affect their occupational profiles.

Learning Activity 13: Dealing With Diversity

1. Interview someone who is a traditionalist. Create an occupational profile of this person, following the guidelines outlined in Chapter 1. What were the main historical events that affected this person's occupational choices?

2. Interview someone who is a Baby Boomer. Create an occupational profile of this person using the AOTA Practice Framework guidelines (2014). How did the historical and political events of the Baby Boomer generation affect this person's occupational history?

3. Suppose an occupational therapist _____ (Choose one: Baby Boomer, Next, Millennial) is assigned to work with a _____ (Choose one: male, female) client who is a _____ (Choose one: Baby Boomer, Traditionalist).

   a. What do you see as the potential cultural differences based only on what you know about each of these generations?

   b. What might be some beliefs and expectations about health care for each?

   c. How would generational characteristics influence your approach to this client as an OT practitioner?

4. For the OT practitioner and client in Question 3, add two different descriptors from the following (African American, Hispanic, Japanese American, Jewish, Muslim, Christian, gay, lesbian, urban, rural, Easterner, Midwesterner, West Coast).

   a. What are some potential conflicts you would predict?

   b. What are some beliefs and expectations about health care for each?

   c. How would both generational and cultural diversity issues affect your approach to this client as an OT practitioner?

5. What would you do if a client from _____ (culture different from your own) expresses bias against you as an OT practitioner? Choose 3 different categories to answer this question and describe below.

   a.

   b.

   c.

   d.

JOURNAL ENTRY (M. C.)

Having taught geriatrics for more than a decade, I have told many stories to my students of Third and Fourth Agers, traditionalists and Baby Boomers, and older clients I have encountered while traveling in Europe, South America, and Australia, often with vastly divergent outlooks on aging, retirement, and the role of health care.

Traditionalists, our older cohorts of clients who may have experienced harder times such as the Great Depression, have a tendency to accept the advice and guidance of health care providers without question. They often don't mind being dependent on doctors, hospitals, or institutions because they trust medical professionals and believe they know what is best. Baby Boomers typically lack such trust and tend to question everything. They double check the facts about health conditions on the Internet, they look up medication alternatives, and they want a second opinion. Because of their firm belief in self-determination, they will probably have a much better transition into the Third Age (retirement) than traditionalists and will fend off the Fourth Age (dependency) for as long as possible. People I've encountered in other countries, such as Costa Rica and Brazil, also have firm roots in the medical model and don't often take the initiative to manage their own aging process. European elders I've met take the opposite stance, taking note of the many viewpoints and choices available to them. Life experiences really do matter; knowing our clients' personal history and cultural background matters if we are to understand why they respond so differently to their own health conditions and to OT interventions.

I automatically think of Third Agers as resilient, innovative, and flexible, and being well able to manage their own aging, to change with the times, and to remain productive. However, there are also many people I know who retire only to become immersed in their own chronic health conditions and unable to escape feeling marginalized and left behind by their former working worlds. These people need the help of occupational therapists, but they remain outside the medical referral pool until an actual health crisis occurs, which, in my thinking, is much too late. Something is wrong with a health care system that does not address wellness and prevention during the predictable transitions of older adulthood.

SUMMARY

The older American population is much too diverse to be categorized according to like characteristics, health status, or occupational preference. However, there are some categories that have been well researched and can therefore help OT students and professionals to better understand and appreciate their older clients. We explored some theories of older adult development that give us insight to the normal life stages and predictable changes of aging. Understanding generations gives us a fuller appreciation for the historical events, eras, and trends that have influenced the life experiences of specific age groups. Rural, urban, and other cultural diversity aspects also impact the varied experiences that make older clients the special people that they are. Occupational therapists also come from generations that have been researched, with certain common characteristics that set them apart from other generations. This background is intended to help occupational therapists to better understand their older clients and to communicate respect and empathy for the changes and challenges they face with aging.

REFERENCES

American Occupational Therapy Association. (2014). Occupational therapy practice framework: Domain and process, 3rd edition. *American Journal of Occupational Therapy, 68*(Supplement 1).

American Psychological Association. (2014). *Lesbian, gay, bisexual and transgender aging.* Retrieved from http://www.apa.org/print-this.aspx.

Adams, K. B. (2004). Changing investment in activities and interests in elders' lives: Theory and measurement. *International Journal of Aging and Human Development, 58,* 87-108.

Adams, K. B., Roberts, A., & Cole, M. (2011). Changes in activity and interest in the third and fourth age: Associations with health, functioning and depressive symptoms. *Occupational Therapy International, 18,* 4-17.

Aranda, M., Villa, V., Trejo, L., Ramirez, R., & Ranney, M. (2003). El Portal Latino Alzheimer's Project: Model program for Latino caregivers of Alzheimer's disease-affected people. *Social Work, 48,* T1.

Atchley, R. C. (1989). Continuity theory of normal aging. *Gerontologist, 29,* 183-191.

Atchley, R. C., & Barusch, A. (2004). *Social forces and aging: An introduction to social gerontology* (10th ed.). New York: Wadsworth.

Averill, J. (2012). Priorities for action in a rural older adult study. *Social Networks and Elders' Health, 35,* 358-372.

Baltes, P., & Smith, J. (2001). *New frontiers in the future of aging: From successful aging of the young old to the dilemmas of the Fourth Age.* Retrieved from http://www.valenciaforum.com/Keynotes/pb.html.

Brokaw, T. (2000). *The greatest generation speaks.* New York: Random House.

Carstensen, L. L. (1992). Social and emotional patterns in adulthood. *Psychology and Aging, 7,* 331-338.

Carstensen, L. L., Isaacowitz, D. M., & Charles, S. T. (1999). Taking time seriously: A theory of socioemotional selectivity. *American Psychologist, 54,* 165-181.

Centers for Disease Control (2012). Deaths: Preliminary data for 2011. National Vital Statistics Reports, Volume 61, Number 6. Retrieved from http://www.cdc.gov/nchs/data/nvsr61_06pdf.

Cumming, E. & Henry, W. (1961). *Growing old: The process of disengagement.* New York, NY: Basic Books.

Diagnostic and Statistical Manual of Mental Disorders—DSM III R (1980). Washington, DC: American Psychiatric Association.

Erikson, E. H. (1963). *Childhood and society.* New York: Norton.

Erikson, E. H., & Erikson, J. M. (1997). *The life cycle completed.* New York: Norton.

Ethics Resource Center. (2010). Retrieved from http://www.ethics.org.

Falcon, A. (2005). Hispanic health and aging in a new century (Preface). *Report of the second conference on aging in the Americas.* Retrieved from www.utexas.edu/lbj.caa.scaia_summary_report.pdf.

Formosa, M. (2010). Lifelong learning in later life: The universities of the Third Age. *The Annual Journal of the Osher Lifelong Learning Institute,* Fall, Volume 5. Retrieved from http://www.um.edu.mt/pub/formosam8.html.

Fredriksen-Goldsen, K. (2012). Resilience and disparities among lesbian, gay, bisexual, and transgender older adults. *Public Policy and Aging Report, 21*(3), 3-8. Retrieved from http://caringandaging.org/wordpress/wp-content/uploads/2012/full-report10-25-12.pdf.

Gelfand, D. E. (2003). *Aging and ethnicity: Knowledge and services* (2nd ed.). New York: Springer.

Hayslip, B., Maiden, R., Thomison, N., & Temple, J. (2010). Mental health attitudes among rural and urban older adults. *Clinical Gerontologist: The Journal of Aging and Mental Health, 33,* 316-331.

He, W., Sengupta, M., Zhang, K., & Guo, P. (2007). Health and healthcare of the older population in urban and rural China: 2000. *International Population Reports, P95/07-2.* Washington, DC: U.S. Census Bureau.

Hicks, J. A., Trent, J., Davis, W. E., & King L. A. (2012). Positive affect, meaning in life, and future time perspective: An application of socioemotional selectivity theory. *Psychological Aging, 27,* 181-189.

Hooyman, N., & Kiyak, H. A. (2011). Aging in other countries and across cultures in the United States (pp. 43-68). *Social Gerontology: A Multidisciplinary Perspective* (8th ed.). Retrieved from www.pearsonhighered.com.

Jetten, J., Haslam, C., & Haslam, S. (Eds.) (2012). *The social cure: Identity, health & well-being.* New York: Taylor & Francis Psychology Press.

Jung, C. G. (1933). *Modern man in search of a soul.* New York: Harcourt, Brace & World.

Krause, N. (2009). Meaning in life and mortality. *Journals of Gerontology Series B: Psychological Sciences and Social Sciences, 64B,* 517-527.

Laslett, P. (1989). *A fresh map of life: The emergence of the Third Age.* Cambridge, MA: Harvard University Press.

Laslett, P. (1997). Interpreting the demographic changes. *Philosophical Transactions of the Royal Society B: Biological Sciences, 352*(1363): 1805-1809.

Leutz, W. (2007). *Immigration and the elderly: Foreign born workers in long-term care.* American Immigration Law Foundation. Retrieved from http://www.immigrationpolicy.org/special-reports/immigration-and-elderly-foreign-born-workers-long-term-care.

Lockenhoff, C. E., & Carstensen, L. L. (2004). Socioemotional selectivity theory, aging, and health: The increasingly delicate balance between regulating emotions and making tough choices. *Journal of Personality, 72,* 1395-1424.

Lyyra, T. M., & Heikkinen, R. L. (2006). Perceived social support and mortality in older people. *Journals of Gerontology Series B, Psychological Sciences and Social Sciences, 61*(3), S147-S152.

McAdams, D. P., Hart, H. M., & Maruna, A. S. (1998). The anatomy of generativity. In D. P. McAdams, & E. de St. Aubin. (Eds.), *Generativity and adult development* (pp. 7-43). Washington, DC: American Psychological Association.

MetLife. (2006). *Out and aging: The MetLife study of lesbian and gay baby boomers.* Retrieved from http://www.metlife.com.

Penningroth, S., & Scott, W. (2012). Age-related differences in goals: Testing predictions from selection, optimization, and compensation theory and socioemotional selectivity theory. *International Journal of Aging and Human Development, 74,* 87-111.

Pew Research Center. (2007). *A portrait of "Generation Next": How young people view their lives, futures, and politics.* Retrieved from http://people-press.org/2007/01/09/a-portrait-of-generation-next/.

Population Reference Bureau. (2008). World population data sheet; World population highlights. *Population Bulletin, 63.*

Prensky, M. (2001, September). Digital natives, digital immigrants: Do they really think differently? *On the Horizon, NCB University Press, 6.*

Rowe, J. W., & Kahn, R. L. (1998). *Successful aging: The MacArthur Foundation Study shows you how the lifestyle choices you make now—more than heredity—determine your health and vitality.* New York: Pantheon Books.

Shmotkin, D., Blumstein, T., & Modan, B. (2003). Beyond keeping active: Concomitants of being a volunteer in old-old age. *Psychological Aging, 18,* 602-607.

Strauss, W., & Howe, N. (1991) *Generations.* New York: William Morrow Publisher.

Strauss, W., & Howe, N. (1997). *The Fourth Turning.* New York: Crown Publishing Group.

Tornstam, L. (1997). Gerotranscendence: The contemplative dimension of aging. *Journal of Aging Studies, 11,* 143-154.

Tornstam, L. (2000). Transcendence in later life. *Generations, 23*(4), 10-14.

Tornstam, L. (2011). Maturing into gerotranscendence. *Journal of Transpersonal Psychology, 43,* 166-180.

United States Department of Health & Human Services, Centers for Disease Control & Prevention. (2011). Deaths: Preliminary Data for 2011. *National Vital Statistics Reports, 61*(6), 1-48.

Vaillant, G. E. (1993). *Wisdom of the ego.* Cambridge, MA: Harvard University Press.

Westermeyer, J. F. (2004). Predictors and characteristics of Erikson's life cycle model among men: A 32 year longitudinal study. *International Journal of Aging and Human Development, 58,* 29-48.

Withnall, A. (2002). Three decades of educational gerontology: Achievements and challenges. *Education and Aging, 17,* 87-102.

Wright, K., & Patterson, B. (2006). Socioemotional selectivity theory and macrodynamics of friendship: The role of friendship style and communication in friendship across the lifespan. *Communication Research Reports, 23,* 163-170.

Xenakis, J. (2010). *Generational dynamics for historians.* Retrieved from www.generationaldynamics.com/D.PL?d=ww2010.book2.

Zimmerman, J. (2012). *Health disparities and depression in rural and urban older adults.* Dissertation Abstracts. Retrieved from http://digital.library.louisville.edu/cdm/landingpage/collection/etd/.

3

Transitions in Older Adulthood

Marilyn B. Cole, MS, OTR/L, FAOTA

Transition is a relative term, with often uncertain beginning and ending points. A life transition implies a carefully orchestrated series of adaptations to major life changes. Transitions include acknowledging, accepting, and coping with change and restructuring the activities that make up daily life. Recently, occupational therapists have focused on some transitions for young adults with disabilities, such as the transition from school to work, from living with parents to living independently, or from institutional to community living. However, there are no such "typical" roles for occupational therapists with the transitions of older adulthood. Some predictable transitions for older populations are as follows:

- Retirement from paid work, changing life structure

- Changes in health status—coping with chronic health conditions

- Relocation—moving and adapting

- Changes in social relationships, grandparenting, caregiving

- Widowhood and coping with loss

- End-of-life care

Without pre-established roles and methods of payment for OT in these areas, we often don't get referrals from medical professionals unless the client happens to also be diagnosed with a medical condition. Potentially, OT community programming for older adult transitions may be publicly sponsored by groups such as Agencies on Aging, and one can find examples of these in the OT or interdisciplinary literature. These might serve as examples for grant-

writing projects, research projects for faculty and students, or community supported programs. In the new provisions of the Patient Protection and Affordable Care Act (2010) or other publicly funded health care initiatives, occupational therapists are well equipped to design preventive programming in any or all of these normal transitions, before they result in loss of function or disability that typically triggers a medically based referral.

Adaptation to changes of any kind requires a kind of mental flexibility and emotional stamina, a quality that has also been called *resilience*, or the ability to thrive in spite of adversity. Occupational therapists have expertise in therapeutic use of self, as well as training in mental health interventions, dealing with difficult behaviors, and group facilitation techniques that can be useful in addressing life's adult transitions.

RETIREMENT: CHANGING LIFE STRUCTURE

In the new millennium, retirement rarely occurs only once, and the age of retirement is largely unpredictable. This contradicts most preconceived notions of one's "golden years" spent golfing, cruising the world, roaming the country in a recreational vehicle, or joining the umbrella girls at the community pool. Currently, American workers first become eligible for Social Security retirement benefits at age 62, but statistics show that a large segment retires before that age. Full retirement eligibility for Social Security

Cole MB, Macdonald KC.
Productive Aging: An Occupational Perspective (pp 33-47).
© 2015 Taylor & Francis Group.

benefits occurs currently at age 66 (and is increasing), yet another large segment works well beyond that age. In a study of Baby Boomers, the majority are projected to reach retirement age financially unprepared, forcing them to continue working at least until age 70 to boost their financial status before applying for Social Security benefits. Nearly 30% of those who do retire from long-term career employment re-enter the work force at least once (Purcell, 2009).

With today's unprecedented budget deficits threatening Medicare and Social Security programs, the U.S. government has funded several large-scale studies in an attempt to predict future retirement patterns. Using the National Institute on Aging's Health and Retirement Study (2009), Warner, Hayward, and Hardy (2010) found that men aged 50 can expect to spend half their remaining lives (16 years) working for pay, and women aged 50 can spend one third, or approximately 12 years working for pay. Although these researchers found a significant spike in the numbers of those retiring at age 62, the earliest eligibility for Social Security benefits, many Americans had retired from career jobs before that age. Some gender differences included the following:

- 50% of all men in the study retired by age 63.
- For women at age 60, 53% are still working, 8% are work disabled, and 33% have retired.
- 16% of men will die while still employed.
- Significantly fewer women die while employed (7%), and few become work disabled (8%).
- 29% of men who retire will re-enter the work force at least once.
- 35% of women who retire will re-enter the work force at least once.

Generally, women's retirement patterns are more highly variable than men's and do not coincide with Social Security eligibility (Warner, Hayward, & Hardy, 2010).

Evidence from the Health and Retirement Study (2008) finds that permanent retirement is currently the exception rather than the rule (Cahill, Giandrea, & Quinn, 2012). These researchers defined "retirement" as exiting from full-time career employment (10-plus years with same job). They found that most retirement is more gradual, often includes "bridge" jobs (60%) or part-time employment, and may involve multiple re-entries and exits. This large-scale study confirms that today's retirement patterns are many and varied, and that retirement from a career job is not a one-time event, but rather a process that takes place over time for the majority of older Americans.

Key Factors in a Good Retirement Transition

George Vaillant (2009), a physician and noted gerontology researcher, suggests four important tasks for a good retirement transition:

1. Create a new social network to replace work colleagues or keep them in another context.

2. Allow yourself to play, an experience many have forgotten during long years at work.

3. Follow your creative instincts by either continuing or learning new forms of creative expression.

4. Engage in lifelong learning, a habit that keeps one positive and young.

"Not everyone's retirement is golden…it can be stressful if it is involuntary or unplanned, if one's home life is unhappy and work has always provided a means of escape, or if it is precipitated by illness or poor health" (Vaillant, 2009, p. 1). Vaillant (2009) culls these four "keys" from over 40 years of research and asking those born between 1910 and 1930 who have reached age 80 what has made their retirement years rewarding. The above tasks mesh nicely with prevailing theories of older adult development, especially the life tasks of Laslett's Third Age. These include finding self-fulfilling occupations, often giving priority to more creative self-expression, as many of our participants did. June, a businesswoman most of her life, took classes in rug hooking and oil pastels. Ken enjoyed learning to play the harmonica, and Signian found joy in finally having time for designing and sewing beautiful quilts. Hans Jonsson (2011), a Swedish OT researcher, found that elders retiring at age 65 often missed the structure and satisfaction of working. He called this the "paradox of freedom," as in the following example: "I had preferred, now when I have the wisdom of hindsight, that I had partly decreased my work, to work just a limited number of hours. Because what one misses is all about having an occupation. Especially… the social part, with friends…I really miss that very much" (Jonsson, 2011, p. 34). Those who made the best transitions to retirement did so by immersing themselves in what he calls "engaging occupations," which are "highly meaningful and important…enjoyable, interesting, and challenging" and which also "reaffirm a person's worth or identity" (Jonsson, 2011, p. 35).

Occupational Therapy Roles in Retirement Transitions

These changing patterns have major implications for occupational therapists seeking to design appropriate interventions for retirement transitions. The roles defined by the AOTA Practice Framework III (2014) may need to be expanded to include other options in the retirement transition, such as adapting employment, and guiding retirees in selecting bridge jobs or seeking other employment alternatives to supplement inadequate income. For Baby Boomers, "encore jobs" represent anything from starting a business to working part time in public service or returning to school for training in an entirely different career (Cahill, Giandrea, & Quinn, 2012).

Retirement preparation and adjustment currently appear under the work area of occupation in the AOTA Practice Framework (2014). The role of OT in this area includes "determining aptitudes, developing interests and skills, and selecting appropriate avocational pursuits" (AOTA, 2014, p. S20). This implies the need to replace the worker role by restructuring one's time (temporal organization) and establishing new performance patterns, routines, and roles. Logical outcomes of this process might be linked with OT's role in the areas of leisure and volunteerism, as well as exploring the possibility of returning to paid work.

Learning Activity 14: Retirement Planning Interview

1. Interview a person who is planning to retire soon.

2. Describe his or her current work role and explore its meaning.

3. How does he or she feel about retiring? Is retirement voluntary or mandatory?

4. How does this person envision life in retirement? What are some goals?

5. In what occupations will he or she participate, and why?

6. What problems does he or she anticipate with this transition?

7. If you were this person's occupational therapist, how would you help with the transition to retirement? Identify three areas of intervention.

   a.

   b.

   c.

CHANGES IN HEALTH STATUS

Accepting one's physical changes and resulting limitations is one of the most difficult parts of aging. No one wants to accept losing strength, endurance, or the ability to fully engage in the activities enjoyed in younger years. Statistics tell us that about 80% of older Americans have at least one chronic health condition (Knight, 2004). Although sadness and anxiety are natural emotional responses to a medical diagnosis, functional disability, rather than the illness itself, is more likely to lead to depression—about 20% in one study (Knight, 2004).

As a transition, adjustment to a medical diagnosis brings a much different response when one is older. Although younger adults experience acute health conditions as temporary, older adults have a different and understandable reaction because, for them, many health conditions are ongoing. As people age, illness often necessitates longer durations of treatment, more frequent medical visits or hospitalizations, more complex rehabilitation, and long-term alterations in life patterns due to functional limitations or adhering to treatment protocols. There are wide variations in emotional and cognitive responses to illness, depending on the seriousness of the diagnosis, the person's state of health prior to illness, the extent to which the illness limits participation in life, and the resilience of the individual. *Subjective longevity*, referring to how long one expects to live, must also be considered (Hesketh & Griffin, 2007), as well as the impact on and influence from significant others: retirees who expect to live longer and who identify more strongly with spouses and families are more likely to "value knowledge relevant goals, and proactively pursue post-retirement work activity and…financial trajectories" (Hesketh, Griffin, & Loh, 2011; Wang, 2007). Ultimately, adaptation to living with a chronic illness depends on the strength of the client's social identity, flexibility, activeness, reactivity, and perseverance—the same as when adapting to occupational transitions (Hesketh et al., 2011).

On the other hand, an unexpected medical diagnosis or health event might trigger a change in an older person's future-oriented estimates of fit—those who come to realize their time is not infinite may change their goals, placing increasing value on meaningful social connections, and spending time with friends and family (Carstensen, Fung, & Charles, 2003). By *fit*, we mean how the older individual's own skills and abilities match the occupations he or she chooses to engage in. For example, paid or unpaid work or lifestyles that entail physical stamina, such as standing, lifting, and long hours of work or travel, may be compromised when health conditions arise, even though one's cognitive capacity, creativity, and intellectual energy remain intact. Fit has to do with social, occupational, and even financial desires, capacities, and expectations, all of which may need to be changed when faced with a newly diagnosed health condition (Hesketh et al., 2011).

Potential Occupational Therapy Roles in Transitions to Altered Health

From what we now know about the multiple factors influencing this important transition, occupational therapists must take the time to fully understand older clients and what might impact their response to illness. We need to know how long they expect to live (subjective longevity), the occupational and social expectations of their significant others, and their important social identities. To what extent can they count on social connections for support? In recognition of these factors, client self-awareness comes first before preferred occupations can be adequately identified and evaluated.

Instead of initially focusing on preferred occupations, OT might best look at how well the client can perform the occupation of self-manager because, ultimately, the best intervention in promoting productive aging is supporting client self-management of chronic illness. A good self-manager takes charge of his or her own aging process, including making lifestyle alterations to reduce risk and increase safety in performing daily activities, adapting environments, and making good choices and decisions about the occupations that will continue or be altered in the face of chronic illness. The following factors could be addressed by OT to support the self-manager role:

- Helping the client to understand the health condition and its effect on daily functioning. Occupational therapists gather evidence specific to the health condition and direct the client to access other sources of reliable information about disease management.

- Establishing the optimum level of independent functioning to avoid overreactions that unduly limit participation or underreactions that compromise safety. For example, can the older adult still drive safely to community activities? How might the client conserve mental energy to continue playing in an afternoon bridge group despite decreased endurance?

- Establish routines for complying with needed medication, exercise, and dietary recommendations relative to managing one's illness. These routines can dovetail nicely with ordinary daily activities, taking into account both health and doing the tasks required within one's social or occupational roles. For example, Sanders and Van Oss (2013) found that older adults were more compliant in taking their prescription medications when they associated this with another daily routine, such as making their morning coffee or watching the evening news.

- Facilitate emotional expression regarding symptoms and discuss their effect on mood and attitude. Explain the difference between real symptoms and depression. Nurture hope, positive thinking, and active problem solving.

- Assist with the coping process of facilitating acceptance and promoting adjustment to change.

- Explore the availability of physical and social resources. Joining a disability support group helps some clients, while others find existing family and social connec-

tions adequately supportive in overcoming obstacles related to illness.

- Explore issues of caregiving when appropriate. What must be done for the client vs. what might the client do for him- or herself with the necessary adaptations?

- Collaborate with the client in establishing a recovery schedule in which lifestyle changes are incorporated gradually and prior occupations are reintroduced with needed adaptations.

- Introduce relaxation training to reduce stress and to promote adequate rest and sleep.

- Provide guidelines for maintaining physical and mental fitness within the confines of safety and encourage social contexts such as groups at a senior center. Self-management strategies should include a list of dos and don'ts relative to one's specific health condition to apply when participating in group exercise.

Home Care Occupational Therapy Interventions for Health Status Transitions

When providing home care, Knotts (2008) suggests that OT practitioners consider the following areas of intervention for older adults coping with chronic illness or the aftermath of acute health events such as a heart attack, stroke, bone fracture, or diabetic episode:

- Fall prevention
- Home modification
- Assistive technology
- Driver screening
- Low vision interventions
- Energy conservation
- Training in activities of daily living and instrumental activities of daily living
- Caregiver support
- Psychosocial issues (adaptations to overcome illness-related emotional reactions)

Many self-management protocols that relate to specific health conditions may be found by searching the Internet. However, care should be taken to make sure the sources of such information are legitimate. Please see Chapter 4 for further discussion of OT's home care role.

Learning Activity 15: Illness Transition Interview

Interview someone who has recently been diagnosed with a serious chronic illness.

1. What is the health condition, and how did this person first experience it?

2. How is the illness being managed or treated?

3. What barriers does it create for the occupations of the person's daily life?

4. How is he or she coping with symptoms/barriers?

5. What is the person's reaction to the role of "patient" or "client"?

Case Example: Pearl

About 1 year ago, Pearl, an English professor, was diagnosed with Parkinson's disease. At the same time, she had to give up driving because of her slow reaction time. She lives in a rural area where driving is necessary to get everywhere she might wish to go, making her dependent on her husband, Bill, for rides. Because of this, Pearl decided to give up teaching, but she was determined not to let it interfere with her social relationships, learning activities, or caregiving role. Pearl and Bill take care of their 18-month-old grandson Hunter every Tuesday and Thursday while his parents are working, an arrangement she began shortly after giving up university teaching. Not surprisingly, running after an active toddler more than satisfies her need for physical exercise. She also enjoys reading to him, and using creative teaching techniques to help him learn.

Pearl had built a lifestyle that included daily outdoor walks of at least 30 minutes. With Parkinson's, she had to compensate for the growing inability to keep her balance when navigating uneven surfaces. Rather than a cane or walker, Pearl has adopted the use of two cross country ski poles, allowing her to traverse the dirt or loosely paved walking trails near her home (Figure 3-1). She writes: "Exercise is important for me…I am able to attend an exercise class for an hour or so while Bill stays with Hunter, and I walk with Bill, slower and for less distance than I used to." However, progression of the disease has also made it impossible for Pearl to climb stairs. Because her bedroom was up a steep flight of stairs, Pearl has now moved her belongings downstairs, where she sleeps on a daybed in the den.

Socially, Pearl keeps lunch dates with colleagues and friends by having Bill drive her to a local restaurant and then having her friend drive her home. She continues to host the book discussion group she helped to organize after she retired. During down times, Pearl still works on scholarly articles, which she hopes to have published. Without her teaching duties, she welcomes the time to finally work on these unfinished projects.

The first step for occupational therapists when encountering clients such as Pearl would be to look up the most recent evidence related to the health condition and its management. A good reference is *Willard & Spackman's Occupational Therapy, 12th edition* (Schell, Gillen, & Scaffa,

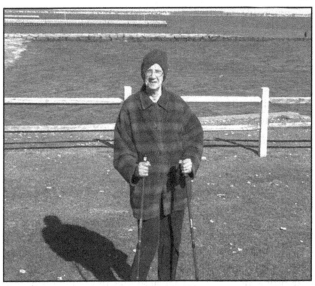

Figure 3-1. Pearl on her daily walk, assisted by cross country ski poles.

2014). See Appendix I for guidelines related to specific health conditions.

In Parkinson's disease, sometimes there is comorbidity with depression or dementia, causing a greater burden for caregivers of older adults with Parkinson's disease. However, Pearl was relieved to learn that this isn't always true. Some suggested OT interventions are as follows:

- Strategies to reduce the effect of tremors (ankle weights, weighted utensils/tools)

- Routines for medication management

- Facilitating joint movement, range of motion, and stretching to avoid contractures

- Education in self-management skills

- Group interventions to maintain/increase function, well-being, and self-esteem

- Promote engagement in productive activities

- Discuss communication difficulties—effect of facial masking and oral rigidity

- Home modification for increased safety and independence

- Encourage participation in support/community groups (adapted from Griffin, 2011)

Learning Activity 16: Occupational Therapy Intervention Managing a Chronic Condition

Considering Pearl's case, answer the following:

1. From the case description, which stage of Parkinson's does Pearl demonstrate? From the source noted previously, you learn that Parkinson's is a progressive,

neurodegenerative disease that affects mostly movement and balance but later affects speech and swallowing. The five stages of Parkinson's are:

a. Mild movement-related symptoms but functionally independent

b. Joint stiffness and resting tremors appear, but balance remains intact

c. Mild imbalance during walking and standing, but functionally independent

d. Motor symptoms more severe, with disabling instability, and changes in speech and swallowing apparent

e. Severe disability, with individual requiring constant care (Griffin, 2011; Hoehn & Yahr, 1967)

Which stage would Pearl best fit into and why? As her occupational therapist, how might you help her to anticipate problems with everyday activities in the next progressive stage, based on just this much information?

2. What would you identify as Pearl's top three occupational priorities? Briefly describe how Parkinson's might create barriers to her participation in these occupations.

a.

b.

c.

3. Pearl is newly diagnosed with Parkinson's, even though she has been experiencing the symptoms for several months. There is often an emotional reaction accompanying anticipation of future loss of function. If you were an occupational therapist working with Pearl in home care, write three questions you might ask to gain a better understanding of her feelings about the progression of the disease and its symptoms and how she is adjusting emotionally to this life transition.

a.

b.

c.

RELOCATION: MOVING AND ADAPTING

According to the AOTA's practice guidelines for productive aging, "to successfully age in place, older adults need to live in an environment that supports their functional abilities" (Leland, Elliott, & Johnson, 2012, p. 31). The continuum of care includes a host of choices for senior housing, from remaining in one's long-time home, to publicly subsidized senior housing, retirement communities (55 and older gated communities), continuing care retirement communities, assisted living residences, transitional care units, inpatient rehabilitation centers, and long-term care (skilled nursing facilities). Some older adults with disabling health challenges may need to change locations to accommodate a higher level of care. This requires a major adjustment and occupational adaptation to deal with the change in environment in addition to declining health (Schkade & McClung, 2001). Other changes in life circumstances can also trigger a decision to move to a new residence, such as reduced mobility, death of a spouse or life partner, reduced ability to manage a home, or financial necessity. Sometimes, as older adults age, their neighbors and friends die or move away, placing them at risk for social isolation should they remain in their long-time home (Knotts, 2008).

Choosing Not to Relocate: Aging in Place

Aging in place (i.e., living independently in one's community), may be the most cost-effective option for older adults, even when they face significant health challenges. Some of the benefits of remaining at home include the following: familiar physical environment, reluctance to abandon neighbors and friends, emotional attachment to belongings and surroundings, or denial or fear of dependency on others (Emlet & Crabtree, 1996). Health professionals need to assist older clients in making the choice to stay in their communities based on the amount of social capital available, as well as their own social networks and connections. When they do remain at home, however, home modification may be necessary for their safety and accessibility when adapting to changes in health or functional status. Home care services, including OT professionals, often provide much support for elders to live safely within the limits of their declining abilities, within their own homes.

Some researchers have recommended aging in place from a sociological standpoint, citing the high cost of most other options, such as assisted living and continuing care retirement communities (Cannuscio, Block, & Kawachi, 2003). However, these authors discuss the current public health dilemma of the diminishing social capital of communities to support the increasing numbers of elderly members with declining functional abilities. The ability of society to meet the care needs of its aging citizens depends, to a great extent, on the availability of social capital. *Social capital* is defined as the resources available to individuals and groups through social connections to their communities (Cannuscio et al., 2003). Although financial capital may be understood as money in the bank, social capital is the collective ability of the citizens of a community to protect the health of its citizens, even those who are socially isolated. For example, communities with a high percentage of available health services, charitable organizations, community-minded businesses, and services such as senior transportation can enable community dwelling seniors to age in place. Without such supports, individuals living alone become vulnerable to a variety of threats to successful aging through limited mobility, social isolation, and lack of access to other needed services.

Fried, Friedman, Endres, and Wasik (1997), in a follow-up to the MacArthur Successful Aging study (Rowe & Kahn, 1998), found that older adults themselves can help build "communities that support successful aging," by participating in volunteer activities within their communities (p. 216). The occupational therapist could encourage older clients to volunteer for efforts that encourage aging in place by making their communities more accessible and inclusive of seniors, thereby contributing to the social capital from which they will eventually benefit. A potential role for occupational therapists might be to consult with community organizations to help them to offer better and more varied opportunities for volunteering or civic engagement for retiring older adults.

Moving in With Family Members

The most frequent move for older adults who have become ill or who have lost their spouse is to the home of a daughter's family (Knotts, 2003). This often entails a great many compromises and adjustments for both. Declining health may put added stress on the caregiver and often the entire household. An occupational therapist can do much to ease this transition by helping to define separate spaces within the household for elder members, and structuring opportunities for them to participate in self-management, self-fulfilling activities, and occupations to help maintain the home, thereby contributing as well as receiving needed care.

Learning Activity 17: Exploring a Relocation Experience

Describe a time when you changed your residence.

1. How did you feel about the move and why?
2. What is involved in moving to new living quarters?
3. How did you decide what to take with you and what to give away?
4. What lessons did you learn that might help you to understand an older adult client going through the same process?

Moving to Long-Term Care

This is probably the most difficult transition of all because usually persons move to long-term care facilities when they have become too disabled to care for themselves and have no other options. In some states or communities, there are waiting lists to get into a reputable facility. Although older residents have the need for a good deal of care, they have difficulty adjusting to the limitations in self-directed choices that many care environments impose on

residents (Crist, 1999). Hersch et al. (2004) studied the process of relocation transitions. They found that greater participation in planning the move, a strong sense of self, and a history of good prior experiences with place transitions increased the likelihood of positive adaptive outcomes. Knotts (2003) developed a series of steps to help with place transitions, including at least three of the following:

- Positive attitude or philosophy of life
- Perform self-care, activities, and occupations
- Develop and maintain supportive relationships
- Define and create one's own personal space

As an OT researcher, Knotts (2008) suggests that familiar occupations and activities can serve as a bridge, both during and after a transition, providing continuity from one setting to another. Occupational therapists need to enable and support bridge occupations that have meaning for clients during difficult transitions whenever possible. Occupational therapists also advocate for more client-centered care in every setting, allowing clients or residents to do as much for themselves as they are able or wish to do.

Learning Activity 18: Relocation Intervention

As an OT, you are asked to design an intervention for an older client with moderate dementia when it becomes necessary for the client to move from a house full of belongings to a single room in a long-term care facility. His two adult children do not live locally but they are both willing to participate for approximately 15 days before and 5 days after the move takes place.

1. List 20 tasks or steps involved with moving to long-term care.
2. Identify who would be responsible for each step.
3. Discuss how you might advise the family to ease this transition for the client.
4. Describe one OT intervention that addresses the emotional issues of downsizing or disposing of belongings, while preserving shared memories for the client and his family.

CHANGES IN SOCIAL RELATIONSHIPS

Many changes in social relationships are possible throughout one's life, and older adulthood is no different. Couples marry, separate, divorce, and remarry. People become parents, raise children, and become caregivers of elderly parents. Families move across the country following the job market and start over again with each move to form friendships, connect with neighbors, and join community groups. As one ages, friends and neighbors may die or move away. When relationships change, a shift in all performance patterns (roles, habits, routines) accompanies the change. Having these experiences at a young age can have an impact on an individual's ability to adapt to relationship changes when people grow older. Here, we will focus on two of the most common relationship transitions: becoming a caregiver for a spouse and becoming a custodial grandparent.

Transition to Caregiving or Receiving Care

Caring for a spouse who is ill can also come to older adults unexpectedly. For spousal caregivers, there are profound changes in the couple's relationship, particularly when one of the pair has dementia. Spousal caregivers mourn the loss of the relationship each time their spouse takes a turn for the worse, and this can make the transition to caregiving an emotionally draining experience. Please refer to Chapter 8 for a review of studies related to grandchild and spousal caregiving.

Grandparents Raising Grandchildren

Becoming a grandparent usually invokes a joyful response; seeing a new life can remind older adults of their own youth or of raising their own children when they were younger with much of their future ahead of them. But what happens when their own children bring their problems back home? Some older adults have adult children who move back in with them, becoming financially dependent on the older adult. Some bring their own children into the household, too. Almost always, taking on responsibility for raising one's grandchildren comes unexpectedly, the result of a crisis with the birth parent, an accident or illness, depression, substance abuse, or the inability to earn enough income to support themselves or their children. Grandparents feel a responsibility and an obligation to help their adult children, but also a desire to be a part of their grandchildren's lives, causing mixed emotions in the best of circumstances. However, older grandparents are known to place themselves at risk because of the added stress, the long hours, and the limitations caregiving brings to their own social and self-fulfilling activities. They often put their grandchildren's needs above their own. They do not take good care of themselves, and they can become socially isolated from their peers.

WIDOWHOOD AND COPING WITH LOSS

Loss of a life partner can be one of the most distressing of all life events, topping the Holmes and Rahe (1967) Stressful Events Scale at 100% at any age. In older adult-

hood, that loss often brings a cascading effect—loss of a caregiving role for a husband or wife with prolonged illness, loss of income or assets due to high medical costs, and profound changes in the rhythms and routines of everyday life that used to be shared. In a recent special edition on widowhood, Lee (2014) writes, "We know much more about the consequences of widowhood now than we did when Holmes and Rahe (1967) made their oft-cited observation about its devastating effects. It does more than just make people sad; it changes their lives in fundamental ways…and the ways in which widows and widowers manage to cope with the loss of their spouses and adjust to the new realities they must face" (Lee, 2014, p. 3).

Sometimes, widowhood also triggers the move to another location, such as moving in with one's adult children, or to smaller, less expensive, and more manageable living quarters; or to some level of institutional residence, such as assisted living, or transitional or senior housing. No matter what, losing someone with whom one has spent many years prompts multiple shifts in one's social relationships. According to one recent study, widowed mothers who were in poor health or older were more likely to co-reside with a daughter or an unmarried son (Seltzer & Friedman, 2014). Widows and widowers no longer socialize as part of a couple. Children and grandchildren, siblings, in-laws, and others have different ways of responding. Sometimes, the death of one parent brings the other closer to family and sometimes it creates distance, depending on the history of those relationships. Not surprisingly, when a spouse of many years dies, a part of the survivor's social identity also dies, leaving the survivor feeling incomplete. This may, in part, account for the 48% increase in mortality risk for widows (Sullivan & Fenelon, 2014).

For example, a longitudinal study examining the relationship between marital quality and psychological adjustment to widowhood found that higher levels of anxiety and yearning occurred with widows who had closer relationships and greater dependency on their spouses/partners prior to the loss. Widows with prior conflicted relationships experienced less anxiety, while those who relied on their husbands for instrumental support (driving, preparing meals, home maintenance) experienced the greatest distress. This study also found that women dependent on their husbands had more difficulty adjusting than men dependent on their wives (Carr et al., 2000).

Most people know Kubler-Ross' (2005) five stages of grieving: denial, anger, bargaining, depression, and acceptance. However, for older individuals, the process has been shown to vary widely. Letting go usually follows earlier patterns of dealing with loss. In other words, when mourning has been avoided or unresolved with earlier losses, or the relationship with the deceased was problematic, grief may become complicated, requiring professional intervention to resolve. However, evidence has shown that depression is not a universal grief response (Knight, 2004). Interventions involving emotional expression with older bereaved persons show lower distress and improved functioning after 1 year (Segal et al., 2001, cited in Knight, 2004). However, the cognitive and affective effects of uncomplicated bereavement can last from 2 to 7 years, with the social role of widowhood and defining a new life for oneself afterward at least as distressing as the death of a spouse itself. In some cases, a spouse's death may actually improve mood and functioning of the one remaining, as might be the case with those who have been caregivers of their spouses through long-term declining health. Not everyone needs grief counseling, but for those still distressed after 6 months, it could be helpful (Knight, 2004).

Some bereaved older adults find bereavement groups helpful, and these can be found locally through hospice, senior centers, or places of worship. Several of our participants reported attending such groups and appreciating the social and community support they found there. Widowhood also brings individual lifestyle changes. For example, when the lost spouse was a breadwinner, the widow may need to find part-time paid work. If he or she handled the finances or did all the shopping and cooking, then the survivor needs to learn some new home management skills. Studies show that, in general, women adapted more easily than men, especially when they engaged in meaningful activities with neighbors and friends. Some men need ongoing advice and support to learn new household tasks (Knotts, 2008).

One recent study addressing social support in widowhood particularly highlighted the role of friendship in early widowhood, including ease of contact and satisfaction with friendship support: greater frequency of contact was associated with negative affective reactions, while higher satisfaction levels produced more positive affective reactions (Vries, Utz, Caserta, & Lund, 2014). Another study helps explain the somewhat puzzling relationship between contact with friends and negative affect, reporting that "loneliness following widowhood cannot be remediated by interventions aimed only at increasing social support. Social support, especially from friends, appears to be most effective if it is readily accessible and allows the newly bereaved an opportunity to express him or herself" (Utz, Swenson, Caserta, Lund, & de Vries, 2014, p. 85). Thus, being alone and being lonely are subjectively different—not all widows feel less isolated when constantly surrounded by other people, and participating in social groups does not always prevent a widowed person from feeling lonely. Rather, a recent widow's loneliness seems to be best remediated by meaningful social relationships in which he or she feels free to express both positive and negative emotional responses.

Case Example: Signian

Signian's husband Ken died unexpectedly at age 68 less than 1 year ago. She has kindly shared some pages from her journal as an example of her experience with the transition to widowhood. She describes what happened within the first few days:

"My husband died 2 months after my mother died. Both on the second day of the month. Ken and I had a wonderful weekend in Philadelphia, where we had taken the train to visit our oldest daughter. I wanted Ken to get used to using the train because it was more relaxing. He had a history of heart disease. He was 10 years post quadruple bypass surgery. We had driven home from the train station and arrived late in the day. We had a late, light dinner. He was in the den, and I was trying on a pair of shoes. He came into the hallway and said 'I cannot handle this' and then his legs gave way and he collapsed to the floor. I was worried he had hit his head on the floor. I ran to him and called his name. I held his head in my arm and then thought to call 911 and went to look for the nitroglycerin to put into his mouth. I remember the 911 person asked me to hold his head in a certain way and then try to do something else with my other hand, which was holding onto the phone at the time. I was angry and told her I could not hold the phone and do what she requested. His face was blue; he felt cold to me even at that early point. His eyes were glazed upward and unfocused. I perhaps knew at that time things were not good. The EMT people came within minutes and the policeman who came with them asked me to step into another room. I am not sure if it was three or four people who worked on Ken. They carried him out on a stretcher and into the ambulance. I remember looking out, seeing the ambulance in the driveway and wondering if the neighbors knew something had happened. The policeman asked if I needed a ride to the hospital and I said yes. I didn't have time to think of even asking anyone for assistance. The policeman was very kind and drove me to the emergency room. Upon our arrival into the ER itself, he asked me if I had someone to call for a ride home. I was unsure, and then a kind onlooker, a stranger, offered me a ride home. The kindness of strangers was like a warm blanket.

"From the ER I started to call people. First, I called my daughter Andrea in Philadelphia. I really do not remember what I said, but she got into her car right away to drive to the hospital or my home. Then I called my sister Janice, who lives about 2 hours away in Massachusetts. She was going either to my house or the hospital. Next I called a friend who was not home, and then family friends who lived nearby. They came to the hospital to bring me home. I am not sure how long I stayed in the ER, but it was not more than an hour. The doctor made it very clear that there was nothing more that I could have done. He was very insistent that I understood this, by saying it several times. They asked me if I wanted to see Ken before I left the hospital with my friends, and I said no. I wish now that I had, but at the time all I could think of was the image of blood and tubes that I just could not cope with. My friend gave me a hankie as I was crying and had a hard time catching my breath. They stayed with me until my sister arrived, I think that was around 1:30 a.m. Then Janice and I stayed up until Andrea arrived around 4 a.m. We all stayed awake and talked for some time. I never talked with [my other daughter] Justine or any other relatives, but phone calls had been made to immediate family. I really do not remember too much about what people said [when they called all through the following day]. The special support of friends will always stay with me.

"The hankie my friend gave me was an old cowboy-style bandana, so faded and soft. It was a treasure I kept with me all the time. The next day, as people learned about Ken's death, it was amazing the support and outpouring. The front steps began to look like a shrine, flowers everywhere. Boxes of food arrived, fruit arrangements, so many containers of soups, stews. Countless people bringing things. My daughter's brother-in-law came on the train from Baltimore with a vegetable lasagna; a friend from school sent a box of bagels and jelly from a wonderful place.

"The next day we three, Janice, Andrea, and me, went to the funeral home and made arrangements for the wake and funeral. I remember being so impressed with the quality of care and attention we received. We then went to look for the floral arrangements, and food for the reception. We went into sort of a work mode, all of us wanting to do what was right for Ken. To honor him and his life. My sister Janice worked with all our photos to create a photo essay of his life. The funeral director was able to scan and burn DVDs with over 250 pictures from early birth throughout his whole life. That was played during the wake, and people were amazed at how beautiful it was. The wake was attended by hundreds of people in spite of a snow storm. The weather was awful. Family from Massachusetts had to work hard to drive through the storm to get to us. I was beside myself that family would not make it. As it was, many dear friends did not make it secondary to the weather. The service was beautiful. Andrea started the program with an incredible eulogy to her father. Then various friends, faculty from the school where he taught, came forward to speak of Ken's life. Even two of his four grandchildren spoke with elegance. Over and over, the message was he was a good man who was modest but brilliant.

"It took me almost a month to read my sympathy cards. I just couldn't do it. When I finally did, they were a comfort and again, the word of what a good person he was came through. I remember Andrea asking for a lock of hair. I remember with horror opening the bag with the cut-up sweater and shirt from the night the EMT made efforts to get to his chest. I remember asking for Ken's ring and watch. A friend whose husband died about 1 year ago visited with me the fourth week after Ken died. She told me it was a long time before she felt anything like 'normal.' That shocked me! The bereavement materials and the group say 2 to 5 years, so the advice would be to take all the time you need to go through the process. My medical doctor wanted me to take antidepressants but I felt like I needed to feel the pain. I feel like it is a process that has no easy steps.

"That *first month* was a struggle to accept the loss. Doing the various tasks helped to provide a focus. Probate took a lot of time, meetings with the lawyer, too. Finding important papers that were needed including titles, bank cards, etc. was a challenge. Canceling the credit cards took a lot of time. I felt at times like I was forgetting things or losing things. I felt shaky, vulnerable, and unsure as to how to proceed. But people kept coming into my life to provide some focus. My sister came for a weekend. Friends from Vermont drove down for a visit. Neighbors had me over for dinner. Book club members provided a food basket. I had to work on keeping Ken's fish tank going, so I had lots of new tasks to learn how to manage. Actually, the first month or so, I just felt numb. Keeping busy with chores felt good. At one point, I noted in my journal that I felt like a baby—needing a good cry two or three times a day. I also noted that I felt like a wounded animal. Later, after my bereavement classes, the idea of being 'ambushed by grief' was an expression that seemed true. You just never knew when you were going to start crying.

"Here are some changes to my lifestyle that unfolded over the next several months:

- Certainly, I had more chores to do. With your partner gone, you have to do it all. So this was a big adjustment. I am not using the grill…Ken was the master grill chef. I miss sharing cooking with Ken. He also did most of the driving. So it is tricky for me now, especially driving at night.

- A friend told me I had to get my 'staff' in order. She is divorced after years of marriage, and that was her advice. So I did arrange for a neighbor to mow the lawn and shovel snow. I paid ahead for 1 year. Mostly I have taken care of everything else. I usually have things that need two people to do…moving lawn furniture, installing air conditioners, for example, so I have my list and whenever someone comes over I ask them to help. I'm planning ahead all the time, with little time to waste. I am trying to cook good food and walk every day.

- My social life with old friends helped me cope and feel less alone. I did not like to meet with couples, like going to a party at a friend's house with couples I did not know.

- My family members all live out of state, so relationships with them have not changed much after the first few months. I visited both my daughters for longer periods of time.

- After 5 months, school started and I took classes and also taught classes in the fall semester. The schedule was full but it helped to keep me grounded, with a regular schedule in my own life in Connecticut. I am trying to claim myself, to discover myself again.

"*Living alone?* Well I have never lived alone, ever. I went from my parents' home to live with Ken. I worried about being lonely. But, I want to learn how to live alone. I don't want anyone trying to tell me what to do. I avoid some friends (one old childhood friend in particular) who are strong-willed people with lots of advice. I feel I could easily be swayed, so I am staying away from folks who have too much advice. I do feel the loss of intimacy. I try to focus on what I need, and I do not think too much about my life without Ken as I find that too sad, too hard to think about, at this point anyway. I worry that I might never feel happy again. I worry that I will turn into a grumpy old lady. I feel sad that I do not have Ken's physical attention. He always made me feel attractive, desirable. Now I just feel old and single. We discussed such feelings often in the bereavement group and yearning for Ken was a strong emotion for me. They said when that feeling starts to diminish it can be a sign that the initial mourning period is coming to an end. But they also warned me *it takes 2 to 5 years to get to the other side of grief.*

"Occupations have provided a focus and a role to help me through this transition. My home manager role has doubled, as I have said earlier. But I am no longer the wife, lover, and companion. So I needed a role to hang onto. The familiar role of teaching was a good one for me. I wanted to have a schedule to keep me on task. I felt it would help me to re-enter the living world. I also took art classes—watercolor painting, Zentangle drawing, cooking classes, exercise classes, bereavement classes, Italian language lessons, and the biology of the honey bee."

Signian is blessed with an outgoing personality, and has developed a fairly large and varied social network. She is the oldest of six children, most of whom live far away, but their relationships remain warm and close. She continues social contact with a large network of former colleagues from her (and Ken's) years of university teaching, as well as several clusters of friends from other areas of life. These friendships and group memberships have supported and facilitated Signian's transition to widowhood, giving her multiple social roles and interaction opportunities (Figure 3-2). Here, she lists the more *formal social groups* she belongs to:

- OC Marsh Fellow at Yale, Peabody Museum—monthly meetings with guest speakers and dinner, reception events

- Bereavement group—once a week get-together

- Succulent/Cactus club—monthly meeting, exhibits, shows

- Osher Lifelong Learning Institute (linked to University of Connecticut)—classes and meetings

- Grange member

- Member of the Cheshire Arts Place

- Professional organizations (Connecticut and national)

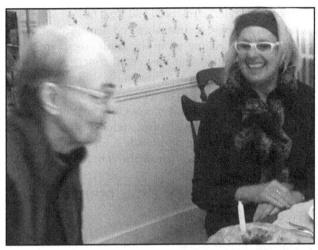

Figure 3-2. Signian made a birthday cake for a widowed friend. Both make a wish for a better year ahead.

- Quilting group—teach classes to students and hospice participants

Theories and research on bereavement say that holidays are the most difficult during the first year after the death of a spouse. These are Signian's plans for the holidays this year: "Thanksgiving I stayed home. I did not want to travel. I had dinner at a family friend's home. Christmas I am going to California to spend the holidays with my younger daughter Justine and her family and will stay a bit longer. This is the first year ever I will not be with Andrea and her children in Philadelphia. So this is a new change and I think it is good. Not doing what Ken and I always did seems right. I'm trying to change with the change.

"*Plans for the future?* Well, I am less sure of the future. I am considering attending an international conference in 2014. I'll visit my brother in Florida, a friend in the Bahamas, a friend in Texas whose husband just died, my daughters in Philadelphia and California. I've been asked to help with a chronic pain course, so will consider that too. I want to take up horseback riding. I have no intention of moving at this time. I am going to start a beehive in the backyard. I want to keep gardening and work on a path in the backyard that Ken and I had started. I want to find the 'right' place for Ken's coral. His turtle heads I am donating in his name to Yale.

"So, it is a long road ahead with sad times, and if you're lucky, good times too. I am still mourning the loss of a future with Ken. I worry that I will not be happy or joyful. I am thinking about what I am thinking. I really still cannot think too much about Ken because then I am sad. I think mostly about what needs to be done."

In this case example, the role of occupations within the grieving and healing process is clear. Occupations give focus, give comfort, and give needed relief and distraction from the episodes of grief that naturally occur in the first weeks and months following the loss. The mechanics of the wake and funeral, the financial and legal tasks, picking up the threads of home maintenance and management, reading and acknowledging sympathy cards, these are tasks that require attention, but they entail concrete steps and completing them moves one forward.

New occupations begin to appear after 3 to 4 months—taking classes in art, Italian, cooking, and beekeeping. Picking up some previous occupations too, such as teaching, quilting, and gardening, all provide bridges to "the other side of grief" (S. McGeary, personal communication, 2013).

Learning Activity 19: Coping With Loss

Consider Signian's case.

1. What occupations smoothed her transition to widowhood?

2. How did her occupations and social connections help her to adapt to living alone?

3. If she did not have such a large social network, how might an occupational therapist help her to build one as part of redefining her life as a single person?

DEATH AND END-OF-LIFE CARE

From a developmental perspective, knowledge that death is near gives new urgency to a person's time left to live. *End-of-life care* refers to care received after giving up hope for a cure from a terminal illness. The growth of hospice, an organization whose mission is caring for people with terminal illness, has decreased the number of older adults dying in hospitals while trying to be kept alive by well-meaning medical personnel. Hospice has its own facilities, but also defines programming for end-of-life care within other facilities and agencies, including home care. They provide palliative care, which describes the total program for designing a "good death," including relative freedom from pain, minimizing symptoms, and maintaining quality of life, enabling the patient to live a meaningful life as long as possible, and to die with dignity.

What Is a "Good Death"?

Younger people prefer to avoid answering this question. Some might even believe that no death can be good. However, as older adults begin to encounter illness and age-related decline, they may give more thought to how they want to die. They also may have experienced the death of peers and family members. Whether avoiding a long and painful illness or not wanting to be dependent and a burden to others, older adults have very diverse ideas about

their own death and its meaning. Carr (2012) looked at the extent of older adults' advance care planning and what motivates them to put those plans in writing. Less than half of all American adults have advance directives—legal documents sometimes called *living wills*—that appoint another person as power of attorney to make health care decisions for them and outlines their specific treatment wishes should they become incapacitated (U.S. Department of Health & Human Services, 2008). Carr's (2012) study found that knowing someone who died at home with end-of-life care, and who used an advance directive served as a positive role model for initiating their own planning. Less significantly, knowing someone who died "badly" (in pain, connection to machines, having mental incapacitation) most often triggered older adults to put their own plans in writing (Carr, 2012).

Beyond making the dying patient physically comfortable by minimizing pain and symptoms and avoiding inappropriately prolonging life, end-of-life care reframes the dying process with some of the following priorities:

- Emotional preparation for death

- Achieving a sense of control and completion, having lived a long, fulfilling life

- Strengthening relationships with loved ones during final days

- Relieving burden on loved ones, especially family caregivers

- Revitalizing spiritual health through continued participation in life as long as possible (Carr, 2003; Pizzi, 2010)

Occupations in the Final Stage of Life

OT practitioners can have an important role in providing adaptations, compensations, and guidance to clients and their families to facilitate the occupations and social roles the client wants and needs to continue, despite terminal illness. Pizzi (2010) advises OT practitioners to use a client-centered approach, beginning with a therapeutic use of self, acknowledging and empathizing with whatever emotions and situations the client faces, without feeling the need to fix anything. Just listening, without judgment, to the client and loved ones and what they want to accomplish prepares both client and therapist for setting occupational goals and structuring everyday tasks within the home, institution, or hospice facility. Some key goals for OT practitioners to ensure quality of life include the following:

- Providing a sense of control over normal daily routines, however the client and family define normalcy.

- Planning ahead to avoid social isolation, designing activities that the client and others can do together (such as preparing and eating meals, playing games, or preserving memories through storytelling or scrapbooking, recording memoirs), or enjoying shared entertainment.

- Adapting tasks and environments to facilitate occupational performance and prevent exacerbation of symptoms during activity. This is important for preserving independence and dignity for as long as possible.

- Preventing complications from immobility through functional positioning or by alternating activity and rest.

- Balancing healthy risk taking with safety when participating in social events. Sometimes the importance of being present at a family event (graduation, wedding, holiday dinner) supersedes the health risks involved, a decision best left to the client and family.

- Facilitating communication through multiple means, such as face to face, telephone, e-mail, letters, and journaling.

- Facilitating the completion of important life projects or creating legacies.

Furthermore, creating a positive end-of-life experience helps with the grieving process for those left behind (Knotts, 2008).

Important progress has been made in the realm of end-of-life issues. Emerging from a taboo or seldom addressed topic, stages of death and dying are now recognized as containing unique occupations. Palliative care offers provision of comfort measures. The occupational therapist has a role to foster continued participation in meaningful activities, environmental adaptations, and interventions designed to decrease pain, fatigue, anxiety, and depression (Keesing & Rosenwax, 2011).

Researchers de Raedt, Koster, and Ryckewaert (2013) studied the viewpoints of older adults related to death and dying. They describe a phenomena in which elders often expressed increases in life satisfaction even with increased awareness of impending mortality. The individuals studied in Belgium displayed a decreasing concern about potentially emotionally stressful topics and an increasingly conscious choice of where to focus their attention. They reported that the fear of death decreased with age, and information about life-threatening conditions was processed quickly but then not focused on. This contrasted with middle-aged adults, who expressed more fear of death and increased attention to a life-threatening condition. The seniors appeared to have a knowledge base and acceptance of changes at that stage of life. Occupational therapists could have increasing roles in supporting realistic viewpoints expressed by their aged clients through supportive acceptance and assistance with planning for occupational engagement for the present time.

The occupation of dying was explored by Upham and Gravenson (2010). They especially noted that family roles became distorted, with family members holding onto the past and avoiding the inevitable future. Recommendations

were related to promoting a means to connect verbally with a dying person to allow for self-expression or quiet times of reconnecting with others through reminiscing. Occupational therapists may work with family members to adjust to the dying process and its continuing changes by suggesting structured, simple activities that create opportunities for meaningful shared time together.

Occupational Therapist's Role in Advance Care Planning

OT practitioners need to be aware of systems of advanced care planning. Anyone may participate in these directives, but with life-threatening or end-of-life issues, family members need to communicate effectively with the patient. Ideally, those would be addressed while clear cognitive skills are present for planning and decision making that reflect the patient's personal choices. Boerner, Carr, and Moorman (2013) review that the "...U.S. Congress passed the Self Determination Act...[in] 1990...[which] requires that federally funded hospitals and nursing homes give patients the opportunity to complete an advance directive..." (p. 246). These include a living will, which is a legal document specifying boundaries of medical treatment, and a durable power of attorney that designates a person to make health decisions if the patient is no longer capable.

The OT might be included in discussions on these topics, which serve to increase an acceptance of the death and dying process and decrease stress for family members. These discussions related to overall family function when encouraged to share in discussions of thoughts, feelings, and joint decision making.

Case Example: Bud—A Dying Sailor's Wish

The oldest of OT clients come from the traditionalist generation, and many of them served in the military during World War II. This story came to me via e-mail from one of our participants, Bob T., who also served as a naval aviator. "After signing my pop, Bud, up for hospice care, the consolation prize I'd given him (for agreeing it was OK to die) was a trip to visit the Navy in San Diego. I e-mailed my friend, who is serving as a Navy public affairs officer...and asked if she had enough pull on any of the bases in San Diego to get me access for the day so I could give Bud, who served on the USS Dewey, a windshield tour. The next day she...invited us down to the ship. We later linked up outside Naval Base San Diego and carpooled to the pier, where we were greeted by a squad size group of sailors. Bud started to cry before the doors of the van opened. He'd been oohing and pointing at the cyclic rate...but when we slowed down and my friend said 'They're all here for you, Bud,' he was overwhelmed.

"After we were all out of the van, directly in front of the Dewey, shaking hands and exchanging pleasantries, an officer introduced himself and said, as the ship's 'sailor of the year' he had the honor of pushing Bud's wheelchair for the day. Unbeknownst to us, they'd decided to host Bud *aboard* the Dewey. And so they carried him aboard, and … [we] were greeted by a platoon-sized group of sailors. To say it was overwhelming is an understatement. These men and women waited in line to introduce themselves to Bud. They shook his hand, asked for photos with him, and swapped stories. It was simply amazing.

"Bud was telling a story when [a sailor] walked up with a huge photo of the original USS Dewey, and Bud yelled, 'There she is!' They patiently stood holding the photo while he told them about her armament, described the way it listed after it was hit, and shared other details about the attacks on Pearl Harbor.

"Bud finally admitted how tired he was after more than an hour on deck. While they were finishing up goodbyes and taking last minute photos, one officer asked if it would be okay to bring sailors up to visit Bud in a few months…I quietly explained the reason we'd asked for the visit…Bud was dying. I told him they were welcome to come up any time they wanted, but I suspected Bud had about a month left to live. Almost without hesitation, he asked if the crew could provide burial honors when the time came. I assured him that'd be an honor we'd welcome. As we headed towards the gangplank, we heard over the loudspeaker, 'Electrician's Mate Second Class Bud ____, departing.'

"Later that night Bud sat in his recliner, hands full of ship's coins, and declared, 'I don't care what you do with my power tools; you better promise you'll bury me with these.' He died 13 days later. For 12 of those 13 days he talked about the Dewey, her sailors, and his visit to San Diego. Everyone who came to the house had to hear the story, see the photos, hold the coins, read the plaques. Those sailors opened their ship and their hearts, and quite literally made a dream come true for a dying sailor" (Bob T., personal communication, Nov. 22, 2013).

Learning Activity 20: Dealing With Terminal Illness

Consider Bud's case.

1. Why do you think visiting the Dewey was so important for Bud?

2. Discuss how his social identity as a sailor during World War II helped him to experience a "good death."

3. How could an OT encourage this type of storytelling, even when an actual visit is not possible?

Learning Activity 21: Coping With Personal Loss

1. Write a brief summary of your own experience with someone close to you who died. What was his or her experience of dying like? Explain.

2. What were your feelings about the death? How did it affect your everyday life?

3. How would you feel about working as an occupational therapist with someone who is dying?

SUMMARY

This chapter reviews some of the predictable transitions of older adulthood: retirement, changes in health, changing residence, grieving over loss of significant others, and issues at the end of life. There are many studies connecting life transitions with health-related issues. Either a decline in health triggers a life-altering transition, such as retirement or death of a spouse, or difficulty coping with a transition lowers the older adult's resistance, and puts him or her at risk for the onset or worsening of health conditions. Either of these occurrences increases the likelihood that an OT will encounter many older clients who face the major transitions reviewed here. Therefore, occupational therapists need to be aware of the evidence that exists and the types of interventions that are effective in dealing with transitions, as well as the health conditions that will become part of the outcome. The occupations that have been important to older clients in the past can often provide comfort and strength, helping older adults to better cope with these inevitable life changes.

REFERENCES

American Occupational Therapy Association. (2014). Occupational therapy practice framework: Domain and process, 3rd Edition. *American Journal of Occupational Therapy, 68*, S1-S48.

Boerner, K., Carr, D., & Moorman, S. (2013). Family relationships and advance care planning: Do supportive and critical relations encourage or hinder planning? *Journals of Gerontology, Series B: Psychological and Social Sciences, 68*(2), 246-256. Doi:10.1093/geronb/gbs161

Cahill, K., Giandrea, M., & Quinn, J. (2012). Older workers and short-term jobs: Patterns and determinants. *Monthly Labor Review*, May, 19-29.

Cannuscio, C., Block, J., & Kawachi, I. (2003). Social capital and successful aging: The role of senior housing. *Annals of Internal Medicine, 139*, 395-399.

Carr, D. (2003). A "good death" for whom? Quality of spouses' death and psychological distress among older widowed persons. *Journal of Health and Social Behavior, 44*, 215-232.

Carr, D. (2012). "I don't want to die like that...": The impact of significant others' death quality on advance care planning. *The Gerontologist, 52,* 770-781.

Carr, D., House, J., Kessler, R., Nesse, R. Sonnega, J., & Wortman, C. (2000). Marital quality and psychological adjustment to widowhood among older adults: A longitudinal analysis. *Journals of Gerontology: Social Sciences, 55B,* S197-S207.

Carstensen, L., Fung, H., & Charles, S. (2003). Socioemotional selectivity theory and the regulation of emotion in the second half of life. *Motivation and Emotion, 2,* 103-123.

Crist, P. A. (1999). Does quality of life vary with different types of housing among older persons? A pilot study. *Physical and Occupational Therapy in Geriatrics, 16,* 101-116.

De Raedt, R., Koster, E., & Ryckewaert, R. (2013). Attentional bias for death-related and general threat-related information: Less avoidance in older as compared with middle-aged adults. *Journals of Gerontology B: Psychological and Social Sciences, 68,* 41-48.

Emlet, C., & Crabtree, J. (1996). Introduction to in-home assessment of older adults. In C. A. Emlet, J. Crabtree, V. A. Condon, & L. A. Treml (Eds.), *In home assessment of older adults* (pp. 1-16). Gaithersberg, MD: Aspen.

Fried, L., Freedman, M., Endres, T., & Wasik, B. (1997). Building communities that promote successful aging. *Successful Aging Western Journal of Medicine, 167,* 216-219.

Griffin, T. (2011). Parkinson's disease. In B. Schell, G. Gillen, M. Scaffa, & E. Cohn (Eds.), *Willard & Spackman's occupational therapy* (p. 1163). Philadelphia, PA: Lippincott, Williams & Wilkins.

Hersch, G., Spencer, J., Schulz, E., Wiley, A., Schwartz, M., Kearney, K., ... Tegethoff, S. (2004). Adaptation to relocation by elders: Evaluation of a model. *Journal of Housing for the Elderly, 18,* 41-68.

Hesketh, B., & Griffin, B. (2007). Work adjustment. In W. B. Walsh & M. L. Savickas (Eds.), *Handbook of vocational psychology vol. 3,* (pp. 245-266). Mahway, NJ: Lawrence Erlbaum Associates.

Hesketh, B., Griffin, B., & Loh, V. (2011). A future-oriented retirement transition framework. *Journal of Vocational Behavior, 79,* 303-314.

Hoehn, M., & Yahr, M. (1967). Parkinsonism: Onset, progression, and mortality. *Neurology, 17,* 427-442.

Holmes, T., & Rahe, R. (1967). The social readjustment rating scale. *Journal of Psychosomatic Research, 11,* 213-218.

Jonsson, H. (2011). The first steps into the Third Age: The retirement process from a Swedish perspective. *Occupational Therapy International, 18,* 32-38.

Keesing, S. & Rosenwax, L. (2011). Is occupation missing from occupational therapy in palliative care? *Australian Occupational Therapy Journal. 58:*329-336.

Knight, B. G. (2004). *Psychotherapy with older adults.* Thousand Oaks, CA: Sage Publications.

Knotts, V. (2003). Creating home: A phenomenological study on place transitions of culturally diverse older women: A dissertation. *Unpublished doctoral dissertation.* Texas Tech University, Lubbock, TX.

Knotts, V. (2008). Transitions for older adults. In S. Coppola, S. Elliott, & P. Toto (Eds.), *Strategies to promote gerontology excellence.* Bethesda, MD: AOTA Press.

Kubler-Ross, E. (2005). On grief and grieving: Finding the meaning of grief through the five stages of loss. New York: Simon & Schuster, Ltd.

Lee, G. R. (2014). Current research on widowhood: Devastation and human resilience. *The Journals of Gerontology, Series B: Psychological and Social Sciences, 69,* 2-3.

Leland, N., Elliott, S., & Johnson, K. (2012). *Occupational therapy practice guidelines for productive aging for community-dwelling older adults.* Bethesda, MD: American Occupational Therapy Association Press.

Pizzi, M. (2010). Promoting wellness in end-of-life care. In M. Scaffa, S.M. Reitz, & M. Pizzi (Eds.), *Occupational therapy in the promotion of health and wellness* (pp. 493-507). Philadelphia, PA: FA Davis.

Purcell, P. (2009). Older workers: *Employment and retirement trends. Congressional Research Service 7-5700.* Retrieved from www.crs.gov.

Rowe, J. W. & Kahn, R. L. (1998). *Successful aging.* New York, NY: Dell Publishing.

Sanders, M., & Van Oss, T. (2013). Using daily routines to promote medication adherence in older adults. *American Journal of Occupational Therapy, 67,* 91-99.

Schell, B. B., Gillen, G., & Scaffa, M. (2014). *Willard & Spackman's occupational therapy* (12th ed). Philadelphia, PA: Lippincott Williams & Wilkins.

Seltzer, J., & Friedman, E. (2014). Widowed mothers' co-residence with adult children. *The Journals of Gerontology, Series B: Psychological & Social Sciences, 69,* 63-74.

Schkade, J., & McClung, M. (2001). *Occupational adaptation in practice.* Thorofare, NJ: SLACK Incorporated.

Sullivan, A., & Fenelon, A. (2014). Patterns of widowhood mortality. *The Journals of Gerontology, Series B: Psychological & Social Sciences, 69,* 53-62.

Upham, E. W., & Gravenson, L. (2010). *In the fullness of time: 32 women on life after 50.* New York: Atria Paperback.

U.S. Dept. of Health & Human Services (2008). Advance directives and advance care planning: Report to congress (online report). Retrieved from http://aspe.hhs.gov/daltcp/reports/2008/ADCongRpt.htm.

Utz, R., Swenson, K., Caserta, M., Lund, D., & de Vries, B. (2014). Feeling lonely versus being alone: Loneliness and social support among recently bereaved persons. *Journals of Gerontology, Series B: Psychological and Social Sciences, 69,* 85-94.

Vaillant, G. (2009). Keys to a healthy retirement. *Harvard Business Review Blog Network/Health and Well-Being.* Retrieved from http://blogs.hbr.org/health-and-well-being/2009/04/keys-to-a-healthy-retirement.html.

Vries, B., Utz, R., Caserta, M., & Lund, D. (2014). Friend and family contact and support in early widowhood. *Journal of Gerontology, Series B: Psychological and Social Sciences, 69B,* 75-84.

Wang, M. (2007). Profiling retirees in the retirement transition and adjustment process: Examining the longitudinal change patterns of retirees' psychological well-being. *The Journal of Applied Psychology, 92,* 455-474.

Warner, D., Hayward, M., & Hardy, M. (2010). The retirement life course in America at the dawn of the twenty-first century. *Population Research and Policy Review, 29,* 893-919. (NIH Public Access Author Manuscript).

4

Continuums of Care

Karen C. Macdonald, PhD, OTR/L and Marilyn B. Cole, MS, OTR/L, FAOTA

The continuum of care for older adults reflects the variety of programs within current and emerging health care systems. They serve as employment opportunities for OT practitioners. These range from well elderly services to rehabilitative or chronic and palliative care (comfort measures only). Therapy services may be offered in primary care, home care, and community programs, as well as traditional rehabilitation and long-term care facilities. Occupational therapists and certified occupational therapy assistants (OTAs) have a vital role in providing interventions that are goal directed and considered preventive, rehabilitative, or restorative. For chronic conditions, therapy may be directed toward maintaining existing skills and preventing deterioration. All are directed toward promotion of independence in self-care and participation in valued activities.

This chapter begins with a basic discussion of the health care systems that now exist: medical, community, and nontraditional models. We then present a continuum of wellness to frail health, with basic descriptions and examples of some of the most common acute and chronic health conditions of older adulthood. The characteristics and severity of different health conditions and subsequent disabilities warrant different levels of care. Therefore, we will next describe the continuum of treatment settings, beginning with prevention and wellness, primary care, aging in place, and descriptions of community-based OT programming. These sections are followed by OT roles in more traditional medical settings available in today's health care system.

In the United States, payment for medical services to older adults is largely dictated by the guidelines of Medicare or Medicaid, with private insurance companies and client copays often supplementing the cost of care. OT practitioners who are employed by medical settings are obliged to follow the reimbursement guidelines of Medicare, including limitations in the timing and duration of treatment, the type of treatment offered, and the assessment and documentation requirements. With the Affordable Care Act, the current system of health care is also changing, and this may open up opportunities for OTs to provide wellness programming and intervention to a greater number of older adults who wish to take an active role in preventing disability from limiting their ability to remain engaged in their chosen productive occupations. Within this broad scope of practice, there are many opportunities for OT interventions, whether in medical or community-based models.

MODELS OF SERVICE DELIVERY

The two prevailing health care models are the medical model and the community-based model. As a brief review, the medical model is seen as reductionistic, focusing on one diagnosis or main area of treatment. Decisions are often determined by a physician with limited input by the client or other health care professionals. The community-based model, in contrast, is client-centered and holistic, with many health care providers jointly deciding team protocols. Client and family member input is valued, along with

Cole MB, Macdonald KC.
Productive Aging: An Occupational Perspective (pp 49-65).
© 2015 Taylor & Francis Group.

consideration of real life functioning expectations in the home and community environments.

Medical Model

Although definitions vary, the medical model commonly refers to traditional Western medicine, with a physician or psychiatrist guiding the intervention of allied health care team members. Medical experts view the human body as mechanistic in nature, meaning the doctors look for the body part or system that is broken (diagnosis) and take steps to fix it (prescription). The result is a narrow focus on a particular symptom, injury, or syndrome. Following examination and diagnosis, referrals may be made to pertinent specialists. Intervention may include medication and/or surgery, with education and support offered to the patient and family members. In recent years, roles have been introduced allowing physician assistants and advanced practice registered nurses to assess and engage in treatment and prescription writing.

In medical settings, the OT typically works directly with a multidisciplinary staff, including nursing, physical therapy, speech pathology, social work, recreation, and dietary employees. In this environment, these professionals share both team- and department-specific goals and communicate through documentation and meetings in an effort to coordinate interdisciplinary services. Most of the services provided in medical facilities are reimbursable according to specified guidelines by third-party reimbursors, such as health care insurance, Medicare, or Medicaid.

Within institutional settings such as hospitals, subacute rehabilitation centers, or extended care facilities, the OT practitioner may also have working relationships with departments such as volunteers and clergy, housekeeping, and maintenance personnel. The occupational therapist may also provide information to these departments about safety and environmental modifications. An example would be providing an in-service session about communication strategies with clients with sensory deficits.

Learning Activity 22: Patient Role Interview

Interview an older adult about an experience he or she had when in a patient role. Discuss the following:

1. What medical condition caused the person to seek medical help?

2. List and describe each step in evaluation and treatment, who was consulted and where, including the time frames and costs involved.

3. What was the diagnosis, prescription, and treatment recommendations?

4. Explore the person's feelings about being a patient. What interactions did he or she have with medical professionals? To what extent did the patient have input, control, or choices with regard to the treatment?

5. What was the outcome and how satisfied was the older adult with the outcome?

Community Model

The other model of practice is labeled in a variety of ways, including community-based, holistic, social, and client-centered models. The essential difference from the medical model may be understood as the difference between a patient and a client. A patient (a medical model term) passively accepts treatment without question and is expected to comply with doctor's orders to overcome a specific symptom or condition. Conversely, clients actively seek medical advice from doctors or other professionals but supplement the advice with their own research, learning also from the experience of friends, family members, or others who have had similar health difficulties. One can immediately see how clients, as independent thinkers who take responsibility for their own health and its treatment, might resist the authoritarian directives imposed by the medical model.

The community-based model also includes environmental and social determinants of illness and disability, as stated by the *International Classification of Functioning, Disability and Health* (WHO, 2001). The cause of a client's inability to participate in life activities or occupations might have nothing to do with his or her health condition, but rather with physical or social barriers. For example, an older person suddenly confined to a wheelchair because of a fractured hip might become housebound, socially isolated, and unable to care for him- or herself (disabled) not because of a lack of motivation, strength, and ability, but rather because he or she cannot get the wheelchair up the steps to the bedroom, through the doorway to the bathroom, or down the gravel driveway to a neighbor's car for a ride to the weekly poker game.

Groups of individuals with disabilities have joined together to advocate for equality and inclusion in mainstream society, including person-first language (e.g., a person with schizophrenia, not a "schizophrenic") and accessibility to public areas, such as town halls, courthouses, parks, public rest rooms, libraries, and schools. Older adults themselves have contested the stigma of ageism, especially in the workplace, but also in other more subtle areas where they are discouraged from participating in certain activities because of advanced age. For example, they may not be allowed to take a class at a university or school or they may be viewed as too old to take on a leadership role or public office in the community.

The community-based model seems like a good fit for the new OT professional paradigm, which is client centered, holistic, and systems oriented. It is also the best fit for OT roles in wellness and prevention with older adults. However, the medical reimbursement system remains an obstacle for many occupational therapists to fully apply their knowledge and skills to promote productive aging in the community.

Nontraditional Models

Complementary and alternative interventions are sometimes referred to as Eastern or nontraditional (Urban, 2013). Although many of these practices could be directed by a medical doctor, they are typically interventions guided by individuals with other specialty training. A broad spectrum of interventions are represented that are client centered and often provided in free-standing clinics or private offices. They may also be available through community or senior centers. Although some may be reimbursable by some form of health insurance, most would be paid for privately by the client. These include practices such as acupuncture, yoga, meditation, tai chi, herbal or vitamin supplements, hypnotism, Feldenkrais, biofeedback, guided imagery, and relaxation techniques. Some of these take place individually—practitioner with client—while others are group sessions. These practices often encompass a holistic philosophy, with consideration to mind, body, and spirit. Individuals are seen as unique, living in a world of varying circumstances. The client is encouraged to envision personal control of his or her personal health, with these interventions guiding self-directed management of symptoms.

The structure of alternative medicine services gives an example of how a nonmedical service might be funded, with clients paying out of pocket or, in some instances, being reimbursed by private insurance policies. As globalization evolves in health care, awareness and interest have developed for the health care practices of other cultures. This reflects a trend for consumers to begin with traditional medicine and then to seek additional intervention through alternative methods. However, many alternative practices remain unsubstantiated by research, yet continue to be used. Anecdotal evidence is often recognized by consumers as valued feedback and as validation of effectiveness.

Occupational therapists often incorporate aspects of these approaches in therapy sessions, regardless of practice setting. A recent position paper from AOTA's Commission on Practice supports the use of complementary and alternative medicine as part of OTs plan of care, either as a preparatory method or a therapeutic activity (AOTA, 2011). For stress reduction, guided imagery and relaxation techniques may be included, along with other interventions. Techniques from yoga, tai chi, or Reiki are "within the scope of occupational therapy as a means to reach goals such as decreasing pain, fatigue, and stress, and promoting a sense of well-being..." (Urban, 2013, p. 9). Some of the practices require certification or other advanced training that an occupational therapist could consider as a stepping stone to community-based practice.

Learning Activity 23: Identifying Health Care Models

1. The following are quotes from a 2014 OT job description: "meets the resident's goals and needs to provide quality care by assessing and interpreting evaluations and test results and determining treatment plans in consultation with physicians and by prescription. Administers therapy statements according to treatment plan approved by the attending physician. Directs treatment given by aides and assistants. Manage (sic) appropriate treatment minutes per RUGS (Resource Utilization Groups, a reimbursement regulation system) categories for residents and patients" (advertisement from www.careerbuilder.com).

   a. If you accepted this position, to whom would you be directly responsible for guidance and direction? To whom would you be giving direction?

   b. Which of the previous models of health care would this job fall under and why?

   c. What type of facility do you think you might be working in? Explain.

2. The following is another 2014 OT job offering: "Responsibilities: a team member for the rehabilitation program, working in a group setting with an interdisciplinary focus primarily for the neurological, orthopedic, and geriatric outpatients. This program provides a continuum of care into the community through education and special therapy aimed at gaining functional independence" (advertisement from www.recruitingsite.com).

   a. If you accepted this position, where do you think you might be working?

   b. Which of the previous models do you think this job would fall under and why?

   c. How might this OT position be different from the first one described?

   d. What are the pros and cons of each of these job descriptions? Which would you prefer and why?

3. Identify some health-altering practices that would be considered alternative.

   a. Describe one in detail, citing your source or website.

   b. Have you ever tried any of these? Why did you try it, and what were your results?

CONTINUUM OF COMMUNITY-BASED PRACTICE SETTINGS

The next two sections highlight some of the traditional and emerging practice settings for OTs and OTAs. Productive aging has been identified as an emerging practice area where OTs are not well-established but are still defining their roles with community agencies, partnerships such as American Association of Retired Persons (AARP) or Agencies on Aging, and positions in primary care. Other, more traditional OT roles exist within medical facilities, such as hospitals, home health agencies, and long-term care facilities.

Aging in Place

Because of the rising cost of institutional long-term care, some national studies have concluded that the most cost effective way to meet the needs of the aging population is to provide supportive services that enable them to remain in their communities, living in their own homes, for as long as possible (MetLife, 2010). This phenomenon is known as aging in place. The MetLife (2010) study states the following three goals for promoting aging in place:

1. Independence: happier, more satisfied older citizens living in homes of their choice with control, dignity, and respect.

2. More economical use of resources: avoiding the high cost of care facilities that provide services that residents may or may not need.

3. The creation of a coordinated, comprehensive, and collaborative relationship between businesses and service providers to support aging in place.

"Planning for long-term care is difficult because no one knows how their health will play out as they age. One in five older Americans faces significant cost associated with long-term care" (MetLife, 2010, p. 2). Additionally, a specific "housing arrangement often becomes a poor match, requiring residents to move multiple times, such as from a home to a hospital because of a health episode, then to a nursing home for rehabilitation, then back to the home, then on to assisted living for longer term care... Moving between facilities is often disorienting, disturbing, and undesirable, not only for the individual, but for the entire family" (MetLife, 2010, p. 2).

However, the services needed to support aging in place currently are fragmented and not organized into an easily accessed and managed system. As more seniors opt to age in place, alternatives to institutionalization have expanded, including home care, home modification programs to accommodate compromised functioning or mobility, senior transportation to community senior centers or medical centers, and adult day care programs. These services allow older adults with increasing health care needs to continue living in their homes and communities for as long as they wish or are able to do so comfortably and safely. For older adults, the intentions are to provide supportive services to enhance "independent living through supported and assisted stages of function gradually transitioning to full care" (MetLife, 2010, p. 2).

Learning Activity 24: Identifying Resources for Aging in Place

Find and briefly describe three web resources that support aging in place in the United States. For each, describe the role OT might play in supporting independent living within its parameters. Which parts of these proposed services come from the medical model and which come from the community model or another source? Explain your reasoning.

1.

2.

3.

Primary Care and Prevention

By primary care, we mean the first tier of health care service delivery, such as the primary care physician's office or walk-in clinic, where an older adult might go for a health check-up, an acute health condition, or to further explore an unusual symptom. For some time, OTs have been encouraged to have a stronger presence within primary care, and to focus on health promotion and prevention activities. "While there is a clear fit between occupational therapy and primary care, there have been too few practice examples, despite a growing body of evidence to support the role" (Donnelly, Brenchley, Crawford, & Letts, 2013, p. 60). According to these authors, the primary reasons for OT's absence from primary care are lack of funding, traditional solo practitioner models, and OT's traditional focus on rehabilitation rather than prevention (Figure 4-1).

With alternate sources of public or private funding outside the current medical reimbursement system, OTs might develop important roles for prevention and wellness within both medical and community settings. An OT might work with a primary care physician in his or her office, which would fall, at least in part, under the medical model of service delivery. For example, this author provided a "protect your back" self-management consultation to patients who received epidural injections for lower back pain in a private practitioner's office, funded by a research grant. Group programs dealing with prevention might be offered in the community, with payment coming from local public funding or from members paying a reasonable fee out of pocket. Examples of community settings are senior centers with matched roommate programs. Some international models have been recognized for their responses to challenging socioeconomic or political environments that led to the development of creative models for senior service delivery. An example from Canada is the Family Health Care Team, into which OT has recently been integrated. This multidisciplinary group shares responsibility with physicians for primary health care of entire families, generally making health care more affordable (Donnelly et al., 2013).

Group Programs for Populations in the Community

According to Fazio (2010), OT programs for community populations have "provided primary service learning opportunities for entry level OT students" (OTs and OTAs). This author suggests a stepwise approach to establishing occupation-based community programs, including the following steps:

1. Idea generation: Based on interaction with patients/clients, other professionals, advocacy groups, or personal experience.

2. Profiling the community: Determining populations, services already available, needs assessment for intended population, focus groups with stakeholders.

3. Researching the evidence for intended interventions, setting appropriate goals, describing theoretical framework.

4. Identifying appropriate leaders, level of expertise or training required, and supervision, including OT students, educators, practitioners, volunteers, client peer leaders, family caregivers, or others.

5. Finding affordable and accessible space, scheduling, supplies, equipment, and budget.

6. Obtaining public or private funding for program.

7. Marketing the program, recruiting participants.

8. Measuring outcomes, designing valid ways to affirm goal achievement.

Some examples of community group programs provided by students for a senior housing project (low income, publically subsidized cluster housing) include senior fitness, memoir writing, scrapbooking, fall prevention, emergency planning, diet and nutrition sessions, and holiday memory sharing. Published programs appear frequently in *OT Practice* magazine. For example, Stepping Stones is a community group OT program established by faculty and students at Texas Woman's University in Denton, Texas, supporting clients with early-stage Alzheimer's disease and their caregivers (Brown & Evetts, 2013). Students at Adventist University in Orlando, Florida, partnering with AARP and AAA, participated in a CarFit and Home-Fit community program, providing education to seniors at a senior living community in Winter Park, Florida, via group

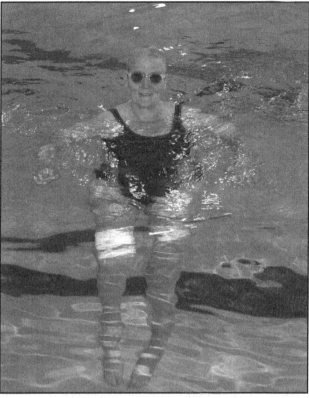

Figure 4-1. Nan enjoys exercising in the pool, a part of her healthy lifestyle in retirement. As a good self-manager, she structures her days with productive occupations that also promote wellness and prevention.

presentations and onsite consultations with seniors in their cars and homes to enhance safety and comfort and facilitate aging in place (Waite, 2013).

Another example of a community-based program, CAPABLE (Community Aging in Place, Advancing Better Living for Elders), involves an interprofessional team—an OT, a nurse, and a handyman—funded by a $4 million, 5-year grant from the National Institutes of Health. Together, the team's purpose is to help low-income older adults in Baltimore, Maryland, with self-identified problems affecting home safety, fall risk, prevention, and carrying out activities of daily living, including home management and caregiving. The OT's role includes social participation, leisure, and functional mobility in addition to the above areas (Bridges, Szanton, Evelyn-Gustave, Smith, & Gitlin, 2013). This program can serve as a model for OTs to provide needed services to productive agers within a community-based model.

TRADITIONAL MEDICAL PRACTICE SETTINGS

The following are more standard tiers of geriatric services at the start of the 21st century.

Hospitals

In the traditional hospital setting, the older adult may be admitted for an acute illness or injury that requires specialized medical diagnosis and intervention. Some patients may also be admitted through the emergency department for symptoms that were not addressed through a primary care physician and then be assigned to a hospital bed.

The OT role has changed significantly in primary hospital care, reflecting shorter stays for patients and early discharge to subacute units or rehabilitation facilities. In some settings, OTs treat conditions such as burns, stroke, cardiac arrest, and postsurgical issues. With in-patients, the OT may complete an evaluation and then provide relevant therapeutic exercise and/or activities, orthotic and positioning products, activities of daily living (ADL) training, functional transfer instruction, and recommendations for discharge planning.

In some hospitals, a geropsychiatric unit is available or older adults may be admitted to a general psychiatric unit. For the duration of a short stay, the patient is assessed for medication needs, safety from harming self or others, and ability to function when returning home to a less structured environment without supervision. Here, the OT would perform an assessment, and utilize individual- and group-oriented strategies for promoting mental health and functional independence. Some goals and approaches may include socialization skills, life skills management, relaxation techniques, cooking groups, and expressive media.

Many hospitals have established outpatient services to provide follow-up for their discharged patients. For example, the following is from an advertisement for a hospital-based OT job: "Evaluates for, organizes, and conducts medically prescribed occupational therapy programs/treatments for outpatients…to restore function and prevent disability following disease or injury. Also directs purposeful activities for self-care, work, play-leisure, and learning. Responsible for helping the patient to reach his/her maximum performance and to assume a place in society, while learning to live within the limits of his or her capabilities" (Advertisement from linkedin.com).

Learning Activity 25: Describing Hospital-Based Occupational Therapy Jobs

Find three advertisements for hospital-based OT positions from employment websites. List them with full job descriptions, salary (if available), and web URL. For each job listing, compose three questions you might ask to clarify the OT's responsibilities in the advertised position.

1.

2.

3.

Subacute Rehabilitation

Following acute hospital care, patients step down to a subacute level, with a focus on promoting greater independence in ADLs. This is considered outpatient rehabilitation and may be located in a section of a hospital or in a separate agency. The older adult needs to arrange for transportation and scheduling for the duration of this phase of therapy. There are also subacute inpatient facilities where Medicare pays for up to 90 days of rehabilitation as an inpatient.

As the individual is healing from the condition that led to hospitalization, rehabilitation services change their focus. As tolerated, progressive strengthening exercises and activities are graded for abilities with motor, cognitive, and social skills. Additional attention is directed toward all aspects of independence in ADLs, including teaching compensatory techniques as needed. With progress, therapy also includes attention to promoting abilities in instrumental activities of daily living (IADLs) including shopping, meal preparation, laundry, and community mobility, among others. A home evaluation may be performed and related to discharge to home care services.

Recent research shows that social support, an often neglected area in rehabilitation settings, has been identified as an "effective rehabilitation strategy that can motivate people with disabilities to participate in meaningful occupation" (Isaksson, Lexell, & Skär, 2007, p. 23). This implies that OTs should consider using group interventions, with persons in the early stages of rehabilitation providing much-needed encouragement for each other, as the above authors found among 23 women with spinal cord injuries. Refer to Section II for examples of these types of groups for clients with physical disabilities.

Home Care

Health services provided in the patient's home, typically provided by a medically oriented agency, include nursing, social work, speech-language therapy, physical and occupational therapy, and aides or assistants with various levels of training and expertise. The patient or client may be seen in the home because he or she is unable to tolerate or travel to outpatient services. Alternatively, home care may be indicated because a higher level of functioning has been achieved in the subacute setting, and therapy is now transferred to "real life" application for ability to manage within the familiar home environment. The OT may conduct a more thorough evaluation of the home and yard, with recommendations for structural changes or safety considerations. Assessments of this nature include attention to all living spaces, stairs, storage, lighting, supplies, emergency procedure preparedness, medications, and meals.

In home care, the OT may work closely with family or paid caregivers, offering suggestions for safe mobility, transfers, communication, memory aids, meal preparation, and promoting self-care skills. The OT may refer the client to community resources or other professionals who may continue with extended home care. Recommendations may relate to architectural considerations, such as widening a doorway to permit wheelchair access, modifying toilets and bathing areas, and installing a ramp for safe entry and exit from the home. A Canadian study of home care services for older adults who had experienced musculoskeletal conditions, including fractures and arthritis, used a variety of ADL and IADL measures (Cook et al., 2013). Their findings confirmed results of prior studies—that home care services led to gains in function, cognition, and quality of life. They suggest that rehabilitation services offered at home by PTs and OTs led to prevention of general decline and falls (Cook et al., 2013).

This setting provides OT practitioners the opportunity to explore the everyday occupations performed by the clients in their usual settings so that together the client and OT can adapt the environment to remove barriers and facilitate independence. The OT practitioner devises individualized treatment plans to match the client's unique abilities, circumstances, and choices. Because skills continue to change with time, the therapist provides ongoing revisions to goals and approaches.

EXPERT'S EXPERIENCE—
JANICE CONWAY, MA, OTR/L

Janice Conway is a professor and academic fieldwork coordinator at Housatonic Community College's OTA program in Bridgeport, Connecticut. She participates in clinical practice through per diem and home care services for adults and older clients. Her experience spans 30 years working with a variety of acute and chronic conditions.

Ms. Conway stated, "In general practice, I have observed and become aware that the people who are active, are out in society, and have friendships…the whole activity piece… these are the people that seem to age well. You can put two 80-year-olds together and they can be so different. One person can be failing health-wise or cognitively and the other looks 60. It makes you think about planning for the future. It almost starts pre-retirement…if you don't belong to something or have any friends, it's hard to get started when you're 80."

Relating to the concept of productive aging, she expressed "…that is when people don't give up on what they can do for themselves…sometimes, when people become ill, they become dependent on other people to do things for them; it seems they hand it over easily and then don't regain it. Occupational therapists need to be aware of the 'learned helplessness' phenomenon. It may be that part of our intervention is to educate caregivers so that they don't easily step in and do too much if they don't need to."

Assisted Living

Assisted living facilities are community-based dwelling in which security, maintenance, and grounds care may be provided. In addition, housekeeping services, meals, laundry, and nursing services may be available. In some of these settings, the resident may choose the extent of assistance provided; in other settings, all services are included in the fees. A higher level of independent functioning is the norm for self-care activities and many residents shop for and prepare some of their own meals.

In some of these communities, there are separate living areas for periods in which a resident needs an increased level of supervision or medical care. These may be temporary or permanent. This is especially beneficial for a couple who has moved to the assisted living facility and one of the pair has a decline in health. This allows for easy contact and visits because they both reside in the same complex. Another positive aspect is that when a member of the community has a health status change, regardless of the level of specialized care, there is a continuity related to the administration and mission of the entire community.

An OT could also serve as a consultant or part-time employee of an assisted living facility, providing recommendations for safety and structural and environmental modifications. Additionally, the OT could recommend interventions for increasing self-management skills of residents. An OTA could be hired as a director of activity programming, or work part-time leading goal-oriented groups. For example, groups could include exercise, meditation, adapted crafts, indoor sports, and special interest celebrations or trips. The OTA would be skilled at providing task analysis and graded activities to increase levels of participation with respect to physical, cognitive, or social challenges.

In assisted living facilities, residents usually have the option to enlist home care services, just as they would if they were living independently. When specialized OT services are needed, these would then be provided by an independent agency and paid for by the resident's own public or private medical insurance.

Adult Day Care

Whether serving a social or medical model, adult day care centers offer a structured environment during daytime hours (Iecovich & Biderman, 2013). Usually designed to match work schedules of family caregivers, participants often arrive by facility-provided transportation. Along with being in a supportive and stimulating environment that promotes well-being for the clients, the centers provide much-needed respite for family caregivers, who then have time to attend to their own needs and responsibilities.

A typical day consists of planned activity groups, both large and small, balanced with quiet rest periods. Lunch, healthy snacks, and beverages are provided. In medically

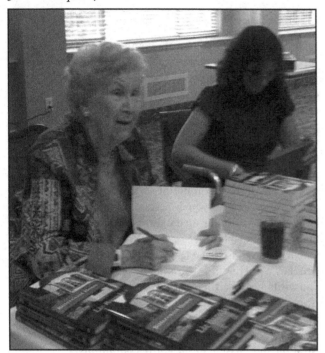

Figure 4-2. Liz enjoys the fruits of her labor, here signing copies of a novel she has written. This event takes place at the extended care facility where she lives.

oriented adult day care centers, medication, health monitoring, and toileting needs are attended to by staff. The staff designs activities to promote and maintain skills, matching levels of functioning. Small groups may include the whole membership, typically from 20 to 40 men and women of varied ages and health conditions. Some centers specialize in care for individuals with dementia. Some activities can be mentally and physically stimulating (group games, line dancing), while others are intentionally passive and calming (watching a film, listening to music).

OTs may have varied levels of involvement in adult day care. Some are part-time employees, offering individual restorative interventions as indicated, consultation for group work, and programming, family education, and home assessments. Some centers have an OT as a director, who is responsible for all administrative, management, and supervisory tasks. An OTA may work as the director of therapeutic activities within the setting, designing and leading groups, attending to scheduling and supplies, and training other activity personnel, aides, and volunteers.

An interdisciplinary team may consist of a director, nurse, social worker, and rehabilitation therapists, with connections to additional services for dietary needs, clergy, and a hairdresser or barber. Some sites are connected to long-term care facilities, while others are free-standing and community based. In some communities, extended hours for evening and weekend programs are also provided.

Long-Term Care Facilities

Throughout the 20th century, long-term care facilities have experienced many changes to reflect family dynamics and responsibilities, health care policies, and resident rights. Negative perceptions often generated dread as older adults feared "being sent to a nursing home." Progressive inspections and regulations led to strict attention to and compliance with laws for services, safety, cleanliness, professional levels of health care delivery from an interdisciplinary team, and quality of life issues. Changing names, such as skilled nursing facility (SNF) or extended care facility accompanied many efforts in recent decades to decrease negative associations of nursing homes. Continuing care retirement communities (CCRCs) offer a stepwise increase in levels of care from minimal to maximum or total care. Currently, whether commercial or not-for-profit, long-term care facilities strive for excellence in individualized services for their residents. Within a given community, many facilities may vie for potential admissions as they publicize an atmosphere of a caring and creative community. The study of gerontology has led to a greater understanding of the unique needs of elders and has led to a growing group of professionals dedicated to ensuring excellence in long-term care for older adults.

Watermark, in Bridgeport, Connecticut, is an example of a CCRC that requires a down payment followed by a monthly fee based on the level of care provided. Liz sold her townhouse and moved into Watermark after her husband died and she began having balance issues, causing her to fall several times. Their professional staff encourages residents to pursue their meaningful occupations within the facility. Liz, a journalist in former years, has turned to creative writing in her retirement. In Figure 4-2, she is pictured reading from and signing her first self-published novel, done through a program sponsored by the facility yet open to the public. Within the community, Liz can function independently and engage in a productive occupation that continues to hold a central place in her life.

Upon admission to extended care, many new residents have long-standing comorbidities of several conditions that have led to a need for 24-hour professional attention related to supervision, safety, personal self-care, and structured activity. In earlier years, individuals who had decreased abilities in home and yard maintenance, shopping for and preparing meals, or driving might have considered moving to a nursing home to be relieved of these responsibilities. Their residents have a wide range, from rather high levels of functioning to very low levels. In more recent years, those individuals with higher functional levels are instead utilizing assisted living communities or home care services. Therefore, current long-term care admissions tend to be more disabled and further along in the progression of symptoms, requiring higher levels of intensive assistance and attention. This reflects today's tendency for older adults to age in place, using home care and community-based services for as long as possible before considering a move to long-term care.

Along with physical limitations affecting mobility and self-care skills, dementia causes many recent referrals for permanent placement in a long-term care facility. Accordingly, many facilities have designed special care units for individuals with cognitive or psychosocial challenges. These are designed to offer consistent behavioral approaches by staff, adapted activities to match levels of skill throughout the day, and specifically structured environments for living and social areas of the unit.

OTs have long held important positions in the rehabilitative departments of long-term care facilities. As health care services evolved, OTs and OTAs have taken prominent roles in many aspects of program design, individual treatment, staff development, and environmental modifications. Some residents are referred to OT for restorative services when they have had a recent change in function, illness, or injury. Skilled services are used to evaluate for and prescribe assistive and adaptive devices for dressing, grooming, and eating. Although certified nurse assistance is available for ADL tasks, most facilities foster a philosophy of promoting maximum independence for as long as possible. The OT offers suggestions for task analysis, sequencing, and graded activities to allow for some optimal levels of independent and successful task completion.

OTs offer instructions for staff, volunteers, and family members related to activity modification, body mechanics, communication strategies, and cognitive behavioral management techniques. Some OTs or OTAs design and lead purposeful, goal-oriented activity groups. Ergonomics are considered along with the least restrictive environment regulations. For residents who are at risk for falling, the rehabilitation department works as a team to design effective means to allow for freedom of movement, yet protection from risk of injury, without the use of physical restraints. Wheelchairs, lounge chairs, and beds are modified to promote comfort and prevent areas of pressure.

Group participation is an important part of daily life for residents in a long-term care facility. Hersch et al. (2012) explored the effects of groups promoting adaptation related to cultural heritage. OTAs lead groups of newly admitted residents for eight weekly sessions focusing on adaptation and social participation. Findings indicated an increase in quality of life.

Learning Activity 26: Health Care Facilities From an Outsider's Perspective

1. Describe an experience that you have had in which you visited an older adult in a health care facility (type of facility, reasons for the visit, others accompanying you)

2. What was the environment like (sights, sounds, smells)? How did it make you feel?

3. Whom did you visit and how do you think they felt about being there?

Hospice Programs

Hospice services for clients with a terminal illness can occur within a hospice facility, a client's home, or assisted living, continuing care, or long-term care facilities. OTs have a developing role in working with terminally ill people, currently referred to as end-of-life care (ELC). The end of life (or dying process) is viewed as a developmental stage, with its own unique life tasks and characteristics. Therapists need both sensitivity and realism when approaching this end of life stage, with its unfamiliar emotions, roles, relationships, and activities.

In palliative care, comfort is provided through medications, relaxation techniques, positioning, client and family support, and expressive modalities. The OT may play a role in designing a therapeutic milieu as an appropriate living environment, engaging individuals in life review or legacy activities, and affirming style strategies. Instruction may be provided for volunteers related to death and dying issues and appropriate supportive verbal exchanges. For most patients, lengthy periods in a bed or a bedside chair are uncomfortable, and the OT may create or recommend specialized seating or padding materials. The OT can have a positive presence while designing or adapting simplified meaningful activities.

Learning Activity 27: Exploring Occupational Therapist's and Occupational Therapy Assistant's Roles

Ideally, going to visit a local facility in each of these categories would be the best preparation for this activity, if time permits. For each of the settings listed next, discuss the possible roles for an OT and a certified OTA. What specific tasks might be a part of their daily responsibilities? Briefly discuss how you would feel about working as an OT in this setting and why.

1. Inpatient Subacute Rehabilitation Center
   a. OT
   b. OTA
   c. Discussion
2. Home Care
   a. OT
   b. OTA
   c. Discussion

3. Adult Day Care

    a. OT

    b. OTA

    c. Discussion

4. Long-Term Care

    a. OT

    b. OTA

    c. Discussion

5. Hospice Care (End-of-Life Care)

    a. OT

    b. OTA

    c. Discussion

CURRENT OCCUPATIONAL THERAPY POSITIONS AND ROLES

Depending on a practitioner's experience and the services available in the community, OT practitioners may choose from a variety of employment opportunities. These range from work environments where there is a team of colleagues to highly independent and autonomous positions. The following is a brief overview that demonstrates that whatever the therapist's time availability, there are possibilities for maintaining active involvement in practice. In each setting, careful determination of issues such as liability protection and scheduling flexibility need to be addressed.

Current Structures for Practice

Direct hire is when a therapist is employed in a public or private setting. As their employee, the therapist is bound to the mission of the organization and its expectations of performance, and they may have a contract specifying a benefits package. In this environment, the OT is often part of a team with strong interdisciplinary connections. The therapist may be part of an organized OT department with layers of supervision available. Therapists might participate in projects assigned to the OT department (e.g., wheelchair ordering and assignment to clients) or in clinical education programs.

Agencies offer other opportunities in which the OT is a subcontractor. The OT works for the agency, which assigns employment positions that may be full- or part-time or per diem (daily, as needed). Assignments may be short- or long-term. In this setting, a therapist may be assigned to several locations, including facilities or home care.

Private practice is an option for OTs who usually have established expertise within a specialty area of practice. This may involve home care or maintaining a private clinic. The private practitioner may work independently or hire

additional staff. In this environment, the OT needs administrative skills to ensure all that is necessary for client referrals; physician orders; an appropriate therapy space with necessary tools, equipment, and supplies; adherence to any local or state regulations; and management of all documentation, billing, and reimbursement systems.

In *community settings*, very few OT positions currently exist for wellness and prevention or for aspects of community integration outside the medical model. Most of the OT programs serving populations such as those who are homeless or have serious mental illness have been provided by students, supervised by educators, and funded by universities or research grants (Kaminsky, 2010). The upcoming generations of OT graduates need to partner with existing organizations, such as agencies on aging or community senior centers, and advocate for more community-based positions for OT to fully reach the profession's centennial vision (AOTA, 2007) in serving the needs of productive agers.

Learning Activity 28: Who Are Health Care Team Members?

Health care teams often include the following in addition to OT practitioners (OTs and OTAs): medical doctors, physician's assistants, registered nurses, nurse practitioners, licensed practical nurses, social workers, dietitians, recreation therapists, physical therapists, physical therapy assistants, speech-language therapists, family members, home health aides, clergymen, and others depending on the facility or level of care for an older client.

1. List five professionals and others who are likely to be members of the health care team for each of the following levels of care. Find some examples on the internet to help you with identifying them, as needed.

2. Describe what role each might play.

3. How do each of their roles differ from that of an OT practitioner?

    a. Long-Term Care Facility (Nursing Home):

        1.

        2.

        3.

        4.

        5.

    b. Home Care Agency:

        1.

        2.

        3.

        4.

        5.

c. Subacute Rehabilitation Facility:

1.

2.

3.

4.

5.

d. Hospice Program:

1.

2.

3.

4.

5.

Learning Activity 29: Productive Aging in Current Occupational Therapy Job Market

1. Look in *OT Practice*, *Advance for OT*, or another OT job listing or website. Find three jobs in the area of gerontology at different levels of care that interest you and describe them below:

a.

b.

c.

For each of the jobs you found, answer the following as best you can or add your own ideas:

1. In what type of facility or setting would you be working?

2. What would be the basis of payment for your services (hourly, per day, salaried, other)?

3. What are a few examples of activities you would perform as an OT doing this job?

4. Do you think this job is medically based or community based? Why?

5. How could productive aging be promoted in this job setting?

REIMBURSEMENT ISSUES FOR OCCUPATIONAL THERAPY IN THE UNITED STATES

The following is a very brief overview of the reimbursement issues for health care in America today. It is included here because reimbursement for OT within the medical payment system creates a major barrier to the expansion of the profession's role with older adults in the community.

Insurance under the fee-for-service system, for example, does not pay for wellness and prevention, seldom pays for group interventions, and excludes OT from primary care settings where they could make a significant contribution.

Fee-for-Service System

This system of payment is simple: provide a service and charge a set fee. Typically, this is the prevailing payment system for medical care for most of the population. Private and employee funded health insurance works this way, paying separately for each medical visit, test, or procedure. As a system, fee-for-service has been held responsible for the inflated costs of health care by creating an incentive for providers to add unnecessary visits, tests, hospital days, or procedures to collect more fees. The profit motive of providers is compounded by the intervention of third-party payers—the health insurance companies—who shield the patients and clients from paying directly, so that most seek more services without regard or even knowledge of their true cost. Some have questioned the ethics of such a system, when health care is considered a basic necessity or a right to which all citizens should be entitled.

The Medicare system began in the 1960s in an attempt to provide elders with needed medical care in their retirement. It also operates under a fee-for-service system but with certain reforms and restrictions.

Medicare Systems of Reimbursement

Currently, adults become eligible for Medicare insurance at age 66, although that age is scheduled to increase gradually in the coming years. To contain the ever-rising health care costs, Medicare has put in place some prospective payment systems (PPS). These are systems that limit the length, frequency, and type of health services that may be reimbursed, in keeping with current evidence about the different diagnoses or disease categories. Theoretically, these would work like health maintenance organizations (HMOs), taking a flat dollar amount (monthly premium), giving an incentive to providers to serve the client's health needs efficiently and without excessive cost. Different facilities must follow unique prospective payment systems in order to be reimbursed by Medicare. Some examples are as follows:

- *Inpatient acute care hospitals* use diagnostic related groups (DRGs); costs and limitations are based on 535 primary diagnoses.

- *Inpatient rehabilitation facilities* use Case-Mix Groups (CMGs) based on patient assessment and impairment categories that consider motor and cognitive skill levels and age.

- *Skilled nursing facilities* (long-term care) use Resource Utilization Groups (RUG III): 58 groups or categories that are based on a comprehensive assessment,

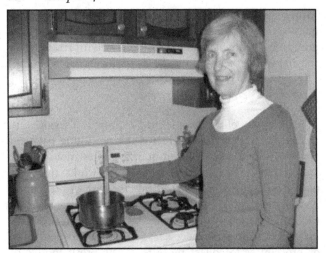

Figure 4-3. Ann tries cooking again as she recovers from a shoulder injury. She worked hard to comply with her rehabilitation program, with a goal of returning to independent function.

the Minimum Data Set (MDS). Each group is paid a specified number of rehabilitation or therapy minutes per week.

- *Home health agencies* use Home Health Resource Groups (HHRGs): 80 categories based on the Outcome & Assessment Information Set (OASIS) that determine number and frequency of home services within each 60-day period.

- *Hospice* uses four care levels for each day: (a) routine home care, (b) continuous home care, (c) inpatient respite care, and (d) general inpatient care (adapted from American Speech-Language-Hearing Association, 2014).

While these cost containment measures limit costs generally, they also restrict the choices afforded to Medicare beneficiaries and often arbitrarily deny needed services, a downfall of the government bureaucracy that oversees the payments without regard to individual differences.

Additionally, some see government regulation as actually increasing costs because of the additional paperwork and recordkeeping service providers must submit, which slows the process and benefits no one.

Fragmentation of Health Care

A recent study states that "high levels of fragmentation characterize health systems in the Americas...[which] can lead to difficulties in access to services, delivery of services of poor technical quality, irrational and inefficient use of resources, unnecessary increases in production costs, and low user satisfaction" (Montenegro et al., 2011, p. 5). For example, Jordan, age 77, falls while walking his dog and has residual pain in his left ribs and shortness of breath. He applies ice packs, takes aspirin, and hopes it will go away. The next day, he makes an appointment with his

primary care physician (PCP), who sees him the following week because it is not an emergency. After a 15-minute office visit (about average for PCP visits), he refers Jordan to an orthopedic specialist (to examine his ribs) and a heart specialist (because of the shortness of breath). A month later, after three MD visits and two tests (x-ray and lab test), Jordan still feels pain but was told the bruises would heal on their own. He receives a prescription for an anti-inflammatory medication.

Learning Activity 30: Exploring an Illness Experience

Recall an injury or acute illness you have experienced within the past few years or, if there are none, interview someone you know who has incurred an injury (Figure 4-3).

1. What happened? Describe the circumstances and how you got medical attention.

2. Who did you see first? Describe the steps involved. What facilities, doctors, tests, and procedures were necessary? How quickly were they accessed?

3. How was your treatment paid for? How much did it cost you? How much was paid by health insurance?

4. To what extent did you experience health care fragmentation?

5. What do you imagine might be a better system for providing health care for this experience?

Occupational Therapy and Health Care Reform

An overview of the Affordable Care Act (ACA) identified at least two areas related to OT in primary care: Accountable Care Organizations and Patient-Centered Medical Home Models (Braveman & Metzler, 2012). "Both will change medical practice dramatically, because the focus will shift from just treating people when they are ill to improving overall health and well-being... The many variations suggested in the ACA...are attempting to facilitate the very kind of contextual, holistic, and coordinated care that is at the center of occupational therapy practice" (Muir, 2012, p. 508). She gives the following examples: "Instead of waiting for elderly patients to fall and sustain a hip fracture, OTs could do a physical assessment in the primary care clinic...complete with a safety assessment of the home. Therapists could then provide a home exercise program, suggest home modifications, and...train in use of adaptive equipment to prevent an injury from a fall, and the related costs.... Therapists could identify common problems within a specific population (and their communities) and develop group education sessions to meet their needs" (Muir, 2012, p. 508).

CONTINUUM OF HEALTH CONDITIONS: WELLNESS-DISABILITY CONTINUUMS

Within the community-dwelling older adult population, there are a variety of considerations for health conditions. An individual may have a genetic condition, an acute illness or injury, or a chronic disease or syndrome that can be managed so as not to interfere with everyday functioning. The onset and severity has strong influence on the impact and meaning of functional challenges to the person. Over the years, the successful ager may experience periods of health challenge or crises requiring intervention by an OT.

The occupational history and profile are the initial steps in the OT process. They include medical history, and provide important information to the OT about whether the client has previous experience with the rehabilitative process. Therapeutic use of self by the therapist conveys sensitivity and empathy to the differences in a client's reaction to a new health challenge vs. exacerbation of symptoms of an existing condition. Please refer to Chapter 3 for a fuller description of the factors influencing a transition to changes in health status.

Acute Health Conditions

Acute conditions are usually temporary and curable. In healthy older adults, an acute condition may lead to many changes in ability, performance, roles, and habits. Conditions of this nature often come on suddenly and unexpectedly, leading to the unfamiliar role as a patient or client. In the midst of what has been a familiar routine and activity schedule, a change occurs that leads to many aspects of healing and coping. Phases of the healing process may mean that the individual progresses through several levels or types of health care services. There are often unknowns about the prognosis and potential for residual changes in function. Table 4-1 lists some examples of acute health conditions potentially affecting physical, sensory, cognitive, emotional, or social skills.

Of the examples listed, some would be a single occurrence and some may have recurrences over time. Some would have a healing period with little or no residual changes, while other conditions with a sudden onset lead to permanent changes in health status or ability.

Sensitivity on the part of the OT practitioner needs to reflect an awareness and appreciation of how an unexpected health change influences the client's ability to establish goals and cooperate for treatment recommendations. An empathetic approach would include helping the client to describe what had been a typical day and to explore occupational history and profile, including family, cultural, and environmental factors. A man with no children living alone

---

TABLE 4-1
EXAMPLES OF ACUTE HEALTH CONDITIONS
• Bone fractures (falls)
• Motor vehicle accidents
• Pneumonia
• Infections
• Injuries (cuts, nerve damage)
• Burns
• Back injury (disks, spinal nerves)
• Myocardial infarction (heart attack)
• Cerebral vascular accident (stroke)
• Congestive heart failure
• Infections (bladder, sinus)
• Spinal cord injury
• Depression (bereavement)
• Traumatic brain injury
• Stress-related illness (panic attacks)
What other acute health conditions can you add to this list?

in a large rural farmhouse would experience a lower back injury very differently from a married woman residing in a suburban condominium with her son and his two children. An assessment of specific problem areas would follow, as a basis for intervention planning.

Learning Activity 31: Acute Health Conditions

1. Describe an episode of an acute health change in your recent life.

2. Where did you go for treatment? Describe what measures you took to cope.

3. How did this condition affect your ability to engage in everyday occupations?

4. What was the most challenging aspect of a change in ability and what were the consequences?

Chronic Health Conditions

Chronic conditions may be treatable, but are generally not curable. Chronic health conditions may have an acute onset of symptoms or a gradual progression leading to eventual diagnosis by a physician. An example of

---

TABLE 4-2

EXAMPLES OF CHRONIC HEALTH CONDITIONS IN OLDER ADULTS

- Dementia (Alzheimer's, vascular, other)
- Heart diseases
- Parkinson's disease
- Multiple sclerosis
- Arthritis
- Amyotrophic lateral sclerosis (Lou Gehrig's disease)
- Post-polio syndrome
- Amputation
- Diabetes mellitus
- Chronic obstructive pulmonary disease
- Emphysema
- Eating disorders
- Lymphedema
- Sensory changes (vision loss, hearing loss)
- Fibromyalgia
- Carpal tunnel
- Neuropathy
- Character/personality disorders
- Developmental/genetic disorders
- Guillain-Barré syndrome
- Repetitive stress/strain

---

acute onset would be acute leukemia, where no signs were evident until an excessive nosebleed indicated a need for blood tests. Progressive types, with hints and signs over time, are represented by conditions such as multiple sclerosis or arthritis. Some conditions defy specific diagnostic measures, and may be diagnosed by exclusion, where other causes are ruled out. This is often the case in diagnosing the chronic condition of Alzheimer's disease. Some common chronic health conditions in older adulthood are listed in Table 4-2.

Combinations of Symptoms and Sequelae

Specialization in geriatric OT practice is often described as challenging and demanding, as well as exciting and stimulating. Although older adults have many things in common from their life history, there are vast individual differences. Many well elders have lived a long and active life with a health condition and are now seen by an OT practitioner for a new or recurring condition. For example, Beth, age 78, has had diabetes for 20 years and is now referred to OT following a hip fracture. Although familiar with many self-management techniques, Beth will now need to learn new rehabilitative and compensatory strategies to be able to return to her two-story home. Her healing may be influenced by her diabetic history. Compare her to Elaine, age 89, who prided herself in taking no medications. She fell while pursuing a dream on her bucket list of hiking on the Appalachian Trail, resulting in a hip fracture. Elaine's first real exposure to the health care system as a patient would require a different approach from her rehabilitation team.

Comorbidities are very common when working with older adults (Wilkie et al., 2013). Several health conditions may exist at once, creating a unique set of circumstances for each individual. When a client has a previously existing condition, OT should explore the client's knowledge, compliance with self-management, coping skills, and adaptive strategies. These may become important strengths for clients with a new health condition because they have experience with healing and managing within the world of the health care delivery system. For other individuals, an added condition may be extremely discouraging, leading to difficulty in finding a new balance in life.

Some other terms relate to symptoms that result in changes in function. These are iatrogenics, residuals, and sequelae. *Iatrogenics* refers to illnesses or increases in symptoms caused by medical intervention. For example, a medication for one condition has side effects that may cause another. Some medications cause constipation and taken long term may cause liver damage. *Residuals* are remaining symptoms that continue after the typical time frame expected for the course of medical treatment. Examples would be continuing upper extremity edema after a mastectomy or an altered gait following a knee replacement. *Sequelae* are changes in function due to residual symptoms. For example, a client with edema in her dominant upper extremity has difficulty with personal grooming, such as styling her hair. The sequelae are of special interest to OTs because they affect a client's performance of preferred activities within his or her home and community environments. Older clients have individual occupational preferences that must be respected. For example, an automobile accident left Ida, age 75, unable to perform her beloved task of doing laundry in her usual way. Miriam complained after a rotator cuff tear and surgery that, "How will I be able to change my curtains for every season and holiday?" Regardless of the cause or course of a health condition, the OT identifies key challenges to function and designs strategies to promote functional abilities.

Acquired infections are another category of symptoms. A client with a compromised immune system or an open wound could be exposed to an infection that is resistant to traditional forms of antibiotics. Infections may be localized or systemic and vary from a chronic annoyance to a life-threatening condition. For example, Matt, age 68 with anemia, cut the forefinger of his left hand on a damaged car door handle. Over the weekend, his left hand became swollen and painful, with red streaks traveling up his left forearm. At a walk-in clinic, he was diagnosed with cellulitis and treated with antibiotics. Within a week, the infection subsided but remained in his system. The doctor told him the slightest injury could trigger a flare up. OTs might discuss with Matt the precautions he needs to consider to avoid a recurrence of this infection or a more serious, antibiotic-resistant one.

Learning Activity 32: Exploring Lifestyle Contributors to Chronic Illness

Many chronic conditions for older adults are the result of lifestyle choices, such as smoking, alcohol abuse, overeating, or lack of exercise. Choose one chronic condition from Table 4-2 and research it. To what extent could this condition have been prevented?

1. List and discuss the lifestyle risk factors that are known to contribute to this condition.

2. What changes could OTs make in the cycle?

3. What are your personal thoughts about the health care system currently supporting long-term treatment for chronic conditions?

4. What could you do in your own lifestyle to protect your body from cumulative strain/stress/injury and other chronic conditions?

Expert's Experience— Ellen Ashkins, Director of Resident Life, Jewish Senior Services

Ms. Ashkins holds a position as Director of Resident Life at Jewish Senior Services in Fairfield, Connecticut. She agreed to be interviewed regarding her perceptions of trends in geriatric services that she has witnessed over time. She has been employed there for 30 years, starting as a music therapist, and then, as Director of Therapeutic Recreation. Formerly known as the Jewish Home for the Elderly, the 360-bed facility has been nationally accredited for continuing excellence. Ms. Ashkins has been involved

with changes and phases of growth and development over the years.

The progressive nature of the facility has been demonstrated because they were pioneers in implementing adult day care, specialized units for dementias, use of creative-expressive therapies, and provision of subacute rehabilitative services. As community and societal needs changed, the facility evolved to determine needs and design specialized services.

Ms. Ashkins reflected on the changes in health care that are impacting their current plans for major restructuring and construction of new styles of dwelling options for seniors. Considerations include recognition of the variety of services that are currently in demand by consumers.

For 40 years, Jewish Senior Services has provided long-term care and skilled nursing services through traditional models of interdisciplinary teamwork, with sharing of roles for holistic intervention. In the past decade, trends shifted toward increased staff role delineation, with specialized certificates and licenses defining boundaries of role performance. Recently, the trend is shifting again for a more expansive team approach and revised job titles. For some duties, many disciplines may participate (e.g., recreation personnel may now assist with the feeding of residents who require assistance).

OT services evolved to include intervention for specialized groups and individual treatment. Additional roles in the facility included a wheelchair management program, inservice training, and involvement with environmental projects. For example, an OT was appointed to head the project of relocation of dozens of residents to a newly completed wing. The "move day" involved coordination of all departments within the facility, with sensitivity to the individual needs of each resident.

As the facility has grown and levels of services expanded, OTs, OTAs, and students continued to assess the needs of the residents, working closely with other rehabilitation professionals. Goals continue for maximum skills in self-care, overall function and safety, participation in meaningful activities, and use of adaptive devices and compensatory techniques.

Jewish Senior Services is currently applying new models for service delivery, and design plans for a new building. They have converted to the concept of a life care community. Previously labeled "nursing units," they are now termed *neighborhoods* to promote an atmosphere of shared community. There is a neighborhood action team that includes a leadership team from a variety of disciplines, including administration and environmental services. There is also a regularly scheduled "community circle" led by a managerial representative. This provides a structured time for an informal gathering related to any topic of choice.

The mission of resident-centered care is labeled "the journey," with a belief that life's journey takes us where we need to go. Activities and preferences are identified by the residents, and the staff attempts to find the methods to accomplish stated wishes and goals. Examples include an all-male trip to Yankee Stadium, including male staff representatives from several disciplines.

A special 10-day trip was arranged in which 11 residents and 8 staff members traveled to Israel. The eldest was 98 years old. Many participating needed wheelchairs for longer periods of mobility. The criteria for participating included independence in toileting and mobility required for stairs and air travel. Ms. Ashkins, who participated, stated that it felt like the pinnacle of her career. She explained that a trip to Israel had been a lifelong dream for those who traveled, and that seeing this example of truly resident-centered care had been a goal of hers throughout her career.

The approach for identifying and addressing residents' personal preferences focuses on several areas. There is an increased awareness and attention to psychosocial needs. There is also an increased variety of the types and levels of activity. The environment has been increasingly designed to appear more homelike. The staff has been encouraged to spend increased amounts of time in direct contact with the residents.

She observed that "the pendulum has swung" recently to return to earlier principles of holism and interdisciplinary care. This is a reflection of many examples of how "the world has changed." She shared that Baby Boomers were expressing that they personally did not want a traditional nursing home for themselves or their parents. The staff and management of Jewish Senior Services developed plans to meet the needs of the current and prospective generation of seniors. Rituals and routines were analyzed, leading to designing methods to implement many changes. Dietary offerings have expanded to match diverse food preferences or unique choices. Snacks are available when requested. Schedules for morning awakening and bedtime at night have been modified to match individual preferences.

When asked about productive aging, Ms. Ashkins explained that the overall themes is to make the facility as homelike as possible and to give people something to look forward to. The residents are to be treated with dignity and respect while therapists purposefully treat the whole person. She continued by stating that "...the residents are coming here to enjoy life. We want to allow the individuals to be who they are and who they want to be."

Ms. Ashkins recalled seeing so many people admitted over the years and observed that, even if the same age, some age better than others. She stated that it didn't seem so much a matter of genes, although she acknowledged that they do play a part. Instead, she has noticed that people do best when the staff makes a real effort to find out about the residents, tune in to what they want, and find a way to give that to them. For example, a resident was offered assistance to sign up for and attend a college course at a nearby university. She

continued, "The goal is to keep the person active with productive and meaningful activities. Some residents try something they never did before, like an art project or attending a play, and discover a new interest...I don't see the person's age or disability. I see their ability and run with it."

Home care services and community-based services have increased in variety and number, leading to fewer admissions to long-term care facilities. Upon admission, many of the current residents are increasingly fragile, requiring increased medical management for multiple conditions. Jewish Senior Services will continue to offer services to these individuals. However, they have been expanding their scope of services to include home care. Plans for the future include a move to a new facility with innovative systems for delivery of care to address varied skill levels.

Design for the building of a new "campus" is in progress. Each floor will represent a "household" with 14 private rooms and bathrooms, with each including a kitchen and living room. With this smaller contained system, there will be a smaller number of assigned staff, with meal and laundry services provided. Because of the location, the construction will be multilevel. Space and services will be provided for four households, which comprise a "neighborhood." These include shared common space, work activity center, café, synagogue, and beauty parlor. They are anticipating the inclusion of child care, adult day care, and a pool.

She stated that in present planning, there may be fewer beds designated for skilled nursing, with increased assisted living and placement for subacute or short-term rehabilitation. Still under discussion are issues of aging in place vs. specializing households for homogeneous specialty needs, such as dementia. The current Jewish Senior Services property will likely be modified significantly. Independent level apartments may be created, as they seek to address multiple levels of care for older adults.

In concluding the interview about shifts in geriatric settings, Ms. Ashkins was asked to comment on three recommendations for future OT practitioners. Her reply:

"Don't be afraid to try something a little different. Don't get stuck in a mold with tunnel vision. Be acutely aware of the essence of the person. What is it going to take to get it done? Think outside of the box. Work with other people to get solutions. Use a team approach. Each of us is an adjunct to helping the whole being" (E. Ashkins, personal communication, September 10, 2013).

SUMMARY

OTs and OTAs have established significant roles in medical model settings and have been increasingly involved in community-based settings. Patients and clients have a variety of physical and mental health conditions, in a range of wellness to illness/injury/disability. OT roles include promotion of health, remediation of conditions that impair functioning, and prevention. Whether seen individually or in groups, clients engage in occupation-based activities that are carefully designed to match the needs of the client's unique goals, circumstances, and living environments. Practitioners are sensitive to the individualized needs of older adults, matching intervention approaches to personal background, interests, and level of skill.

OTs who specialize in geriatric practice often comment on their rewarding and creative career. Working with elders offers continual exposure to special older individuals who are often inspiring due to their life experiences and ongoing perseverance. Each patient has a different set of conditions and goals, leading to individualized considerations for intervention. Offering support and suggestions to family and staff members also promotes a sense of accomplishment for practitioners when able to see concrete outcomes of recommendations.

REFERENCES

American Occupational Therapy Association. (2007). AOTA's Centennial Vision and executive summary. *American Journal of Occupational Therapy, 61,* 613-614.

American Occupational Therapy Association. (2011). Complementary and alternative medicine position paper. *American Journal of Occupational Therapy, 65,* S26-S31.

American Occupational Therapy Association. (2014). The AOTA practice framework: Domain and process (3rd ed.). *American Journal of Occupational Therapy, 68,* S1-S48.

American Speech-Language-Hearing Association. (2014). *Medicare prospective payment systems: A summary.* Retrieved from: http://www.asha.org/practice/reimbursement/medicare/pps_sum.htm.

Braveman, B., & Metzler, C. (2012). Health Policy Perspectives: Health care reform implementation and occupational therapy. *American Journal of Occupational Therapy, 66,* 11-14.

Bridges, A., Szanton, S., Evelyn-Gustave, A., Smith, F., & Gitlin, L. (2013). Home sweet home: Interprofessional team helps older adults age in place safely. *OT Practice, 18*(16), 9-13.

Brown, D. P., & Evetts, C. L. (2013). Stepping stones: An occupation-based community support group for clients with early-stage Alzheimer's disease and their caregivers. *OT Practice, 18*(11), 13-17.

Cook, R. J., Berg, K., Lee, K. A., Poss, J. W., Hirdes, J. P., & Stolee, P. (2013). Rehabilitation in home care is associated with functional improvement and preferred discharge. *Archives of Physical Medicine and Rehabilitation, 94,* 1038-1047.

Donnelly, C., Brenchley, C., Crawford, C., & Letts, L. (2013). The integration of occupational therapy into primary care: A multiple case study design. *BMC Family Practice, 14,* 60.

Fazio, L. (2010). Health promotion program development. In M. Scaffa, S.M. Reitz, & M. Pizzi (Eds.). *Occupational therapy in the promotion of health and wellness* (pp. 195-207). Philadelphia, PA: F.A. Davis.

Hersch, G., Hutchinson, S., Davidson, H., Wilson, C., Maharaj, T., & Watson, K. (2012). Effect of an occupation-based cultural heritage intervention in long term geriatric care: A two-group control study. *American Journal of Occupational Therapy, 66,* 224-232.

Iecovich, E., & Biderman, A. (2013). Use of adult day care centers: Do they offset utilization of health care services? *The Gerontologist, 53,* 123-132.

Isaksson, G., Lexell, J., & Skär, L. (2007). Social support provides motivation and ability to participate in occupation. *Occupational Therapy Journal of Research, 27,* 23-30.

Kaminsky, T. (2010). The role of occupational therapy in successful aging. *OT Practice, April,* 11-14.

MetLife. (2010). The MetLife report on aging in place 2.0: Rethinking solutions to the home care challenge. *MetLife Mature Market Institute.* Retrieved from www.metlife.com.

Montenegro, H., Holder, R., Ramagem, C., Urrutia, S., Fabrega, R., Tasca, R., et al. (2011). Combating health care fragmentation through integrated health service delivery networks in the Americans: Lessons learned. *Journal of Integrated Care, 19,* 5-16.

Muir, S. (2012). Health policy perspectives—Occupational therapy in primary health care: We should be there. *American Journal of Occupational Therapy, 66,* 506-510.

Urban, M. (2013). Using complementary and alternative medicine in occupational therapy practice. *OT Practice, Sept. 23,* 9.

Waite, A. (2013). Occupational therapy students help with CarFit-Home Fit Event. *OT Practice, Nov. 4,* 19-21.

World Health Organization. (2001). *International Classification of Functioning, Disability, and Health.* Geneva: Author.

Wilkie, R., Pilagojevic-Bucknall, M., Jorden, K. R., Lacoy, R., & McBeth, J. (2013). Reasons why multi-morbidity increases the risk of participation restriction in older adults with lower extremity osteoarthritis: A prospective cohort study in primary care. *Arthritis Case and Research, 65,* 910-919.

5

Occupational Therapist's
Roles in Productive Aging

Karen C. Macdonald, PhD, OTR/L and Marilyn B. Cole, MS, OTR/L, FAOTA

"Engagement in meaningful occupation supports health and leads to a productive and satisfying life."
(US DHHS, 2010).

In this emerging practice area, OT practitioners will use their heightened understanding of productive aging from an occupational perspective to serve new generations of older clients whose goals far exceed the management of symptoms of illness and disability. Participation in productive occupations becomes a realistic and desired goal, not only for the well elderly, but also at every step along the continuum of care. The OTPF III (AOTA, 2014) embraces many evolving changes in the health care system, and these will guide OT evaluation and intervention with future productive agers. This chapter focuses on applying the OTPF III with interpretations that specifically address productive aging.

TEN OCCUPATIONAL THERAPY STEPS IN SUPPORT OF PRODUCTIVE AGING

To understand the OT's role with productive aging, it may be helpful to break the OT process down into steps (Table 5-1). Steps 1 through 6 represent the OT process and will be modified as needed with the OT practitioner's experience in consideration of different client needs and situations. The steps apply equally across the continuum

of care. Steps 7 through 10 are applied as needed to guide OT group interventions, education, and consultation for community organizations and populations. Issues of professionalism further clarify the role of OT practitioners in productive aging.

Step 1: Establish a Therapeutic Relationship

No matter how the client is defined—whether a single individual, a group, an organization, or a population—establishing a personal relationship precedes OT service delivery. Engaging the person (or persons) seeking services in a dialogue defines the relationship with the following purposes:

- Makes personal introductions
- Opens lines of communication
- Establishes trust
- Defines and confirms the value of what OT can offer
- Creates mutual understanding of the problems to be solved
- Defines the therapeutic process to follow
- Recognizes the client's role as a therapeutic partner

Cole MB, Macdonald KC.
Productive Aging: An Occupational Perspective (pp 67-94).
© 2015 Taylor & Francis Group.

TABLE 5-1
TEN KEY STEPS FOR OCCUPATIONAL THERAPY SUPPORT OF PRODUCTIVE AGING
Step 1: Establish a therapeutic relationship
Step 2: Create an occupational profile
Step 3: Set collaborative goals
Step 4: Analyze occupational performance (assessment)
Step 5: Design individual OT interventions
Step 6: Evaluating outcomes
Step 7: Design OT group interventions
Step 8: Education and training roles for OT practitioners
Step 9: OT advocacy roles
Step 10: OT consulting roles

On first meeting, the OT practitioner faces the client, making sure both are comfortably seated or positioned, and makes eye contact during verbal introductions. Ideally, the context during this initial meeting should be quiet, free of distractions, and, if possible, without barriers such as a desk, table, or laptop computer shielding the client or therapist from full view. During this initial session, the OT practitioner gathers information for the occupational profile, and begins to explore the client's occupational priorities. However, the first priories in establishing rapport are to listen carefully to what the client is saying and to convey an understanding of his or her concerns through the expression of empathy or recognition of the emotional content of the message, as well as the thoughts and descriptions.

Therapeutic Use of Self

An important agent in the therapeutic relationship is the intentional and conscious use of self. *Therapeutic use of self* is a cherished aspect of what makes an OT unique. Through careful and conscious self-awareness and structuring of one's own skills, strengths, personal attributes, and a caring attitude, the OT practitioner's own creativity and insights contribute to both the art and science of OT intervention.

According to the OTPF III, this "integral part of the OT process...allows OT practitioners to develop and manage their therapeutic relationship with clients by using narrative and clinical reasoning, empathy, and a client-centered, collaborative approach to service delivery" (AOTA, 2014, p. S12). The therapeutic relationship has been defined as "A trusting connection and rapport established between therapist and client through collaboration, communication, therapist empathy and mutual understanding and respect" (Cole & McLean, 2003, p. 49).

Intentional Relationship Model

The process of developing a therapeutic relationship has many labels, including establishing rapport, developing a therapeutic alliance, or developing a collaborative partnership. Taylor's (2008) intentional relationship model outlines the six modes of therapist interaction that encompass therapeutic use of self:

1. Advocating mode: Facilitating access to resources, referring to peer networks, and building client understanding and skill in navigating the health care system to get his or her own needs met.

2. Collaborating mode: Shifting decision-making power to the client and encouraging client choice, all critical aspects of continued autonomy in self-management.

3. Empathizing mode: Striving to understand the client's perspective through questioning and summarizing statements that validate the client's emotional expressions; interactions that build trust between therapist and client.

4. Encouraging mode: Instilling hope, emphasizing client strengths, and highlighting positive situations and progress made. Such encouragement empowers clients to believe in their own ability to engage in actions that improve health and well-being, and to manage their own health conditions effectively.

5. Instructing mode: Guiding and structuring therapy, educating client and caregivers, providing corrective feedback about performance, and setting limits when necessary. Client education provides the foundation for good self-management, which can then be personalized through feedback about client abilities and limitations, as well as possible ways to adapt or to overcome barriers to engagement in occupation.

6. Problem-solving mode: Weighing consequences, asking strategic questions that allow the clients to analyze their options, verbalizing pros and cons needed for making good self-management decisions (adapted from Taylor, 2008).

According to the OTPF III, OTs incorporate therapeutic use of self throughout the therapeutic process. Many of the older clients who seek OT services may not have the same strong self-management skills as the PAS participants demonstrated. OT practitioners, to encourage productive aging for clients at every level of care, are advised to first establish rapport that supports self-management and collaboration. The process of engaging in the therapeutic relationship continues throughout the next section, and beyond.

Communicating With the Elderly

Some special needs the OT practitioner should consider when working with older adults involve basic communication abilities. As people age, their vision, hearing, and other sensory perceptual abilities may be compromised. Even healthy elders may have sensory impairments that influence how a professional should communicate with them. Other areas of attention relate to respecting an individual as unique, and recognizing how social and environmental contexts impact responses.

- Auditory: Make sure that the technique of "low and slow" is used, with the deliberate use of a lower tone of voice and slower speed during conversation. Face a person when speaking and determine that you have the individual's attention. Check to see if hearing devices are present and in working order.

- Visual: Does the individual make eye contact? Use glasses? When necessary, use visual aids in addition to verbal cues, especially when asking questions regarding specific functions or offering directions. This may include hand-over-hand demonstration, showing by example, or written directions for follow-up reminders. Keep written materials clearly labeled and organized by category, with representative graphics if possible.

- Tactile: Some older adults may be uncomfortable with types of casual touch that are socially acceptable to others. This could include a caring touch on the forearm or shoulder, or a squeeze of the hand. Others welcome such interaction. The therapist should determine what is comfortable for the individual and precede handling or transfer techniques with a verbal statement about what is about to happen. For example, "I am going to demonstrate with you a safe way to maneuver as you move from using the walker to get into your bathtub."

- Gustatory: Related to eating, drinking, and food issues, the therapist should always be aware of any precautions. This may include restrictions such as thin liquids, salt, or sugars. For some clients, a certain type of food preparation is required, such as pureed or chopped. Allergies and religious dietary restrictions should also be noted.

- Olfactory: In some situations, an olfactory clue signals danger or a need for action. If this is an area of impairment, compensatory techniques need to be in place. For example, if food is burning on the stove and would be undetected by odor, the person may need to adapt by careful use of timers or making sure to not leave the stove unattended.

- Vestibular: For a healthy adult who is temporarily residing in a hospital or care facility, wheelchairs are often used for transport to appointments. If moved or turned quickly, this can elicit very uncomfortable dizziness for the client, adding to a sense of discomfort and frustration of being dependent on others. Make sure that the client is moved in a forward direction, allowing him or her to face the environment.

- Motor: Well elders often express shock at how quickly one's strength and endurance decreases after a hospital stay or a change in health that required bed rest. The OT may make helpful recommendations for preventing this decline and for returning to former physical status.

- Emotional: When seen by an OT, by definition, the client is in a state of change, coping, healing, and possible confusion or pain. Because the OT has an intimate level of relating with the individual while working on important personal self-care goals, there is an opportunity to explore the client's emotional state. This provides information to share with colleagues about possible need for further assessment for depression or anxiety. The OT offers unconditional positive regard, empathy, motivational strategies, and supportive counseling.

When interviewing residents in a rehabilitation facility or nursing home, it is important that the above factors be considered. There will be no therapeutic relationship established without the ability to communicate effectively with the older client. Observation during the interview can sometimes also serve as a preliminary evaluation, or can alert the OT to potential problems that may need further evaluation.

Applying Cultural Sensitivity and Competence

Respect for cultural diversity will be increasingly important as the "melting pot" of America ages and requires rehabilitative intervention. When working with older adults, their lifelong habits and routines need to be recognized and understood as influential to their self-identity and constructs of health and illness. Kozub (2013) recommends that practitioners first need to develop an awareness of their own cultural beliefs and values. In interaction with clients, the therapist should avoid stereotypes and attempt to view the client's current health experience from his or her unique perspective. Through direct interaction, the therapist seeks to understand the meaning of health challenges and relationship to goal setting toward independence. For example, in some cultures, following a stroke maximum efforts would occur for self-directed return to full independence. In other cultures, an immediate transition occurs in which full dependence on family members is expected.

Sensitivity to cultural diversity may be demonstrated through efforts for assisting with language barriers, use of bilingual assessment tools, empathy with experiences of immigrants, and recognition of varied possible fears or suspicions related to the health care system (Niemeier, Burnett, & Whitaker, 2003). Therapists should seek additional training and insights into potential issues to avoid any offensive

TABLE 5-2
OCCUPATIONAL PROFILE CONTENT
• Why are clients seeking service, and what are their current concerns relative to engaging in occupations and daily life activities?
• In what occupations do clients feel successful, and what barriers are affecting their success?
• What aspects of their environments or contexts do clients see as supporting or creating barriers to engagement in desired occupations?
• Describe clients' occupational history and important life experiences.
• What are clients' values and interests?
• What are clients' daily life roles?
• What are clients' patterns of engagement in occupations, and how have they changed over time?
• What are clients' priorities and desired targeted outcomes related to occupational performance, prevention, participation, role competence, health and wellness, quality of life, well-being, and occupational justice?
Adapted from American Occupational Therapy Association. (2014). Occupational therapy practice framework, 3rd edition. *American Journal of Occupational Therapy, 68,* S1-S48.

behaviors related to nationality, race, ethnicity, or religion. For example, in some religions, a man is not permitted to touch a woman.

Other general sensitivities are helpful when working with an older population. Cheah and Presnell (2011) explore perceptions of older adults experiencing acute hospitalizations. A therapist needs to be empathetic in recognizing the individual's unique reaction. Their research revealed perspectives of the older adults who reported that hospitalization was not a normal part of life; hospitalization was undesirable but accepted as necessary. Hospitalized elders reluctantly accepted present limitations as temporary setbacks in relation to recollections of prior life changes. They resented decision making by professionals and expressed an urgency to return to prior home life. This is all in contrast to a therapist who may have preconceived notions that most seniors are hospitalized at some point and are pleasantly accepting and cooperative for imposed recommendations by professionals.

Abreu (2011) reminds OTs of the importance of a humanistic approach, optimism, and focusing on clients' strengths. She encourages avoidance of depersonalization and promotes skills for the therapist to recognize the client's emotional state and to carefully communicate and encourages planned use of self as a motivational agent for change. Individuals need to be recognized as participants in their own unique personal and social circumstances.

Step 2: Create an Occupational Profile

The occupational profile answers the question, "Who is the client?" In today's practice, both the person with a health condition and his or her spouse or family caregiv-

ers may together become the recipient of OT services. The "client" may also be a group of people, such as individuals with mild dementia at an adult day care center, a senior fitness group at a community center, or a group of residents recovering from stroke in a rehabilitation facility. These are populations as clients. Organizations may also be clients with whom OTs consult, such as a local Agency on Aging or a chapter of the American Association of Retired Persons (AARP). When serving such groups, the OT will create a "community profile," often posing questions with focus groups of representatives of the community group seeking services.

The OTPF III defines an occupational profile as "a summary of a client's occupational history and experiences, patterns of daily living, interests, values, and needs" (AOTA, 2014, p. S13). The areas of information for the occupational profile are defined in Table 5-2. The desired outcome of the occupational profile will lead to identifying client occupational priorities, and answer the question, "What does the client want and need to do?"

In gathering the identifying information, the OT has the opportunity to establish initial patterns, including therapeutic use of self, interest and empathy, and respect for client-centered concerns. Depending on the client's level of self-report skills, insight, and communication skills, "wrap up" questions may be posed, such as: "What activities or experiences have contributed to your identity and define who you are today?" The findings from the occupational profile are related to several dimensions of the OT domain, including client factors, performance patterns, and context and environment. The content represents "Who is this person, and what is important, related to his or her background patterns and present abilities?"

TABLE 5-3
EXAMPLES OF OPEN-ENDED QUESTIONS RELATING TO OCCUPATIONAL PROFILE

- Describe a typical day. What types of activities do you do throughout the day?
- What special habits or routines do you prefer? Please describe them further.
- What occupations have been important to you in the past? Currently?
- What did you do for work to support yourself?
- Who are the most important people in your life? How are they related to you?
- Related to your present referral to OT, how long have these issues been present?
- What types of assistance do you need each day (caregiver, durable medical equipment, assistive devices, adaptive equipment)?
- What activities do you feel are most challenging to you (further ADL and IADL formal assessment would follow in the same or subsequent session)?
- What would be your priority areas to increase your ability to participate in activities (self-care, home management, work/volunteer caregiving, education, social, leisure)?
- What concerns do you have about safety (falls, emergency situations)?
- What else should I know about your functioning in your home or community settings?
- What are your questions about OT services? How do you think OT could be helpful to you (regarding specific activities/occupations)?
- What would you identify as three priority goals for OT intervention?

Created by K. C. Macdonald, 2015.

Designing a Semi-Structured Interview

The occupational profile is a general guideline to be converted by the OT practitioner into a semi-structured interview format. The OT uses professional judgment for the selection of questions to match the apparent level of functioning of the client. For a lower level of functioning, questions may be modified or referred to family members. The process of gathering data about past and present occupations provides valuable opportunities for the OT to observe sensory, cognitive, and emotional skills. For example, difficulty hearing, short attention span, and low self-esteem may become evident.

In gathering specific information, the OT may ask both closed and open questions. When factual information is needed, asking a closed question may be more direct: "Are you married? When did you fall? Who takes care of you at home? Do you use a cane or walker? Can you read these instructions?" However, when seeking to gain an understanding of the person's values, perspectives, or meaning of life experiences, open-ended questions can generate more in-depth information. Older people can sense when you are truly interested in what they are saying. Prompting clients to continue or embellish their answer ("give me an example," "tell me more about ____") will communicate your genuine interest in getting to know them and help establish trust in the therapeutic relationship.

Learning Activity 33: Open-Ended Questions

Open-ended questions are those that cannot be answered with a "yes" or "no" but require a more thoughtful answer. In considering the information needed for an occupational profile, write one open question for each category listed in Table 5-2. Try to think of questions that are different from those listed in Table 5-3, which are questions that could assist the OT in gathering information for the occupational profile.

1.

2.

3.

4.

5.

6.

7.

8.

Because many older clients are traditionalists, they learned from childhood to be polite, speak with courtesy and respect, expect the same from others. They especially expect these traits in trained health professionals. Appearance does make a difference, no matter which generation the OT practitioner comes from. Therefore, the therapist's clothing and jewelry should not convey any specific cultures, religions, or nationalities (in some settings) or have any other feature that would create a distraction from the rapport building that should occur during an initial session.

Learning Activity 34: Attending to the Client

For a brief exercise, imagine you are meeting a client for the first time.

1. After completing the open-ended questions learning activity, choose a partner to practice your open-ended questions and answers, taking turns being the "client" and "therapist."

2. Set the stage for an initial interview and role play the OT, complete with an introduction and a brief explanation of what OT does. Allow 15 to 20 minutes for this exercise (doing the same with a client may take longer).

3. On a scale of 1 (poor) to 5 (excellent), how would you rate yourself on the following:

   ○ Friendly hello and personal introduction

   ○ OT and client positioned comfortably with no barriers

   ○ Explain occupational therapy

   ○ Eye contact—avoid prolonged gaze at laptop

   ○ Professional dress, jewelry, makeup/grooming, hair. No gum or facial jewelry

   ○ Prepared and organized

   ○ Respectful of uniqueness of individual, including communication style

   ○ Body language—not bored, impatient, fatigued

   ○ Good listener, encouraged elaboration of important points

   ○ Express understanding and empathy

   ○ Limit interruptions as much as possible (no cell phones)

   ○ Effectively manage time for session

   ○ Explore issues related to ethnic or cultural diversity

   ○ Offer the opportunity for the client to ask questions

   ○ End session with wrap-up and discuss follow-up

OTs have a reputation for being empathetic and truly connecting with and caring about their clients. Because we work with clients on their most intimate issues and impor-

tant goals, we often connect on a deep, interpersonal level. Some of the behaviors listed previously help to establish rapport, communicate respect, and acknowledge the client as a valued and unique person. The OT may create a form to offer prompts for focusing these types of questions. Usually, the intended tone would be conversational, avoiding the appearance of a formal structured questionnaire.

Adapting the Occupational Profile for Productive Aging

Taking current evidence and the PAS into account, OTs can now refine the OTPF III's occupational profile for older adults. We suggest the following additions or refinements, posing questions more specific for older adults who wish to age productively.

- What occupations and social roles make up the client's social identity? Knowing which generation, religious, or ethnic groups and the most valued occupational and social life roles the client most identifies with can give OTs a better appreciation for who the client is.

- What is the client's level of self-awareness and insight? People cannot identify their occupational priorities until they have a good understanding of what their occupations are, their role in the ebb and flow of everyday life, and their role in maintaining life satisfaction, health, and well-being. This often takes some introspection and self-reflection and may involve therapeutic use of self on the part of the OT practitioner.

- What are the client's skills and strengths as a self-manager? We now know that being able to direct one's own aging process is an important key to productive aging. Some of the factors contributing to self-management are self-awareness, self-discipline, lifestyle habits, motivations, positive attitude, and cognitive abilities, such as reasoning, organizing, planning, decision making, and problem solving.

- What are the client's social connections? Evidence has shown that strong social identities and connections provide older adults with protection against physical and cognitive decline, as well as disability and even premature death (Holt-Lunstad, Smith, & Bradley Layton, 2010). Therefore, it is imperative that OTs recognize that their clients' productive occupations are embedded in and cannot be separated from, the social connections that support them. Some specific social factors are life partners, friendships and family relationships, membership in social groups and community organizations, frequency of participation, and quantity and quality of social interactions.

- What are the client's self-fulfilling occupations? What activities matter most and how can the client overcome barriers to doing them? Our perspective adds the following factors: importance of continuity, developmental stages, creativity, pursuit of lifelong learning, and the ability to adapt one's interests to accommodate changing abilities and circumstances.

The results of the occupational profile form a foundational background for developing meaningful and purposeful directions in treatment planning. They serve as background guidance for selecting appropriate assessment tools.

Step 3: Set Collaborative Goals

Goals must be set as a focus before further assessment of occupational performance, facilitators, and barriers can take place. Theoretical rationale and frames of reference may be selected as clinical reasoning develops. The intervention plan is then designed in collaboration with the client, establishing operational goals, projected timeframe, and consideration of discharge plans.

This step offers the OT and client an opportunity to further define the parameters of their relationship. As implied by the term *partnership*, OTs and clients work as a team, each contributing their own expertise to the discussion. The OT respects the clients' expertise about their own occupations; their life history, patterns, and style; their culture, beliefs, and values; and their experience of illness, injury, or disability. In a client-centered approach, "only clients can identify the occupations that give meaning to their lives and select goals and priorities that are important to them" (AOTA, 2014, p. S13). The OT practitioner offers expertise differently, using knowledge, skills, current evidence, clinical reasoning, and professional experience to educate, support, and enable the clients' choices for occupational participation. In a client-centered partnership, both the client and therapist have equal power, with neither attempting to dominate the other. Family members and significant others may also be involved in this collaborative partnership.

Client-Centered Goals

A client-centered approach avoids the issue of *compliance or noncompliance* because both the client and OT are equally invested in the therapeutic process, but with the client identifying the direction of treatment according to his or her own occupational priorities. Clients may be naturally motivated to work toward goals they have set for themselves, and the OT becomes a resource and facilitator, offering strategies, addressing safety issues, and encouraging self-management and engagement in collaborative problem solving.

Some clients may still look to the OT practitioner to set goals for therapy. This situation implies that the client does not take responsibility for self-management and may depend on significant others in his or her life to make the right decisions. The OT could take this opportunity to explore client autonomy or the extent to which the client wishes to self-direct his or her own life. The research shows that persons who engage in the occupation of self-management are more likely to reap the benefits of productive aging, including continued health, well-being, and longevity (DeRosa, 2013). Those who have a sense of their own subjective longevity, make future plans, and continue to engage in meaningful social relationships will be the best collaborators in setting meaningful yet realistic OT goals.

Goals as Motivation

Goal setting has been identified as a motivational strategy for behavior change within Bandura's (1997) social cognitive theory. Interdisciplinary literature demonstrates the beneficial effects of goals on behavior in organizational and health settings (Hall, Crowley, Howard, & Morey, 2010; Kelley & Abraham, 2004). These studies emphasize that the most important outcomes of health-related goals are self-reported outcomes, including individually meaningful milestones (self-selected goals) leading to client satisfaction in the ability to perform valued activities. A group of physical therapy researchers affirm the importance of personal objectives; they developed the Personal Functional Goals (PFG) interview protocol to assess and track personal functional goals in older adults in the context of an exercise intervention (Bearon, Crowley, Chandler, Robbins, & Studenski, 2000). Its use has shown that self-selected functional goals are a motivating factor, increasing participation and satisfaction. Furthermore, "asking individuals to self-identify meaningful goals is a form of engagement with some power to inform, motivate, and personalize the behavior-change process. Health care practitioners may want to consider working with patients to identify goals and monitor both subjective and performance-based progression toward those goals as part of a treatment regimen" (Hall et al., 2010, p. 448).

In the case of clients with cognitive limitations, the involvement of family members or other important individuals in their lives contributes to the important process of selecting and prioritizing goals. Using a client-centered approach, the therapist seeks to understand the individual's unique identity, priorities, and goals. Once goals are set, OTs follow up with assessments of the specific domains that may be creating barriers to successful occupational performance or targeted outcomes.

Setting Behavioral Goals

Goals that are *behavioral* can be observed and measured. By definition, they are specific in nature, with implied parameters for measuring progress. In determining behavioral goals, discussion may include the content of occupational performance, and what factors inhibit or facilitate capacity for independent functioning. Specifics are reviewed about daily tasks that pose challenges: "Why is it difficult for you to make your own lunch?" might be answered by, "I can't reach into the refrigerator/dishwasher/pantry to get what I need." Goal setting includes anticipated outcomes of successful achievement: "I want to go out to lunch with my friends." Then, the OT explores specific actions necessary for overcoming barriers to that goal, such as inability to drive, lack of sitting tolerance, impaired eating skills, or inability to follow a conversation and respond appropriately. Assessment will become the next step, looking more specifically at the skills, abilities, contexts, and levels of assistance necessary to reach a desired goal.

Long-term goals are not always observable and measurable nor are they always achieved during the OT process. While the long-term goal might be chosen by the client, such as the performance of a specific activity or occupation, the OT's contribution to the partnership will likely be a reality check based on evidence, both from research and from the results of careful assessment of the parameters involved. Thus, goals are determined with the client, both short and long term, with a determination of anticipated needs for frequency and duration of OT visits and for what time period. For example, "client will be seen twice a week for 45 minutes for a 6-week period."

Goal Setting for Productive Agers

In setting goals for older adults, OTs must explore the occupations that clients consider productive. This can begin with simply identifying the activities clients have been doing or wish to continue to do after recovery from illness or injury. The OT might ask which of the following the client has recently engaged in: home management, caregiving, paid work, volunteering, and lifelong learning. Social roles might be viewed as separate from but equally important to identity. A discussion allows the OT to discuss the evidence contained in this textbook about the importance of productive occupations to health and well-being in aging. Goals for establishing new occupations may be added to form a healthier lifestyle.

In keeping with the PAS, the importance of self-management cannot be understated. The first step involves determining to what extent older clients are self-directed. Are they able to manage their own aging, structure a healthy lifestyle, continue to be engaged with social groups, and be motivated to be involved with their community? Supporting self-management means not only managing symptoms or chronic conditions, but also supporting a client's ability, and right to choose and engage in, the meaningful occupations and concurrent social connections. It requires the OT to assess not only the clients' functional abilities, but also their ability to structure their time and make rational decisions based on reliable information. Good self-managers should be able to maintain a positive outlook, demonstrate good judgment, plan for the future, intentionally initiate social connections, and give priority to their own self-fulfilling occupations, whatever those might be. Some ways that OTs can encourage self-management in goal setting include the following:

- To what extent is the client self-determined (vs. passive or led by others)?

- Evaluate the client's ability to gather information to make informed choices.
- Determine the client's level of self-awareness and insight.
- To what extent does the client think positively?
- What are the client's plans for the immediate future? Distant future? Are plans realistic?
- Determine and encourage intentional social connections, maintaining relationships.
- Identify which occupations offer the client self-fulfillment.
- Assist the client in exploring the meaning of activity choices. Are there better choices available? Do choices afford desired socialization?
- To what extent is the client willing and able to advocate for himself or herself?

Step 4: Analyze Occupational Performance (Assessment)

After completing an occupational profile for the client, an assessment may consist of screening tools, clinical observations, standardized assessment tools, or site-specific (designed to match the clientele population of a particular setting) evaluation of function. The OT may evaluate client factors, performance skills, or any other aspect of the OT domain. Short- and long-term goals are identified, and ongoing assessment continues through the course of treatment. Upon discharge, outcomes for efficacy of services and client satisfaction need to be determined. This may include documentation of client self-report for progress in personal ability and quality of life. In some settings, the OT is treating current challenges of altered ability while also anticipating needs as the client makes progress and is discharged (or moved) to another level of care. For example, the OT might make recommendations for home care following discharge from a subacute care facility. Therefore, the analysis of occupational performance may be ongoing as the client moves through the process of intervention, learning, healing, and recovery.

The challenge for OTs with the analysis of specific occupations is to retain a holistic perspective while also focusing on the evaluation of skills, abilities, task demands, and contexts to establish a baseline from which to measure progress toward occupational goals. According to the OTPF III, analysis of the client's ability to execute tasks or activities included as goals is accomplished through "assessment tools designed to observe, measure, and inquire about factors that support or hinder occupational performance" (AOTA, 2014, p. S14). Some evidence-based screening and assessment tools have been compiled by Leland, Elliott, and Johnson (2012) (Table 5-4). Doucet and Gutman (2013)

TABLE 5-4

EXAMPLES OF STANDARDIZED SCREENING TOOLS AND ASSESSMENTS

SCREENING TOOLS AND ASSESSMENTS	REFERENCE
Occupational Performance/Participation Assessments	
Activity Card Sort (ACS)	Baum, C. M., & Edwards, D. (2008). *Activity card sort (ACS)*. Bethesda, MD: AOTA Press.
Canadian Occupational Performance Measure (COPM)	Law, M., Baptiste, S., McColl, M. A., Carswell, A., Polatajko, H., & Pollock, N. (2005). *Canadian Occupational Performance Measure* (3rd ed.). Toronto, Ontario, Canada: CAOT Publications CAE.
National Institutes of Health Activity Record (ACTRE)	Gerber, L., & Furst, G. (1992). Validation of the NIH activity record: A quantitative measure of life activities. *Arthritis Care Research, 5,* 81-86.
Occupational Questionnaire	Smith, N. R., Kielhofner, G., & Watts, J. H. (1986). The relationships between volition, activity pattern, and life satisfaction in the elderly. *American Journal of Occupational Therapy, 40,* 278-283.
Assessment of ADLs and IADLs	
Assessment of Living Skills and Resources (ALSAR)	Williams, J. H., Drinka, T. J. K., Greenberg, J. R., Farrell-Holtan, J., Euhardy, R., & Schram, M. (1991). Development and testing of the Assessment of Living Skills and Resources (ALSAR) in community-dwelling veterans. *The Gerontologist, 31,* 84-91.
Assessment of Motor and Process Skills (AMPS)	Doble, S. E., Fisk, J. D., Lewis, N., & Rockwood, K. (1999). Test-retest reliability of the Assessment of Motor and Process Skills (AMPS) in elderly adults. *Occupational Therapy Journal of Research, 19,* 203-215.
Melbourne Low Vision ADL Index	Haynes, S. A., Johnson, A. W., & Heyes, A. D. (2001). Preliminary investigation of the responsiveness of the Melbourne Low Vision ADL Index to low-vision rehabilitation. *Optometry and Vision Science, 78,* 373-380.
Performance Assessment of Self-Care Skills	Rogers, J. C., & Holm, M. B. (1989). *Performance Assessment of Self-Care Skills (PASS-Home)*. Unpublished tests. Pittsburgh, PA: University of Pittsburgh.
Work Assessments	
Blankenship System (TBS) Functional Capacity Evaluation	Narro, P., & Clarke, E. (2007). The sensitivity and specificity of the Blankenship FCE System's indicators of sincere effort. *Journal of Orthopaedic and Sports Physical Therapy, 37,* 161-168.
DSI Work Solutions Functional Capacity Assessment	Isernhagen, S. J. (n.d.). *A brief history of the Isernhagen–DSI Work Solutions Functional Capacity Assessment.* Retrieved from http://dsiworksoiutions.com/history.htm
Workwell Systems Functional Capacity Evaluation	Soer, R., Van der Schans, C. P., Geertzen, J. H., Groothoff, J. W., Brouwer, S., Dijkstra, P. U., & Reneman, M. F. (2009). Normative values for a functional capacity evaluation. *Archives of Physical Medicine and Rehabilitation, 90,* 1785-1794.
	(continued)

TABLE 5-4 (CONTINUED)

EXAMPLES OF STANDARDIZED SCREENING TOOLS AND ASSESSMENTS

Leisure Assessments	
Idyll Arbor Leisure Battery (IALB) Leisure Assessment Inventory	*Idyll Arbor Leisure Battery.* (2010). Retrieved from http://www.idyllarbor.com/agora.cgi?pJd=A145&xm=on
Older Americans Resources and Services (OARS) Multidimensional Functional Assessment Questionnaire (OMFAQ)	Fillenbaum, G. G. (2005). *Multidimensional functional assessment of older adults: The Duke Older American Resources and Services Procedures.* Hillsdale, NJ: Lawrence Erlbaum.

Social Participation and Quality of Life Assessments	
Satisfaction with Performance Scaled Questionnaire	Yerxa, E. J., Burnett-Beaulieu, S., Stockin, S., & Azen, S. P. (1988). Development of the satisfaction with performance scaled questionnaire. *American Journal of Occupational Therapy, 42,* 215-221.

Performance Skills: Motor Assessments	
Activities-Specific Balance Confidence (ABC) Scale	Poweli, L. E., & Myers, A. M. (1998). The Activities-Specific Balance Confidence (ABC) scale. *Journal of Gerontology, Medical Sciences, 50*(1), M28-M34.
Disabilities of the Arm, Shoulder and Hand (DASH)	Institute for Work and Health. (2006). *The DASH outcome measure: Disabilities of the arm, shoulder and hand.* Retrieved from http://www.dash.iwh.on.ca/conditions.htm
Dynamic Gait Index	Shumway-Cook, A., & Woollacott, M. (1995). *Motor control theory and applications.* Baltimore, MD: Lippincott Williams & Wilkins.
Falls Efficacy Scale (FES)/Falls Efficacy Scale International (FESI)	Tinetii, M., Richman, D., & Powell, L. (1990). Falls efficacy as a measure of fear of falling. *Journal of Gerontology, 45,* 239.
Fall Risk for Older People-Community setting (FROP-Com)	Russell, M. A., Hill, K. D, Blackberry, I., Day, L. M., & Dharmage, S. C. (2008). The reliability and predictive accuracy of the falls risk for older people in the community assessment (FROP-Com) tool. *Age and Ageing, 37,* 634-639.
Fullerton Advanced Balance (FAB) Scale	California State University, Fullerton, Center for Successful Aging. (2008). *Fullerton Advanced Balance (FAB) Scale.* Retrieved from http://hhd.fullerton.edu/csa/CenterProducts/center prod ucts_assessment.htm
Functional Reach	Duncan, P. W., Weiner, D. K., Chandler, J., & Studenski, S. (1990). Functional reach: A new clinical measure of balance. *Journal of Gerontology, 45,* M192-M197.
Modified Clinical Test of Sensory Interaction in Balance	California State University, Fullerton, Center for Successful Aging. (n.d.). *Modified Clinical Test of Sensory Interaction in Balance.* Retrieved from http://www.patientsafety.gov/SafetyTopics/ fallstoolkit/resources/educational/Balance_Assessment_Handbook.pdf
Senior Fitness Test	Rikli, R. E., & Jones, C. J. (2001). *Senior fitness test manual.* Champaign, IL: Human Kinetics.
6-Minute Walk Test	Enright, P. L., McBurnie, M. A., Bittner, V., Tracy, R. P., McNamara, R., Arnold, A., & Newman, A. B. (2003). The 6-Minute Walk Test: A quick measure of functional status in elderly adults. *Chest, 123,* 387-398.

(continued)

TABLE 5-4 (CONTINUED)	
EXAMPLES OF STANDARDIZED SCREENING TOOLS AND ASSESSMENTS	
Timed Up and Go (TUG)	Podsiadlo, D., & Richardson, S. (1991). The Timed Up and Go: A test of basic functional mobility for frail elderly persons. *Journal of the American Geriatrics Society, 39,* 142-148.
Performance Skills: Psychological Assessments	
Caregiver Strain Index	Robinson, B. C. (1983). Validation of a Caregiver Strain index. *Journal of Gerontology, 38,* 344-348.
Short Comprehensive Assessment and Referral Evaluation (SHORT–CARE)	Gurland, B., Golden, R. R., Teresi, J. A., & Challop, J. (1984). The SHORT CARE: An efficient instrument for the assessment of depression, dementia, and disability. *Journal of Gerontology, 39,* 166-169.
Geriatric Depression Scale	Sivrioglu, E. Y., Sivrioglu, K., Ertan, T., Ertan, F. S., Cankurtaran, E., Aki, O.,...Kirli, S. (2009). Reliability and validity of the Geriatric Depression Scale in detection of poststroke minor depression. *Journal of Clinical and Experimental Neuropsychology, 31,* 999-1006.
Performance Skills: Cognitive Assessments	
Executive Function Performance Test	Baum C. M., Connor L. T., Morrison T., Hahn, M., Dromerick A. W., & Edwards, D. F. (2008). Reliability, validity, and clinical utility of the Executive Function Performance Test: A measure of executive function in a sample of people with stroke. *American Journal of Occupational Therapy, 62,* 446-455.
Montreal Cognitive Assessment	Nasreddine, Z. (2011). *Montreal Cognitive Assessment* (MoCA). Retrieved from http://www.mocatest.org/
Short Blessed Test	Katzman, R., Brown, T., Fukd, P., Peck, A., Schechter, R., & Shimmel, H. (1983). Validation of a short orientation–memory–concentration test of cognitive impairment. *American Journal Psychiatry, 140,* 734-739.
Performance Patterns: Assessments of Roles, Habits, and Routines	
Role Change Assessment	Rogers, J. C., & Holm, M. B. (1989). *Performance Assessment of Self-Care skills* (PASS–Home). Unpublished tests. Pittsburgh, PA: University of Pittsburgh.
Context and Environment	
Home Assessment Profile (HAP)	Chandler, J., Duncan, P., Weiner, D., & Studentski, S. (2001). The Home Assessment Profile—A reliable and valid assessment tool. *Topics in Geriatric Rehabilitation, 16,* 77-88.
Home Environment Assessment Protocol (HEAP)	Gitlin, L. N., Schinfeld, S., Winter, L., Corcoran, M., Boyce, A. A., & Hauck, W. (2002). Evaluating home environments of persons with dementia: Interrater reliability and validity of the Home Environmental Assessment Protocol (HEAP). *Disability and Rehabilitation, 24,* 59-71.
Home Falls and Accidents Screening Tool (Home Fast)	Mackenzie, L., Byies, J., & Higginbotham, N. (2002). Reliability of the Home Falls and Accidents Screening Tool (HOME FAST) for measuring falls risk for older people. *Disability and Rehabilitation, 24,* 266-274.

(continued)

TABLE 5-4 (CONTINUED)
EXAMPLES OF STANDARDIZED SCREENING TOOLS AND ASSESSMENTS

Safety Assessment of Function and the Environment for Rehabilitation (SAFER)	Oliver, R., Blathwayt, J., Brackley, C., & Tamaki, T. (1993). Development of the Safely Assessment of Function and the Environment for Rehabilitation (SAFER) tool. *Canadian Journal of Occupational Therapy, 60,* 78-32.
Westmead Home Safety Assessment (WeHSA)	Cooper, B., Letts, L., Rigby, P., Stewart, D., & Strong, S. (2005). Measuring environmental factors. In M. Law, C. Baum, & W. Dunn (Eds.), *Measuring occupational performance: Supporting best practice in occupational therapy* (2nd ed., pp. 326-327). Thorofare, NJ: Slack.

Reprinted with permission from Leland, N. E., Elliott, S. J., & Johnson, K. J. (2012). *Productive aging for community-dwelling older adults.* Bethesda, MD: AOTA Press.

describe the need for research and development of effective means to quantify function. They provide the design and use of standardized, reliable, and measurable means to measure aspects of function, such as body impairment, activity limitation, and participation restriction. They remind practitioners that reimbursement sources seek this type of documentation and evidence for assessments and measurement of progress. Recommendations are made to avoid "site-specific" tools and to avoid using evaluation measures borrowed from other disciplines. While this may not always be true in practice, OTs should work toward this goal, as it is likely to affect future reimbursement for OT services.

Step 5: Design Individual Occupational Therapy Interventions

The OTPF III identifies types of OT interventions to include "the use of occupations and activities, preparatory methods and tasks, education and training, advocacy, and group interventions to facilitate engagement in occupations to promote health and participation" (AOTA, 2014, p. S29). The OT practitioner designs interventions to address the occupational goals that have been collaboratively determined by the client and therapist together. Using a client-centered approach, the OT also discusses options for intervention with the client, sharing knowledge, expertise, evidence, and experience about which strategies have the best chance of success for a specific individual.

Applying the OTPF III Intervention Process

To assist OT professionals in focusing on enabling productive aging for all of their clients, we have reconfigured the OTPF III domain as a "spool" model to structure our thinking. When OT and OTA students are learning about the OTPF III (AOTA, 2014), they are often both impressed and overwhelmed at the comprehensive universe of OT

considerations for evaluation and intervention. OTs work in a variety of settings with individuals and groups and across a continuum of wellness and illness to promote independence and function. Types of interventions are designed to address a unique combination of client-centered occupational issues.

The Spool Model of OT Interventions (Figure 5-1) is designed to visually combine elements of the OTPF's Domain and Process. A symbolic image of a spool was used to represent the clinician's "unwinding" of information and data about the client, which evolves into the "merging" of critical thinking, clinical reasoning, and ongoing collaborative treatment planning.

Basic function is defined as the performance skills and client factors required as foundational abilities to participate in selected tasks. The OT practitioner could focus on increasing strength, range of motion (ROM), balance, coordination, self-esteem and expression, planning and sequencing, or visual tracking, to offer diverse examples. Intervention may consist of purposeful activities, such as manipulative table top tasks, or preparatory techniques, such as exercise, massage, splinting, or hot packs.

Applied function relates to the performance of actual life tasks or occupations. The areas of occupation delineated in the OTPF III are the real life activities that individuals engage in—some daily, some weekly, and some annual, seasonal, or as appropriate. The large spectrum of activity categories shows the breadth, depth, and importance of OT as a profession dedicated to promoting "real life" abilities. The OTPF III includes the following occupations: ADLs, rest and sleep, work, play, leisure, and social participation. Appreciating the large scope of OT practice, Karen offered her students the slogan "Occupational therapists assist with adapting any activity to match any ability for any age."

Considerations for applied function include elements of client education for most approaches. Examples include ergonomics, energy conservation, or consultation and sup-

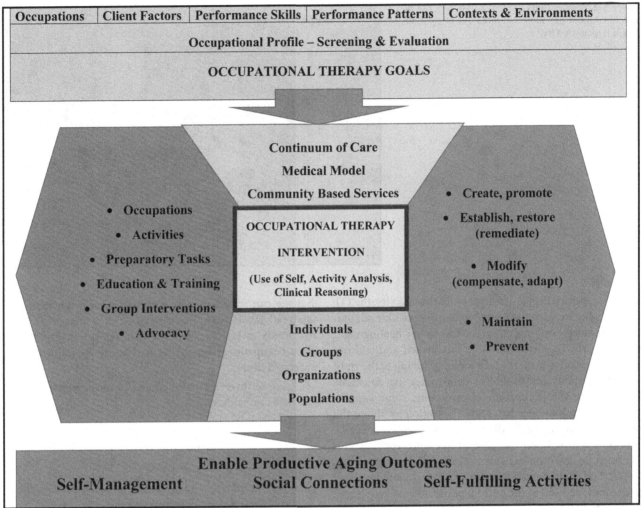

| Occupations | Client Factors | Performance Skills | Performance Patterns | Contexts & Environments |

Occupational Profile – Screening & Evaluation

OCCUPATIONAL THERAPY GOALS

Continuum of Care

Medical Model

Community Based Services

- Occupations
- Activities
- Preparatory Tasks
- Education & Training
- Group Interventions
- Advocacy

OCCUPATIONAL THERAPY

INTERVENTION

(Use of Self, Activity Analysis, Clinical Reasoning)

- Create, promote
- Establish, restore (remediate)
- Modify (compensate, adapt)
- Maintain
- Prevent

Individuals

Groups

Organizations

Populations

Enable Productive Aging Outcomes

Self-Management   Social Connections   Self-Fulfilling Activities

Figure 5-1. Spool Model of OT Interventions, designed to integrate OTPF III domain and process with Productive Aging Study themes. (M. Cole & K. Macdonald, 2015).

port to family caregivers regarding prescribed assistive or adaptive devices.

The general scope of practice also extends beyond hands-on strategies. Other aspects of intervention include roles in consulting, education (client, family, facility, community), and advocacy. An example of the latter would be involvement in an organization promoting occupational justice for an underserved population of older adults with limited incomes.

Intervention usually addresses priority occupations. What is a typical day? Prior to being seen for therapy, what were the person's usual routine, habits, and patterns? Daily and weekly schedule? Responsibilities?

Knowing the variety of combinations of performance patterns, the OT designs a treatment program to anticipate current and future needs for engagement and performance.

How to Use the Spool Model

In Figure 5-2, Peggie, age 78, wants to plant a tree that has grown too big for the patio. Peggie could be your home

care client following a right knee replacement that prevents her from squatting or bending her knee more than 90 degrees. On the spool model (see Figure 5-1), begin at the bar at the top: the *occupation* selected is gardening, the *client factor* in question is lower extremity strength and mobility related to the task. Peggie uses previously learned *knowledge and skills* about gardening regarding how deep the hole must be dug and what fertilizers to mix with the soil. The *contexts* include a warm sunny day, rather dry hard earth to dig in, and the presence of her husband Jack as helper. Moving to the left side of the spool, OT intervention is the activity itself, planting a tree. The problem-solving strategies for this task are addressed to both client Peggie and her spouse, Jack. To *prepare for the task*, Jack has purchased fertilized topsoil, borrowed a wheelbarrow, and dug a hole in the desired location. Peggie has dressed appropriately for outdoor work and donned some gloves. To *prepare* Peggie physically, the OT suggests some stretching and limbering exercises for her lower extremities, warming up her muscles to prevent injury. Some *education* might also be

Figure 5-2. Peggie wants to plant a tree. Jack has dug a hole but cannot get some old roots out of the hole, so Peggie is giving it a try.

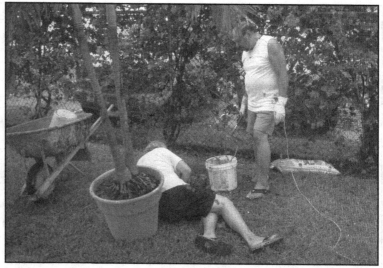

advisable. Before Peggie attempts to do this activity, the OT may collaborate with the couple to discuss possible adaptations for safety and injury prevention to her healing right knee. Clearly, Peggie wants to do this herself and will not accept Jack's offer to do the task for her. Moving to the right side of the spool model, the OT determines that to enable Peggie to do the occupation of gardening, some *adaptations* to the task are needed, and her position for doing the task must be *modified*. To dig the hole deep enough, Peggie cannot squat or kneel; because of her knee replacement, she must lie down on her side to reach into the hole with a trowel. She props herself up with an elbow to add fertilizer to the loosened soil at the bottom of the hole. When Peggie gets ready to stand up, Jack should be on hand to steady her. The tree is too large for one person to lift, so the couple will lower it into the hole together to *prevent injury*. However, the goal is not fully achieved when the tree is planted. The OT's assistance has enabled Peggie to realize she must take some precautions and accept some help if she wishes to continue participating safely in the occupation of gardening. This OT intervention uses an occupation both as a goal and as a means. In terms of productive aging, the OT supports the self-manager role in advising Peggie on ways to manage a chronic health condition, to enlist and accept available social support (Jack), and to adapt or modify the circumstances that will allow her to continue a meaningful, self-fulfilling occupation. For practice, try applying the spool model with the following learning activity.

Learning Activity 35: Applying the Occupational Therapy Spool Model of Intervention

Your home care client, Sara, has low vision that interferes with her ability to cook her own meals, which is a priority occupation for her. Upon evaluation, you discover that she can see adequately with increased brightness and can read labels with the assistance of a magnifier. She also needs to build confidence that she can still perform these occupations, which she had given up following an unrelated illness.

1. Choose three activities related to meal preparation to focus on with Sara.

    a.

    b.

    c.

2. What preparatory tasks should precede each of these tasks to increase safety and success?

3. What adaptations will Sara need for her work area to enable occupational performance?

4. What education or training can you suggest for Sara when she shops for groceries?

5. What task modifications can you suggest for Sara when cleaning up and storing cooking equipment and supplies?

6. How could you incorporate social participation into this occupation-based intervention?

The OT process clearly includes an ongoing process of therapeutic use of self, analysis of activities, and clinical reasoning, applied throughout the course of intervention. Outcomes that were defined at the outset can be continually evaluated and modified with clients' response to treatment.

Therapeutic Use of Self in Supportive Counseling and Dealing With Emotions

When dealing with clients in various transitional states, the OT needs to find ways to evaluate the clients' motivations, emotions, and abilities to cope and adapt. Clients who have taken responsibility for their own life and aging process make the best collaborators in setting occupational goals and achieving them. However, many clients have not fully understood or accepted the impact of an illness or disability or may have emotional issues that prevent them from making good choices with regard to prioritizing occupations. In these situations, OT in mental health training comes into play. Throughout the therapy process, OTs need some advanced communication skills to deal with such issues, which may involve lack of trust, lack of insight, or inability to resolve interpersonal conflicts.

- *Immediacy* brings the therapeutic relationship itself into focus. It is probably not a good idea to use this skill during the initial stages of rapport building but can help explore emotional roadblocks involving trust between client and OT partners as treatment progresses. Begin with an observation, such as "I've noticed that you haven't followed through with my suggestions to actively build your strength between our sessions." Then, ask the client to explain: "What seems to be interfering?" or "What difficulties are you having about my recommendations?" It is important for the OT not to show negative emotions or judgments, but rather to define the observation as a discrepancy between the clients' verbalized goals and their behaviors or actions. In a client-centered partnership, it is not the OT practitioner's position to judge the client's behavior, but rather it is to ask questions to gain a better understanding of what is occurring within the relationship.

- *Therapeutic self-disclosure* is another way to encourage clients to think more deeply about their own doubts, motivations, or emotions without conveying any negative judgment. For example, when clients doubt their own ability to perform an activity, the therapist might give a brief personal example: "Last year, right after a death in my family, I found it hard to find the willpower to get up and exercise before work like I had been doing before. I had to give myself a break for a few weeks before I could get back to my routines." The disclosure should always be brief and to the point, and followed up by, "Could that be happening with you?" The disclosure is individualized to each client's circumstance, and its purpose should always be to increase the client's own self-awareness, as well as to encourage further trust in the therapeutic relationship.

- An *advanced empathy* response also encourages deeper self-understanding and can be effective when dealing with the client's negative emotions, such as anger, hostility, fear, or anxiety. For example, a client may wish to get back to driving after his license is taken away following a health condition affecting vision. He is angry, demanding the car keys from his son, who has taken them for his father's own good. The OT practitioner, hearing his anger, might ask, "You sound very angry at your son. What might be his reasons for taking your

keys?" or "If you did drive, what if you hit someone crossing the road because you couldn't see him or her?" The goal for this skill is to peel away the layers of emotion so that the client can see what lies beneath. In using this skill, the OT takes care not to expose the client to emotions he or she may not be ready to handle. However, when the therapeutic relationship is well developed, clients will be more likely to reveal the emotions that may be interfering with progress in therapy. Another goal of advanced empathy is to encourage client awareness of the choices or alternate solutions to problems. In the above situation, the OT might ask, "What might be another way for you to get downtown to have coffee with your buddies, without driving yourself?" or "Where is it you need to drive, and who else might be going there too?" or "What transportation services does your community offer for seniors who cannot drive?" These questions get beyond the anger and frustration and build self-management by helping the client to identify social or community connections that might assist him in overcoming the problem of an inability to drive.

- *Confrontation* focuses on discrepancies between the client's verbal statements and his or her behaviors. "You've told me you want to go back home, but you have missed the last two therapy sessions addressing your ability to increase your mobility and strength. How might the lack of exercise affect progress toward your goal of preventing another fall?" In a client-centered relationship, the OT never jumps in to solve a problem that the client is capable of solving. The OT's role in supporting self-management always encourages client problem solving and respects the client's ability to use his or her own reasoning and coping ability to resolve problems. In this way, the client builds self-confidence, with resources and guidance from the OT practitioner.

(For more information about these skills, see Cole's *Group Dynamics in Occupational Therapy*, 2012.)

Learning Activity 36: Evaluating Client Self-Determination

Suppose you are interviewing an 80-year-old man with multiple sclerosis as a home care OT, along with his wife who is also his main caregiver. After the third session, progress is stalled. When inquiring about progress, you note that the wife dominates the discussion and the husband, who can and should be speaking, remains passive, always deferring to his wife.

1. How might you change the structure of your interview to get the husband's opinions and answers without offending the wife? Which of the previously mentioned skills might be helpful in this situation?

2. What three questions could you ask the husband to find out how motivated he is to direct his own life?

   a.

   b.

   c.

3. What three questions might you ask the wife to better understand her dominating attitude with regard to caregiving?

   a.

   b.

   c.

4. What three questions might you ask them as a couple to determine what meaningful occupations they might do together?

   a.

   b.

   c.

Step 6: Evaluate Outcomes

Outcomes are "the end result of the OT process: they describe what clients can achieve through occupational therapy intervention. The outcomes of OT can be described in two ways. Some outcomes are measurable and are used for intervention planning, monitoring, and discharge planning. These outcomes reflect the attainment of treatment goals that relate to engagement in occupations" (AOTA, 2014, p. S34). They may or may not include the achievement of occupational goals, but the measures of progress should have been identified at the outset of OT intervention. When the goal of performing a priority occupation is set, the specific barriers to that performance would have been identified, along with baseline measurements. Therefore, both the occupational therapist and client can chart progress along a specific continuum, such as building tolerance for sitting up to 1 hour to enable social participation in going out to eat dinner with friends. The goal may also be achieved another way, such as using positioning aids to compensate for lost strength or balance. Therefore, the goal may be achieved but the original methods may have changed along the way.

The second type of outcome defined by the OTPF III is "experienced by clients when they have realized the effects of engagement in occupation and are able to return to desired habits" (AOTA, 2014, p. S34). Performance of an occupation involves the "dynamic transaction among the client, the context, and the activity. Improving or enabling skills and patterns in occupational performance leads to engagement in occupations or activities (adapted in part from Law et al., 1996, p. 6)" (AOTA, 2014, p. S34). For example, a goal of returning to part-time employment will need to be broken down into components as the client and OT identify problems and barriers to be addressed. For this goal to be achieved, the older worker's skills, as well as the physical and social contexts of the employer and adaptation of the work activities and tasks, would have to be measured and changes documented as part of the outcome evaluation.

The OTPF III (AOTA, 2014) further defines possible outcomes within the following categories, which are not intended to be all-inclusive:

- Occupational performance: The actual in-vivo performance of an occupation set as a goal, such as entertaining at home by cooking and serving dinner for a few close friends (home management, social connections).

- Improvement: Reflecting increased quality of occupational performance that was previously limited, such as working up to full participation in a yoga class to increase flexibility (self-management, lifelong learning).

- Enhancement: Reflecting improved performance with no previously identified limitation. An older adult working toward greater fitness will increase energy level and be better able to perform a volunteer job or provide care for a loved one.

- Prevention: Increased safety, risk reduction, and avoidance of health conditions or symptoms, which enables clients to continue their most meaningful occupational roles.

- Health and wellness: Therapeutic or educational efforts aimed at maintaining health, including encouraging and enabling good self-management.

When working toward productive aging, outcomes for older clients should always include autonomy in self-management, continued social connections, and engagement in self-fulfilling activities. The evidence shows that these components have a high probability of resulting in an outcome of successful and productive aging.

Step 7: Design Occupational Therapy Group Interventions

Therapeutic groups have a long and varied history in OT. At one time, group interventions were mainly used in mental health settings, but that has changed in recent decades as OTs have become aware of the importance of social aspects of activities and co-occupations. The OTPF III (AOTA, 2014) has added group interventions (absent from the previous two versions of the Framework). They are defined as "use of distinct knowledge and leadership techniques to facilitate learning and skill acquisition across the lifespan through the dynamics of group and social interaction. Groups may also be used as a method of service delivery" (AOTA, 2014, p. S31).

Mosey (1986) describes levels of group functioning in a therapeutic setting. Parallel project, egocentric, coopera-

	TABLE 5-5

COLE'S 7 STEPS FOR CLIENT-CENTERED GROUP LEADERSHIP

GROUP SESSION STEPS	DESCRIPTION AND EXAMPLES
1. Introduction	Names, warm-up, timing, purpose, and goals
2. Activity	Tasks the group will do (e.g., worksheets, drawings, writing, communicating, occupation/preparation, role playing, reminiscence, games, educational information, group problem solving)
3. Sharing	Every member speaks to the group about the activity (e.g., reading aloud what they have written, describing their drawings)
4. Processing	Describing feelings about the activity, the leader, or each other
5. Generalizing	Members talk about what they learned from doing the activity
6. Application	Each member describes how he or she will apply the lessons learned in his or her own life outside the group (e.g., practicing social skills with family members)
7. Summary	Members or leader reviews the session, highlighting positive responses; leader gives homework and/or announces next session

Adapted from Cole, M. (2012). *Group dynamics in occupational therapy* (4th ed.). Thorofare, NJ: SLACK Incorporated.

tive, and mature are described as stages of possible group development. Social roles for dyadic interaction are presented as family, associate, authority, chum, peer, intimate, and nurturing. Through use of purposeful leisure activities, the OT may facilitate insight, interpersonal awareness, and aspects of group dynamics.

Related to other conditions, Paleg and Jangsma (2000) identify group intervention with both short- and long-term objectives. Using behavior-based principles, their group approach is similar to classroom education. A specified diagnosis is explored with sharing of feelings and personal history and experiences. Peers offer information and compare results of strategies used. They explore the impact of the condition on their broader lives, including work, relationships, sleep, diet, medications, and communication skills, and coping strategies for emotions. OTs integrate real life and purposeful activities, including leisure, to accompany many of these strategies.

In Howe and Schwartzberg (2001), classic theorists related to group work are reviewed for identifying curative factors in group work, including hope, universality, altruism, corrective recapitulation of the family group, social techniques, imitative behavior, catharsis, existential factors, cohesiveness, and interpersonal learning. Mosey (1981) describes activity groups as consisting of homogeneous or heterogeneous membership, with types of groups listed as evaluation, task oriented, developmental, thematic (learn new skills), topical (apply skills in real life setting), and instrumental. The OT's role is to evaluate individual and group skills and goals, design and lead activity groups, and offer leadership and feedback.

Client-Centered Group Guidelines for Occupational Therapy

Groups designed to promote productive occupations should be kept to a maximum of 8 to 10 participants, with a series of at least six sessions. The facilitator uses a client-centered approach by following Cole's (2012) 7-step format to assure that every member has input, participates in a group activity or exercise, and reflects on the activity's meaning and application within his or her own life (Table 5-5). Group activities should address the specific issues expressed by members, to ensure the intervention's relevance for them. More importantly, facilitating group interaction during the session builds reciprocal relationships among members, allowing them to empathize with and feel supported by one another as the sessions continue. OTs through the years may have underestimated the importance of social aspects of occupations and interventions.

Learning Activity 37: Designing a Group Session for Self-Management

Design a group session for one of the suggested topics to support self-management, listed in Chapter 1. State the purpose and goals of this session. Include a group activity lasting about 20 minutes. Write three discussion questions for each of the following steps of group leadership: processing, generalizing, and application. Refer to Table 5-5 for descriptions of these steps.

1. Title and brief description of activity with instructions

2. Purpose and goals of the session

3. Processing questions

   a.

   b.

   c.

4. Generalizing questions

   a.

   b.

   c.

5. Application questions

   a.

   b.

   c.

Please refer to Cole (2012) for a more in-depth description of how to design a group session.

Learning Activity 38: Designing a Series of Occupational Therapy Groups for Self-Fulfilling Activities

As an OT consultant to a senior center, imagine that you are asked to design an OT group for newly retired community dwellers to help them to identify meaningful activities to replace their worker role. Using the previous evidence as your guide, create a series of six exploratory sessions for the group that focus on remembering the activities that have brought members self-fulfillment in their past. Give group members an opportunity to teach each other by sharing their own activity preferences with others. Discuss ways to adapt, expand, or otherwise continue some form of the preferred activities as part of their planned lifestyle in retirement. The sessions can be structured using worksheets, drawing, or journal style writing, or trying out different types of crafts, games, sports, educational, or volunteer activities. Social aspects such as joining interest groups, volunteering, or taking classes might figure into future plans. Briefly describe the goal, structure, activity, and desired outcome for each of six group sessions centered on this theme.

   Session 1:

   Session 2:

   Session 3:

   Session 4:

   Session 5:

   Session 6:

Step 8: Education and Training Roles for Occupational Therapy Practitioners

The OTPF III (AOTA, 2014) defines OT education and training roles as follows:

- Education: "Imparting knowledge and information about occupation, health, well-being, and participation that enables the client to acquire helpful behaviors, habits, and routines that may or may not require application at the time of the intervention session" (p. S30).

- Training: "Facilitation of the acquisition of concrete skills for meeting specific goals in a real-life, applied situation. In this case, skills refers to measurable components of function that enable mastery. Training is differentiated from education by its goal of enhanced understanding, although these goals often go hand in hand (Collins & O'Brien, 2003)" (AOTA, 2014, p. S30).

Teaching as an Intervention

OTs have an important role in teaching clients and their caregivers about techniques to promote safety, comfort, and maximum ability. The therapist applies principles of task analysis to match a client's learning needs and style to the characteristics of the activity and performance environment. The therapist gauges use of his or her own volume, positioning, and pacing of instructions or recommendations through aspects of therapeutic use of self. Awareness of the desired successful task completion includes steps, supplies, sequence, and means of grading for simplicity or complexity.

An ongoing assessment coincides with demonstrated occupational performance. The therapist uses this important data from clinical observation to determine the effectiveness of intervention techniques, evaluate activity tolerance, and consider need for subsequent sessions and discharge. The therapist, with experience, builds a repertoire of instructions for techniques, with assorted "how to" approaches to match varied client needs for learning and follow through.

Client education often includes a program for follow-up or homework to promote carryover of skill development and progress between sessions. These assignments need to be carefully designed for clarity and realistic compliance.

Some aspects of client education may include teaching about the client's health status or condition. This might review the typical progression of a condition, or make referrals to resources for independent research. The latter may include community organizations, such as libraries and agencies, or online sites. As therapy progresses, feedback is offered to the client about levels of progress or pending plateaus related to functional status. The client may wish to learn about expected patterns of healing or recovery.

Due to reimbursement regulations for services, most current rehabilitative therapies are short term and limited in scope. The OT may have an increasing role in teaching universal concepts of adaptation, adjustment, and compensatory techniques for the clients' ongoing efforts to self-manage after discharge.

Understanding Client Learning Needs

Because individuals have different learning abilities and styles, the OT needs to consider cognitive, visual, and auditory skills. Some clients will need extensive reinforcement of main points. Some prefer fine details to be offered only after broad strokes are described. The therapist needs to informally test for comprehension, retention, and application of instructions. Key words may need to be repeated, with care to avoid information overload. From session to session, a review may be necessary to remind the client about some elements and explore for feedback about his or her experiences.

Teaching Methods

The OT utilizes many methods for instruction. Verbal instruction offers description of a procedure. Observation by the client may be effective as he or she watches a role play or demonstration of a technique. "Hand over hand" techniques may be beneficial to physically guide a client through a specific motion or movement. In general, the therapist creates the structured situation for performance, the client attempts a technique, and together adaptations may be determined to promote successful experiences. Throughout, methods of positive reinforcement are helpful to recognize efforts and promote ongoing engagement.

Some clients need considerable encouragement from the therapist to initiate participation in a therapeutic recommendation. This may relate to a tendency to resist trying new or novel approaches, lack of self-confidence, or emotional influences that interfere with performance. The therapist uses assorted strategies to offer support and to justify the recommendations offered for attempting proposed therapeutic strategies. A willingness to learn new or adapted methods may be promoted by carefully repeated explanations about how the suggested intervention is designed to match the client's personal goals.

Written instructions are often offered by the OT. This may include a description of techniques with diagrams or photographs. Handouts are helpful for follow through with reminders of tips for positioning, pacing, time elements, and any precautions. Some therapists provide publications or professionally prepared pamphlets about a condition, such as procedures following a hip replacement. Virtual education is available in many forms, including shared exploration of search engines on a topic, such as Google, or viewing YouTube videos about other clients' experiences.

Another valuable form of client education is through peer comparison, whether formal or informal. Formal is guided sharing while cotreating clients, or a therapist-led support group for individuals with depression. Here, clients relate to one another as equals and share helpful discoveries from their own journey toward function and health. Informal sharing often takes place in the waiting room of a clinic or anywhere in the community where peers discuss health issues and compare notes for successful intervention. The OT may be asked for a professional opinion on such topics, such as the wearing of a copper bracelet to prevent or reduce symptoms or arthritis.

Teaching Family Caregivers

Many older adults have involved family members who will assist in the follow-up of therapeutic recommendations. Careful description may be provided for ADL or IADL techniques for the client. Caregivers are instructed about attention to their own body mechanics, energy conservation, and joint protection techniques because they may be assisting with transporting or transfers.

Family members may be helpful in providing insight into how the client best learns and applies new information. They may be asked to learn techniques and have responsibilities for promoting practice and follow-up. The OT may need to instruct family members about calibrating their own level of involvement and assistance. They may be taught principles of levels of assistance, ranging from maximum to moderate to minimum. A continuum of independence-to-dependence may be described, explaining the client's unique level of need for assistance, supervision, guidance, and cuing.

Instructing Professional and Paid Caregivers

Interdisciplinary team members and aids have training in health conditions and promoting basic function and safety for clients. However, OTs specialize in an in-depth program to encourage maximum independence, and communicate their recommendations to others in an effort for consistency of approaches by all team members. Because staff members may rotate daily, or perhaps over three shifts in a long-term care facility or home care setting, it is important to establish and share recommended approaches for all to apply. Printed recommendations with clear graphics are important for assisting others with follow-through of an OT plan. For example, for proper positioning in bed, diagrams or photographs may be made available. Simple labels of "Do" and "Don't" may be effective. To avoid a hospital-like environment in a home setting, printed directions and recommendations may be organized into a single notebook or electronic file rather than displayed on walls. A communication book may be a resource for all involved caregivers to write comments to promote continuity.

OTs offer in-service training to interdisciplinary team members, aides, and volunteers in many settings. Consistency is sought for all caregivers to apply techniques for promoting autonomy in self-care and other areas of function for the client. Clients are often learning a new approach to a familiar task, like dressing. Although it may be much faster for a home health aide to quickly dress the individual, a client may be focusing on the re-development of self-dressing ability while using assistive devices like a reacher and a zipper pull.

In providing information to colleagues and other paid caregivers, the OT needs to modify communication styles by avoiding OT jargon, considering the person's professional background, and determining ways to evaluate their understanding and ability to implement recommendations. The latter would include discussion about how realistic OT recommendations might be, considering ideal and real staffing situations in some settings. The OT needs to be able to modify recommendations to fit the needs of the caregivers who will be implementing them, while maintaining the priority of the client's needs.

OTs spend a considerable amount of their professional life in a teaching role, whether to clients, family members, or professional caregivers. Materials must be presented at a level that considers ability to learn, is clear and concise, and has realistic potential for compliance. As intervention proceeds, the therapist gains insights about the client's learning needs and adapts the ways in which instructions and recommendations are offered. Follow-up is necessary to evaluate whether the materials taught have been effective or need further review and reinforcement or modification.

Learning Activity 39: Teaching and Learning

Self-reflection: Recall a time when a health care provider offered instruction and recommendations to you.

1. How was it provided? Verbal? Printed materials? Critique the effectiveness: did you understand? Was it clear?

2. Were you able to follow through effectively? What was successful or unsuccessful about the approaches used?

3. What would be the ideal way for you to learn a new technique or follow-up recommendation?

4. Consider your experiences with any fieldwork exposure of an OT practitioner relating to a client with directions or instructions. Briefly describe the encounter.

5. How was the therapist using therapeutic use of self to engage attention and interest, offer explanation, and determine understanding when communicating with the clients?

6. What did you notice about the therapist's listening skills?

7. How do you feel about being in the role of a teacher? What strengths or challenges might this professional behavior pose for you?

8. How might you develop strengths and resolve challenge areas?

Step 9: Occupational Therapist Advocacy Roles

Participation in advocacy initiatives occurs on many levels for the OT. This may begin as an OT student, corresponding with local officials regarding attention to a public health issue. As a professional, therapists are encouraged to be knowledgeable and proactive about issues related to policy development or changes. As a practitioner, the OT may address advocacy issues on several levels: personally advocating for a client's rights, promoting self-advocacy skills for a client or client group, and personal participation in projects to create policy change.

Whether in student or professional roles, advocacy relates to promoting the special interests and rights of consumers or organizations. In general, it consists of raising awareness about a proposed change in policy or procedure or it may relate to requests for increased enforcement of existing regulations. For example, a class of OTA students may approach their college administration to advocate for increased campus accessibility to public restrooms for individuals who use wheelchairs. A group of practitioners may work with board members of an arthritis organization to advocate for town funding of a health and wellness program to be offered at a local senior center. Advocacy includes defining a problem, need, or issue, and suggesting proposals for change. This could include program development, protection of patient rights, or involvement in policy change efforts.

Promoting Professional Issues

OTs may rally resources to promote increased or expanded services. For example, through the AOTA's Political Action Committee, lobbyists participate in efforts to protect and promote OT service delivery, both for individuals and group intervention.

As emerging areas of practice evolve, advocacy is needed to justify OT expertise and differentiate OT's unique roles from other professionals competing for the same reimbursement dollars. This may include work with local, regional, or national political representatives to create appropriate bills, laws, or regulations. Whether pursuing new legislation or protecting existing laws, advocacy efforts may also include work to increase public awareness about the issues. If congressional or community votes are involved, OTs may participate in campaigns to promote support for their special interests.

Representing Client Interests

Another level of advocacy is acting on the behalf of clients. In general, this would include advocating for quality assurance in services and enforcement of the principles of patient rights. OTs are expected to maintain continued competency for their area of clinical practice. This would include an ongoing awareness and knowledge of gerontology, such as advances in treatment approaches, research related to conditions, and public policy for funding of health services. With this knowledge, OTs have an extensive background to assist in understanding and promoting services for older adults.

The OT might also serve as a resource and referral person as another dimension of advocacy. At interdisciplinary conferences, the OT may advocate for the client by recommending that services be provided by additional disciplines.

Learning Activity 40: Offering Referrals

Imagine that you are working in home health with a recently widowed 80-year-old woman who had a fall and fractured her dominant wrist. She feels especially alone and vulnerable after the fall, and cannot focus on OT intervention due to increasing grief and anxiety.

1. To which professionals would the OT refer the client for assistance in coping and emotional regulation?

2. What are some community resources to recommend?

3. If the client was computer literate, what suggestions may be offered for online education and support?

Enabling Client Self-Advocacy Skills

A client may have a goal of personally advocating for change. This could be related to a number of topics, such as patient rights, quality of care, privacy, extending reimbursable treatment sessions, or enhanced health insurance. Issues may be based on positive suggestions for improvements but may also reflect goals to prevent negative practices. Advocacy may be related to abuse, neglect, unethical issues, or noncompliance with regulations. In this area, the client may be advocating on his or her own behalf or to prevent similar negative experiences from occurring to other individuals.

Advocacy efforts require a commitment of time and energy as well as assertiveness. The OT may assist a client with the following:

- Discussing methods for defining an issue.

- Educating about the parameters of patient rights and service system policies.

- Designing communication pathways and methods to relevant contacts.

- Establishing a networks of contacts.

- Providing introductions to involved administrators or other officials.

- Providing referrals to local agencies.

- Connecting with other individuals with similar concerns to develop support and a larger base of support for action.

- Joining or contacting representative groups with experience and resources for addressing issues, such as the AARP, or national organizations serving a particular client population, such as those with Parkinson's disease or multiple sclerosis.

- Devising methods for preparing clear, realistic, and focused letters, e-mails, text messages, or phone calls.

- Referrals to a local ombudsman who specializes in problem solving for individual cases.

- Assisting with effective techniques to connect with local agencies regarding economic assistance for specific needs.

- Collaborating with family members to advocate for awareness and research needs for a condition through fundraising efforts. An example would be a walk-a-thon for breast cancer.

- Promoting client's understanding of rights and responsibilities to report illegal or unethical practices.

The process of advocating for or against an issue may be a short-term or a very long-term effort. The role of the OT would be to identify the areas of interest or concern; investigate and contact possible individuals, networks, or responsible parties; document ongoing efforts; follow up as needed; and track progress toward ultimate results. This is typically beyond reimbursable billing units. Instead, it is often performed on a volunteer basis by the individual or groups of therapists who share an objective of promoting occupational justice.

Through carefully prepared efforts, a single client or therapist can make a difference in policy affecting larger populations. Working in conjunction with others to promote goals for the profession of OT can potentially lead to state and federal law changes to increase service delivery for client populations. Therapists interested in participating in advocacy projects may become involved in their own local or state OT associations through government affairs committees or by serving as a state representative for the AOTA.

Step 10: Occupational Therapist Consulting Roles

Consultation refers to the indirect provision of OT services through education and guidance given to groups, organizations, populations, or governmental entities. Two types of consultation are reviewed here: (1) promotion of health and well-being with populations, and (2) supporting occupational performance and health in community organizations and agencies.

Health Promotion With Populations

According to a recent AOTA position paper, "to be effective, health promotion efforts cannot focus only on intervention at the individual level. Because of the inextricable and reciprocal links between people and their environments, larger groups, organizations, communities and populations may also benefit from occupational therapy intervention (AOTA, 2008; Law, 1991; Wilcock, 2006)" (AOTA, 2013, p. S52). Prevention can be divided into the following 3 types:

1. *Primary prevention* has the objective of deflecting onset by reducing the incidence of unhealthy conditions, diseases, or injuries before they occur. Efforts include identifying risk factors, and reducing or eliminating them. For example, evidence shows that modifying the homes of frail elderly to eliminate hazards, combined with education regarding fall risk and recovery, use of assistive devices and regular exercise to maintain strength and sustain balance can prevent injury due to falls (American Geriatrics Society, 2010).

2. *Secondary prevention* typically includes screening, early detection, and intervention after disease has occurred, with the goal of disrupting the disabling process. Persons who have been diagnosed with a chronic health condition or who are already identified as disabled have a higher risk for developing secondary conditions. OT practitioners can educate and provide strategies to groups and populations with specific conditions, "limiting the development of secondary conditions and their subsequent impact on function and quality of life" (AOTA, 2013, p. S49). For example, the OT designs a group intervention for older adults who have survived a stroke to promote upper body strength and ROM, broaden visual attention and perception, increase self-awareness regarding driving safety, and assess their readiness to resume the occupation of driving (Hunt & Arbesman, 2008; Kua et al., 2007; Leland et al., 2012; Strong et al., 2008).

3. *Tertiary prevention* stalls or slows the progression of a health condition. OTs target outcomes at this level toward promoting "equal opportunity, full participation, independent living, and economic self-sufficiency (Patrick, Richardson, Starks, Rose, & Kinne, 1997)" (AOTA, 2013, p. S49). For example, OTs may consult with assisted living facilities to structure and adapt sports, games, or other group activities to accommodate functional limitations due to chronic or acquired health conditions of residents. The goal of this intervention would be to increase participation in chosen occupations that will maintain social connections, support health and well-being, and protect against functional decline.

Outcomes related to OT intervention for productive aging include occupational performance, prevention, health and wellness, quality of life, participation, role competence, well-being, and occupational justice. At a population level, some possible topics for consultation might be the following:

- Fall prevention programs for community dwelling seniors.

- Musculoskeletal injury prevention and management.

- Education and training regarding eating habits, activity levels, and prevention of secondary disability due to obesity.

- Stress management training and adaptive strategies following mood or post-traumatic stress disorders.

- Leisure participation groups for older adults with dementia, to prevent or slow further decline through socialization and quality of life.

- Social and educational opportunities for older caregivers of persons with dementia, stroke, or other disabling conditions.

Learning Activity 41: Groups for Secondary Prevention

Choose a specific health condition common to older adulthood (e.g., Parkinson's disease, Alzheimer's disease, diabetes, cardiopulmonary obstructive disorder, or osteoarthritis). Design a group intervention that will provide education and training in secondary prevention, using an occupational focus.

1. Briefly describe the population and some typical problems you would expect to find.

2. Describe the purpose and goals for the OT group intervention.

3. Design and describe six group sessions dealing with both education and preventive strategies:

    a.

    b.

    c.

    d.

    e.

    f.

4. Define the expected outcome for this group. How would you measure or evaluate this outcome?

5. Design a four- or five-item rating scale to measure member satisfaction with the outcome.

OT prevention opportunities are expected to become available with the implementation of the Affordable Care Act of 2010, which provides funding for prevention and public health programs, education and outreach, community-based prevention and wellness programs, and personalized prevention plans for older clients within primary care settings (AOTA, 2013). The AOTA (2013) suggests that OT practitioners "seize opportunities to participate in the provision of health promotion and prevention services under the ACA by becoming a member of the primary care team and the patient's medical home. Failure to integrate OT into these arenas could severely limit the profession's future growth" (p. S53).

Consulting With Community Organizations

Attention to the development of community-based services has been a theme throughout this text. This includes home care and other outpatient or specialty services available through senior centers or other organized agencies. Accessibility to these services raises issues of funding, access to services (transportation), and resource allocation. Some communities offer significant health and social services, while others do not. Where shortages of OT personnel exist, parts of the OT's role are often delegated or divided among other personnel, often with considerably less training. Concepts of distributive justice are described by Carrier, Levasseur, and Mullins (2010). Future OTs need to recognize where gaps in service exist that could appropriately be met by occupational therapists. Local and state OT associations need to become aware of shortages in availability of qualified OTs and get involved in recruitment efforts so that other professionals do not get hired to fill OT positions.

Community programs have a variety of funding sources: government agencies, foundations, nonprofit organizations, insurance companies, and large corporations, among others (AOTA, 2013). For example, the Bridgeport, Connecticut, area Agency on Aging established an OT part-time consulting position to design and run a support group for grandparents raising grandchildren (Anne Golensky, 2013, personal communication). A university OT program pays a faculty member to supervise OT students designing physical and mental fitness group activities as a Fieldwork I experience at a senior housing project (Elm Terrace) in Stratford, Connecticut. OT practitioners can partner with specific disability organizations to design programs for elders with disabilities and their caregivers.

Two well-elderly studies (Clark et al., 1997, 2011) provide ample evidence that OT group interventions with community dwelling older adults have significantly reduced health-related problems and their subsequent costs. However, taking this evidence to community organizations, such as insurance companies, senior centers, or other publicly funded senior service programs, requires some creativity on the part of the OT. New or recent graduates could collaborate with more experienced OTs to design and market group programs addressing topics that relate to productive aging. The results from the PAS suggest that these topics should appropriately address self-management, social connection, and self-fulfilling activities, especially within the productive occupations of home maintainer, volunteer, caregiver, paid worker, and lifelong learner.

Fazio (2008) has written a workbook to assist OT practitioners in planning and designing community programs. Some of the steps she suggests were described in Chapter 4. For example, a retired OT practitioner has an interest in memoir writing. Writing memoirs benefits older adults by strengthening social identity through preserving shared memories of important events—both world events and family histories. There is ample evidence that sharing one's memories with others, both by writing and story-telling, increases the feeling of social connectedness and self-esteem and decreases isolation. The OT visits a local senior center to explore the programs that already exist and to discuss her ideas with the center's directors. She learns that other specialized professionals charge a nominal fee for classes offered at the center, such as yoga, aerobics, woodworking, and line dancing. The OT was invited to design and advertise the memoir writing group program, set a fee, and recruit volunteers to attend a 10-week class. Fifteen people signed up, and the OT was given a space and put on the schedule for the weekly sessions. This example demonstrates that community programs do not have to be complicated or time consuming. However, they do need to be well thought out and answer an acknowledged need for the people they serve.

Learning Activity 42: Profiling the Community

It has been strongly recommended that OT practitioners, anticipating future opportunities for community consultation, become well informed about the resources and workings of their communities. Choose a community—a small town or a section of a larger town or city—and explore the following:

1. What are the demographics? How many people reside there, and what is the average income? What is the breakdown by ethnic background, religion, and place of residence? If available, how many people are over 65 and where do they reside (own homes, rented apartments, assisted living facilities, long-term care facilities)?

2. What medical services exist in this community? Identify the following:

   a. A senior center

   b. A hospital

   c. A rehabilitation center (residential or outpatient)

   d. Assisted living and extended care facilities

   e. Adult day care centers

   f. A walk-in clinic for emergency care

g. A public transportation system

h. Home health agencies or services

i. Number of medical doctors and their specialties

j. Other services specifically for seniors, such as wellness clinics or geriatric centers

3. What social services exist in the community? (Most towns have websites that list these.)

a. A public transportation system? Senior or handicapped transit services?

b. A town hall? Police stations? Fire stations?

c. A senior center? What programs take place there?

d. Recreational facilities such as parks, hiking trails, sports complexes, swimming pools, golf courses, country clubs, beaches. Which are public, which are private?

e. Which charitable or volunteer organizations are located there?

f. Public library? What is available there?

g. Public schools? What adult education classes are offered?

h. Public or private universities?

4. Locate or print a road map of the community. Choose a random street where an older adult may be living alone. Draw a circle on the map representing a 1-mile radius around this imaginary house. Locate each of the following within the circle, if available:

a. A primary care physician who accepts Medicare patients.

b. A grocery store, a bank, a barber, or hairdresser.

c. A drug store or pharmacy.

d. A Christian church, Jewish temple, or other place of worship.

e. A place where people would go to vote in a local, state, or national election.

5. Describe where you would go in this community to find productive agers. How would you go about gathering information to identify problems or unmet needs for the well elderly population?

The following section relates to other areas that help delineate the roles OTs play in productive aging in current practice.

PROFESSIONALISM

Whatever the setting, the OT practitioner is expected to maintain high standards of professional behavior. This includes many types of personal responsibility, such as time management throughout the day, respect for individuals, confidentiality, and responsiveness to supervision, ongoing continued education, and appropriate documentation.

Self-Management for the Occupational Therapy Practitioner

Regardless of the area and level of expertise, OT practitioners need to embrace many elements of professionalism. Taking responsibility for your own protection includes maintenance of personal health and wellness through careful therapeutic use of self, such as positioning, body mechanics, avoiding repetitive strain, and preventing harm to self when working with agitated individuals. Infection control procedures need to be identified and adhered to. Recommended vaccinations and physical examination should be adhered to. Working as an OT can be physically and mentally challenging, and therapists need to follow their own recommendations about a healthy and balanced lifestyle.

Working as an OT exposes the practitioner to many physical, emotional, sensory, and cognitive demands. The practitioner needs to attend to preventive measures for safety risks and personal injury through careful attention to potential hazards. This would include attention to lighting and floor surfaces, as well as careful body mechanics when assisting a client with a transfer.

Time management skills are especially important, because many facilities expect the practitioner to see a defined number of clients per day. This reflects the realities of health care as a business, with attention to reimbursable units calculated to determine the facility's income, and to reflect a therapist's efficiency. Evaluations must be focused and streamlined, with careful delineation of goals and suggested approaches. A treatment session includes the process of scheduling, potentially arranging for transport to and from the clinic, chart review, touching base with other professionals before or after a session, actual contact with client, and possible follow-up with family members. Documentation is a vital summary that reflects attention to the treatment plan, comments on progress, and revising of a plan for subsequent sessions. Time required for assessment and documentation are often not considered billable units of time. This leads to challenges for therapists to use documentation methods that clearly reflect client performance in a concise yet clear manner. Goals are intended to be observable and measurable. New systems are in development for electronic medical record keeping.

Sessions typically range from 30 to 40 minutes, with longer time required for assessment and discharge sessions. Some therapists also need to schedule travel time to home care clients.

Occupational Therapist's and Occupational Therapy Assistant's Role Divisions

OTs and OTAs share many responsibilities but do have a division of labor for direct and indirect treatment. Client interaction is scheduled within additional clinical responsibilities of the OT. OTAs would typically spend the bulk of their day providing direct treatment, with some time for assisting with a department's administrative or clerical work. The OT has additional responsibilities including attending required meetings for interdisciplinary client care, scheduling, billing, providing in-service staff education, and meeting family members. OTs also supervise assistants, aides, fieldwork students, and volunteers. Their role includes use of documentation systems, ordering and maintaining an inventory of equipment and supplies, and promoting awareness of potential OT services to match the needs of the facility.

In each setting, role delineation may vary somewhat for both therapist and assistant according to the quantity of the staff. Delineation of duties is also variable between the health care professionals, with clarification required to identify the responsible professional. This collaborative team approach may vary between settings for OT, physical therapists, speech pathologists, nurses, social workers, and recreational staff workers. With careful and continuing dialogue related to which department is responsible for what aspect of care, the optimum in holistic interdisciplinary treatment is realized.

Co-Treatment and Other Professionals

Some clients are now seen in co-treatment with physical therapists. For example, the physical therapist initiates a session with stretches and exercises or a physical agent modality for pain reduction. This is directly followed by the OT practitioner, who, now that the client is "warmed up," proceeds with mobility training for bed or toilet transfers. Some clients are seen at the same time by one therapist, with one client resting momentarily while another is engaged directly with the therapist. Special attention to documentation is required in this situation, delineating whether it is considered to be an individual or a group session.

OTs work within a broad system of other professionals. Referrals for an OT evaluation may be initiated by the therapist, physician, nurse, or other rehabilitation team members. Ongoing communication should be offered to these potential referring services related to the range of potential types of OT intervention. Conversely, OTs must have an extensive knowledge of facility and community services; referrals from physicians allow OT to enter into other treatment services or community programs.

Commitment to Theory and Research Across Practice Settings

New evidence emerges frequently, especially in the area of productive aging. Continuing education is a vital part of any OT practitioner's journey in lifelong learning. Required for maintaining licensure and certification, workshops, seminars, and conferences offer new ideas and perspectives. Online opportunities are available for short courses or specialty types. Many gerontology-focused topics are available in the course of a year. Continuing education credits may also be earned through teaching. The OT professional should carefully maintain a portfolio of all evidence of professional development and continued participation. This is helpful when a resumé needs to be updated.

Even if the clinician does not have an inclination for participating in research, the professional expectation is that each practitioner is a consumer of research publications. Many articles reflect meta-analysis or systematic reviews of content areas that would be relevant to clinicians seeking to provide evidence-based care. Murphy (2010) describes a 2-year review of geriatric studies, some provided information about effectiveness and efficacy; others were basic research, often descriptive in nature, shedding light on a particular phenomenon. Instrument development and testing procedures were discussed. Murphy (2010) stated that the research presented was still of a foundational level and confirms a need to justify provision of services based on quality research.

Examples of helpful findings that translate directly to clinical practice are available. Forster, Lambley, and Young (2010) studied the effectiveness of physical rehabilitation for long-term care residents. Through an intervention of exercise and a measurement of level of activity restriction, results showed an increase in ability and distance, and a lesser finding of increase in ADL functioning. Landa-Gonzalez and Molnar (2012) studied the results of OT intervention on self-care, performance satisfaction, self-esteem, and role functioning for arthritic older Hispanic women. Using preparatory methods of heat, massage, ROM, and strength exercises, results demonstrated an increase in self-care, homemaking, and leisure skills.

DePalma et al. (2013) studied the topic of hospital readmission for older adults. Upon discharge from a hospitalization, many patients have newly developed challenges with aspects of self-care performance. They referred to this as "...needing home help or equipment to complete the tasks" (DePalma et al., p. 454). When these needs were unmet, the patient was at increased risk for readmission to the hospital. Unmet needs result from lack of help available when needed or caregivers incapable of offering correct amounts of assistance. This could result in skin breakdowns, decrease in nutrition, falls, and decreased mobility. They highlight "...Section 3026 of the Affordable Care Act describes the Community Care Transitions Program which provides funds for implementation of evidence based care transition interventions for adults who are vulnerable for readmission..." (Patient Protection and Affordable Care Act, 2010; DePalma et al., 2013, p. 455). They summarize by stating a need for comprehensive discharge planning and adequate home care.

This is an example of how OTs can identify themselves as ideal candidates for providing these types of home care services. New graduates are urged to be familiar with all current health policy, identify potential OT roles, seek employment, and continue the cycle with shared program description and further research.

Specialized types of intervention are often the basis for research, exploring the effectiveness of use, or contrasts in types of populations. For example, several studies describe investigation of the use of reminiscence. Cappeliez and O'Rourke (2006) measured several behavioral functions when related to positive (identity, problem solving) and negative themes (boredom) of reminiscing. They found that review of self-functions contributed to physical and mental health. Cappeliez and Robitaille (2010) explored styles of coping related to psychological well-being as related to positive versus negative reminiscing about the self. They found that reminiscing led to "protective mechanisms through which the self-system constructs continuity of meaning over the life course" (Cappeliez & Robitaille, 2010, p. 818). Korte, Bohlmeijer, Westerhof, and Pot (2011) studied the relationships of themes of reminiscing and their effect on depressive symptoms. They recommended avoiding recollections that recall bitterness for clients with depressive symptoms, and attention to problem-solving reminiscences for clients with anxiety symptoms.

Recent graduates are encouraged to develop lifelong habits of accessing, reviewing, and applying results of research. The AOTA offers numerous sources for general and specialty topics related to gerontology. Practitioners also benefit from regular review of materials from the related health care professions to determine trends and developments in services and programs.

EXPANDING NEEDS FOR OCCUPATIONAL THERAPY SERVICES AND EVOLVING PRACTICE SETTINGS

OT service provision must adapt to match shifting models of health promotion and treatment services. This does not mean dropping traditional practices for any new "fad" that is developed. However, progress is inevitable in terms of equipment, technology, and possibilities for therapeutic approaches. Practitioners need to welcome change with skilled clinical reasoning and critical thinking related to

the needs of their particular clients and practice setting. We also need to respect and reflect the evolving expectations of our clients and their caregivers as consumers.

Primary Care Settings

Currently, developments are evolving related to provision of services for the frail elderly. De Stampa et al. (2013) studied working relationships between primary care physicians, case managers, and geriatricians providing services for a community-dwelling population. Ideally, an integrative care model was promoted to provide a comprehensive assessment, joint care planning, and regular patient and family contact and support, with increasing numbers and types of disciplines offering direct care services. OTs need to effectively define and promote their unique role and services, even with a frail population. Issues of positioning, medication management, and pursuit of adapted meaningful leisure activities could promote quality of life for even the most infirm.

Wellness and Prevention

Section II of this textbook explores aspects of function and interventions related to the continuum of care. This includes issues from wellness and prevention to considerations of the frail and dying. Hildenbrand and Lamb (2013) raise the topic of prevention of chronic disease as a key future area of practice. They urge OTs to initiate connections to work in organizations and communities to increase awareness of OT's role in prevention and wellness. They see wellness as its own continuum, including maximizing wellness and reduction of limitations when illness or disability is present. Techniques include healthy lifestyle support, attention to ergonomics, and promoting remaining skills through compensatory techniques.

Occupational Therapist's Roles in Discharge Planning

Gamble, Abate, Wenzel, and Ducharme (2011) describe how the rehabilitation team needs to increase readiness for discharge in those individuals who need customized strategies. OTs may have a lead role in developing trust and rapport, promoting confidence in a change in living environment, and recommending for appropriate settings. OTs may contribute to team decisions about discharge readiness, and measuring levels of independence in self-care and work. They also must work sensitively with family members who may be resistive to potentially increased roles in caregiving. Ethical issues related to discharge planning are described by Durocher and Gibson (2010) in a single subject case study. They describe an independent woman, who, after a fall, experienced a downward spiral of decreased skills. Her goal was to return home from a rehabilitation setting as soon as possible, but the staff felt she was at an increased risk for further injury. Patients, in order to preserve their autonomy and self-determination, may fear truthfully describing their actual challenges. They fear they won't be permitted to return home. Team members may have conflicting views in regard to respecting client choice versus protection from harm. The authors promoted developing a compromise in which occupational identity is preserved through prioritizing values and interests, in balance with risks to safety. They remind practitioners of the obligation to respect beneficence, in which the therapist contributes to positive actions and prevents harm.

In general, OTs frequently communicate with significant others and family members, offering support and education about symptoms and adaptive strategies. Family members often have a heavy responsibility for all follow-up care recommended and for therapy "homework." Baucom, Porter, Kirby, and Hudepohl (2012) specifically promote attention to the couple relationship. The OT needs to be attentive to the family caregiver, answering questions, encouraging expression of thoughts and feelings, and acknowledging changes related to altered roles and abilities.

New graduates must embrace the critical role that OTs have in discharge planning (Duxbury, DePaul, Alderson, Moreland, & Wilkins, 2012) Following a stroke, many clients are eager to be discharged home, yet do not realize the magnitude of changes in function until after they are discharged. The impact of new limitations led to reported unmet needs for intervention for self-care. This was especially prevalent for individuals who had some limitations prior to the stroke. The authors promote stronger roles for the OTs to collaborate with administrators and policy makers related to anticipating and providing for post-acute care needs.

OTs, independently partnering with other health professionals, may have an increasing role in advocating for client rights. This could include availability and quality of services. Future roles for OT practitioners may increasingly include extensive awareness and involvement in social, political, and legislative issues.

SUMMARY

As we approach the centennial of the AOTA, professional leaders have reflected upon our past growth and anticipated future needs. In the specialty field of geriatrics, efforts in recent decades have redefined important roles in long-term care, subacute care, and home care services. Roles in acute hospitalization have declined, with shorter stays and increased in- and outpatient services. OTs have had additional specialization in dementia care, orthotics, driving, home modification, low vision, fall prevention, and mental health or geropsychiatry.

National OT leaders envision the profession as capable of matching society's ever-changing needs to promote health, ability, and function. They coordinate efforts with state leaders and the representative assembly to identify and interpret needs for health care policy reforms. Specialists in the AOTA's Political Action Committee participate in lobbying to ensure promotion of and protection of funding for OT services. Regional and local leaders and clinicians work in tandem to address gaps in service delivery in underserved areas. The new graduate is entering a career that goes beyond an 8-hour shift and encourages a commitment to expanding the profession.

REFERENCES

Abreu, B. C. (2011). Accentuate the positive: Reflection on empathic interpersonal interactions. *American Journal of Occupational Therapy, 65,* 623-634.

American Geriatrics Society. (2010). *2010 AGS/BGS clinical practice guideline: Prevention of falls in older persons.* Retrieved from http://www.americangeriatrics.org/files/documents/health_care_pros/Falls.Summary.Guide.pdf.

American Occupational Therapy Association. (2014). Occupational therapy practice framework, 3rd edition. *American Journal of Occupational Therapy, 68,* S1-S48.

American Occupational Therapy Association. (2013). Occupational therapy in the promotion of health and well-being. *American Journal of Occupational Therapy, 67,* S47-S58.

American Occupational Therapy Association. (2008). The occupational therapy practice framework, 2nd edition: Domain and process. *American Journal of Occupational Therapy, 62,* 625-683.

Bandura, A. (1997). *Self-efficacy: The exercise of control.* New York: W.H. Freeman.

Baucom, D. H., Porter, L. S., Kirby, J. S., & Hudepohl, J. (2012). Couple-based interventions for medical problems. *Behavior Therapy, 43,* 61-76.

Bearon, L., Crowley, G., Chandler, J., Robbins, M., & Studenski, S. (2000). Personal functional goals: A new approach to assessing patient-centered outcomes. *Journal of Applied Gerontology, 19,* 201-222.

Cappeliez, P., & O'Rourke, N. (2006). Empirical validation of a model of reminiscence and health in later life. *Journal of Gerontology, 61,* 237-244.

Cappeliez, P., & Robitaille, A. (2010). Coping mediates the relationships between reminiscence and psychological well-being among older adults. *Aging in Mental Health, 14,* 807-818.

Carrier, A., Levasseur, M., & Mullins, G. (2010). Accessibility to occupational therapy community services: A legal, ethical and clinical analysis. *Occupational Therapy in Health Care, 24,* 360-376.

Cheah, S., & Presnell, S. (2011). Older person's experiences of acute hospitalization: An investigation of how occupations are affected. *Australian Occupational Therapy Journal, 58,* 120-128.

Clark, F., Azen, S., Carlson, M., Mandel, D., Zemke, R., Hay, J., ... Lipson, L. (1997). Occupational therapy for independent living older adults: A randomized controlled trial. *Journal of the American Medical Association, 278,* 1321-1326.

Clark, F., Jackson, J., Carlson, M., Chou, C., Cherry, B., Jordan-Marsh, M., & Azen, S. (2011). Effectiveness of a lifestyle intervention in promoting the well-being of independently living older people: Results of the Well Elderly 2 Randomized Controlled Trial. *Journal of Epidemiology and Community Health.* Retrieved from http://jech.bmj.com/content/early/2011/06/01/jech.2009.099754.abstract.

Cole, M. (2012). *Group dynamics in occupational therapy* (4th ed.). Thorofare, NJ: SLACK Incorporated.

Cole, M., & McLean, V. (2003). Therapeutic relationships re-defined. *Occupational Therapy in Mental Health, 19,* 33-56.

Collins, J., & O'Brien, N. P. (2003). *Greenwood dictionary of education.* Westport, CT: Greenwood Press.

Depalma, G., Xu, H., Covinsky, K. E., Craig, B. A., Stallard, E., Thomas, J., & Sands, L. P. (2013). Hospital readmission among older adults who return home with unmet need for ADL disability. *The Gerontologist, 53,* 454-461.

DeRosa, J. (2013). Providing self-management support to people living with chronic conditions. *OT Practice, 18*(Sept 23), CE 1-8.

de Stampa, M., Vedel, I., Bergman, H., Novella, J. L., Lochowski, L., Ankri, J., & Lapointe, L. (2013). Opening the black box of clinical collaboration in integrated care models for frail, elderly patients. *The Gerontologist, 53,* 313-325.

Doucet, B. M., & Gutman, S. A. (2013). Quantifying function: The rest of the measurement story. *American Journal of Occupational Therapy, 67,* 7-9.

Durocher, E., & Gibson, B. E. (2010). Navigating ethical discharge planning: A case study in older adult rehabilitation. *Australian Occupational Therapy Journal, 57,* 2-7.

Duxbury, S., DePaul, V., Alderson, M., Moreland, J., & Wilkins, S. (2012). Individuals with stroke reporting unmet need for occupational therapy following discharge from hospital. *Occupational Therapy in Health Care, 26,* 16-32.

Fazio, L. (2008). *Developing occupation-centered programs for the community* (2nd ed.). Upper Saddle River, NJ: Pearson/Prentice Hall.

Forster, A., Lambley, R., & Young, J. B. (2010). Is physical rehabilitation for older people in long-term care effective? Findings from a systematic review. *Age and Aging, 29,* 169-175.

Gamble, K., Abate, S., Wenzel, K., & Ducharme, J. (2011). Promoting readiness for discharge for long-term state hospital residents. *Psychiatric Rehabilitation Journal, 35,* 133-136.

Hall, K., Crowley, G., Howard, T., & Morey, M. (2010). Individual progress toward self-selected goals among older adults enrolled in a physical activity counseling intervention. *Journal or Aging and Physical Activity, 18,* 439-450.

Hildenbrand, W. C., & Lamb, A. J. (2013). Occupational therapy in prevention and wellness: Retaining relevance in new healthcare world. *American Journal of Occupational Therapy, 67,* 266-271.

Holt-Lunstad, J., Smith, T. B., & Bradley Layton, J. (2010). Social relationships and mortality risk: A meta-analytic review. *PLoS Med 7*(7): e1000316. Doi:10.1371/journal.pmed.1000316. Retrieved from www.plosmedicine.org.

Howe, M. C., & Schwartzberg, S. L. (2001). *A functional approach to group work in occupational therapy.* Baltimore, MD: Lippincott Williams & Wilkins.

Hunt, L., & Arbesman, M. (2008). Evidence-based and occupational perspective of effective interventions for older clients that remediate or support improved driving performance. *American Journal of Occupational Therapy, 62,* 136-148.

Kelley, K., & Abraham, C. (2004). RCT of a theory-based intervention promoting healthy eating and physical activity amongst outpatients older than 65 years. *Social Science & Medicine, 59,* 787-797.

Korte, J., Bohlmeijer, E. T., Westerhof, G. J., & Pot, A. M. (2001). Reminiscence and adaptation to critical life events in older adults with mild to moderate depressive symptoms. *Aging and Mental Health, 15,* 638-646.

Kozub, M. L. (2013). Through the eyes of the others: Using event analysis to build cultural competence. *Journal of Transcultural Nursing, 24,* 313-318.

Kua, A., Korner-Bitensky, N., Desrosiers, J., Man-Son-Hing, M., & Marshall, S. (2007). Older driver retraining: A systematic review of evidence or effectiveness. *Journal of Safety Research, 38,* 81-90.

Landa-Gonzalez, B., & Molnar, D. (2012). Occupational therapy intervention: Effects in self-care, performance, satisfaction, self-esteem/self-efficiency and the functioning of older Hispanic females with arthritis. *Occupational Therapy and Health Care, 26,* 109-119.

Law, M. (1991). The environment: A focus for occupational therapy (Muriel Driver Memorial Lecture). *Canadian Journal of Occupational Therapy, 58,* 171-179.

Law, M., Cooper, B., Strong, S., Stewart, D., Rigby, P., & Letts, L. (1996). Person-Environment-Occupation Model: A transactive approach to occupational performance. *Canadian Journal of Occupational Therapy, 63,* 9-23.

Leland, N. E., Elliott, S. J., & Johnson, K. J. (2012). *Productive aging for community-dwelling older adults.* Bethesda, MD: AOTA Press.

Mosey, A. C. (1981). *Occupational therapy: Configuration of a profession.* New York: Raven Press.

Mosey, A. C. (1986). *Psychosocial components of occupational therapy.* New York: Raven Press.

Murphy, S. L. (2010). Geriatric research. *American Journal of Occupational Therapy, 64,* 172-181.

Niemeier, J. P., Burnett, D. M., & Whitaker, D. A. (2003). Cultural competence in the multidisciplinary rehabilitation setting: Are we falling short of meeting needs? *Archives of Physical Medicine & Rehabilitation, 84,* 1240-1245.

Paleg, K., & Jongsma, A. E. (2000). *The group therapy treatment planner.* New York: Wiley & Sons, Inc.

Patient Protection and Affordable Care Act (PPACA). (2010). Pub. Law 111-148, #3502, 124 Stat. 119, 124.

Patrick, D. L., Richardson, M., Starks, H. E., Rose, M. A., & Kinne, S. (1997). Rethinking prevention for people with disabilities, part II: A framework for designing interventions. *American Journal of Health Promotion, 11,* 261-263.

Strong, J., Jutai, J. W., Russell-Minda, E., & Evans, M. (2008). Driving and low vision: An evidence-based review of rehabilitation. *Journal of Visual Impairment and Blindness, 102,* 410-419.

Taylor, R. (2008). *The intentional relationship model: Occupational therapy and use of self.* Philadelphia, PA: F.A. Davis.

Wilcock, A. (2006). *An occupational perspective of health* (2nd ed.). Thorofare, NJ: SLACK Incorporated.

U.S. Department of Health and Human Services (2010). *Healthy People 2020* (Brochure). Retrieved from www.healthypeople.gov/2020/TopicsObjectives2020/pdfs/HP2020_brochure_with_508.pdf.

Section II

Productive Occupations in Older Adulthood as Defined Through Productive Aging Study (PAS)

This section focuses on the main findings of the PAS. Based on 40 interviews, this qualitative study explored the meaning of productive aging for older adults who were currently and regularly engaged in at least three of five productive occupations: self-manager, home manager, caregiver, paid worker, and/or lifelong learner. These occupations were derived from a previous study by Knight et al. (2007). Our premise in doing the study was to provide new evidence upon which to base our textbook. We wished to learn what has worked for successful agers, so that we could use this information to assist older adults who might be struggling with age-related issues. It is our observation from doing this study that older adults choose to engage in productive occupations because this makes them happy and gives their lives meaning. There is also ample evidence that remaining active and connected to others through continued social roles and being engaged in self-fulfilling occupations preserves health and well-being, and delays the onset or severity of physical or mental disability.

Following the overview of the PAS qualitative study, we further explore the three main themes: **Chapter 6: Self-Manager**; **Chapter 12: Social Connections: Participation and Strategies**; and **Chapter 13: Self-Fulfilling Activities**. The additional productive occupations that PAS participants defined within the context of self-management are covered in **Chapter 7: Home Manager**; **Chapter 8: Caregiver**; **Chapter 9: Volunteer**; **Chapter 10: Older Worker**; and **Chapter 11: Lifelong Learner**. We included these as separate chapters because each produced a differ-

ent set of participant perspectives, body of research, and guidelines for application to OT practice.

FORMAT OF SECTION II CHAPTERS

The format for most of Section II remains consistent. First, we provide a brief introduction with basic definitions. We then summarize PAS participant perspectives, with quotes and stories they have provided through interviews. A literature review follows, presenting related interdisciplinary research, statistics, and evidence on each productive occupation and theme. Our key research topics reflect themes identified by the participants. There is a great deal of research in each one of these areas, and our literature review is not intended to be all-inclusive, but rather, to capture the current trends, and summarize the evidence upon which we can base OT interventions. The next three sections in these productive occupations chapters also summarize research in specific areas of practice. *Applications for Continuum of Care* looks at how specific occupations of older adulthood might be addressed at the various levels of care: communities or aging in place, retirement communities, assisted living, and long-term care. *Implications for OT Practice* includes an overview of OT approaches and published studies. When available, published program examples have been included. Sometimes, we have interviewed colleagues, clinicians, or experts who work with older adults in these areas. We also share some of our own

Cole MB, Macdonald K.
Productive Aging: An Occupational Perspective (pp 95-96).
© 2015 Taylor & Francis Group.

professional experiences. Within each chapter, we include suggested learning activities to help students and professionals to think about and to integrate the information presented.

Throughout this section, we apply a top-down approach, beginning with the occupations clients choose to do. OT begins at the top, with the client's occupational goals, and works backward from there to address challenge areas or barriers to occupational performance—both client factors, such as foundation skills or physical capacities, and contextual factors, such as social support or adapted physical environments (Weinstock-Zlotnick & Hinojosa, 2004). Because OT professionals understand that the occupations clients have engaged in over their lifetimes have become a part of their personal and social identity (Christiansen, 2001), OTs collaborate with clients to discover facilitators and barriers to continued or desired occupational performance. When health conditions create barriers, OT professionals use a client-centered approach to help clients remediate, adapt, or compensate for the necessary skills and to adapt the various contexts or environments.

Any of the occupation-based models currently in use can support the top-down approach such as the following, Person-Environment-Occupation (PEO) (Law & Dunbar, 2007), Person-Environment-Occupational Performance (PEOP) (Christiansen, Baum, & Bass-Haugen, 2005), Ecology of Human Performance (Dunn, Brown, & McGuigan, 1994), Occupational Adaptation (OA) (Schkade & Schultz, 1992a, 1992b), or Model of Human Occupation (MoHO) (Kielhofner, Forsyth, & Barrett, 2003). All of these approaches take a holistic view of clients within their current circumstances, focusing on the transactions between persons, environments, and occupations when assessing and treating occupational performance issues.

From the results of the PAS study as well as current aging research, it became clear that interventions for older adults should ideally begin much earlier than they currently do, while they are still in the Third Age, in which they are retired but still relatively healthy and socially engaged. All of the successful agers we interviewed for PAS fit the criteria for Laslett's (1989, 1997) Third Age. This is not to say they were all free of disease or disability, but rather that they were good self-managers who made the necessary adaptations so that they could continue to do the occupations most meaningful for them. Prevention and wellness programming at the community level, or through organizations such as AARP or senior centers, would best meet the needs of Third Agers, especially those who might not be as good at self-management as the PAS participants have been. There are many valuable lessons from the PAS, as well as collected evidence to guide OT practitioners working with new retirees, those who are newly widowed, or persons with newly acquired health challenges, about how to remain productive and age successfully. Most of the current OT geriatric practice begins when clients have already begun their final stage of life, Laslett's Fourth Age. Because the current health care system is medically oriented, the onset of illness or disability usually triggers an OT referral.

REFERENCES

Christiansen, C. (2001). Defining lives: Occupation as identity: An essay on competence, coherence, and the creation of meaning. *American Journal of Occupational Therapy, 53*, 547-558.

Christiansen, C., Baum, C., & Bass-Haugen, J. (Eds.) (2005). *Occupational therapy: Performance, participation, and well-being.* Thorofare, NJ: SLACK Incorporated.

Dunn, W., Brown, C., & McGuigan. A. (1994). The ecology of human performance: A framework for considering the effect of context. *American Journal of Occupational Therapy, 48*, 595-607.

Kielhofner, G., Forsyth, K., & Barrett, L. (2003). The model of human occupation. In E. Crepeau, E. Cohn, & B. Schell (Eds.), *Willard & Spackman's occupational therapy* (pp. 212-219). Philadelphia, PA: Lippincott Williams & Wilkins.

Knight, J., Ball, V., Corr, S., Turner, A., Lowis, M., & Ekberg, M. (2007). An empirical study to identify older adults' engagement in productivity occupations. *Journal of Occupational Science, 14*, 145-153.

Laslett, P. (1989). *A fresh map of life: The emergence of the third age.* Cambridge, MA: Harvard University Press.

Laslett, P. (1997). Interpreting the demographic changes. *Philosophical Transactions of the Royal Society B: Biological Sciences, 352*, 1805-1809.

Law, M., & Dunbar, S. (2007). Person-environment-occupation model. In S. Dunbar (ed.). *Occupational therapy models for intervention with children and families* (pp. 27-50). Thorofare, NJ: SLACK Incorporated.

Schkade, J., & Schultz, S. (1992a). Occupational adaptation: Toward a holistic approach to contemporary practice, Part 1. *American Journal of Occupational Therapy, 46*, 829-837.

Schkade, J., & Schultz, S. (1992b). Occupational adaptation: Toward a holistic approach to contemporary practice, Part 2. *American Journal of Occupational Therapy, 46*, 917-926.

Weinstock-Zlotnick, G., & Hinojosa, J. (2004). Bottom-up vs. top-down evaluation: Is one better than the other? *American Journal of Occupational Therapy, 58*, 594-599.

Self-Manager

Marilyn B. Cole, MS, OTR/L, FAOTA

"Self-management is good medicine." (Bandura, 2004, p. 143)

Self-management, the first of three main themes in our productive aging study, may be understood as taking care of oneself on a personal level, performing ADL, as well as making self-directed choices based on one's own priorities within the wider spectrum of social contexts. From the broader perspective, self-management encompasses the selection and development of all of the other social and productive roles discussed in this section: working, volunteering, caregiving, maintaining a home, and lifelong learning. Family and social relationships that have developed over a lifetime have also resulted from choices made along the way. Maintaining social roles and relationships in older adulthood, as participants in our study have repeatedly told us, takes intentional effort after retirement, and thus becomes another important aspect of self-management. Furthermore, the overarching self-determination of our participants in setting goals and organizing their life structure around their own priorities acted to preserve their existing self and social identities.

In this chapter, we will first explore self-management from the perspective of our participants. Next, we review the literature on self-management from different disciplines and compare this with our findings. Then, we examine how self-management is being supported within the current continuum of care, with community dwelling older adults, acute and chronic health care settings, assisted living, and long-term care environments. Finally, we suggest strategies to expand OT's role in supporting self-management across the spectrum of contexts and stages of older adult development.

Learning Activity 43: What Makes You a Good Self-Manager?

1. Describe a typical day, including what you are doing each hour, from the time you get up to bedtime. Are weekdays different from weekend days? How?

2. Which parts of the day are routines (bathing, grooming, dressing, meals, work tasks, cleaning up, maintenance of surroundings and belongings)?

3. What occupational roles currently guide your daily/weekly schedules (work role, student role, family or caregiving role, team or group member, friend)? Name at least three roles.

4. What are the long-term goals that drive your daily/weekly schedules? Name at least three goals.

5. What daily activities and choices contribute to maintaining your physical health? Mental health? Spiritual well-being?

6. How do you prepare for the day's activities? When do you take time to plan ahead?

Cole MB, Macdonald KC.
Productive Aging: An Occupational Perspective (pp 97-114).
© 2015 Taylor & Francis Group.

7. How do the people with whom you interact each day support or create barriers to your successful self-management?

8. Which activities do you consider to be productive?

9. What do you do to relax or recover from stress?

10. How do you manage your finances, and to what extent do you control spending and save for the future?

Participant Perspectives

Our participants defined self-management as an "essential" productive role that continues throughout life, guided by their *self, social, and occupational identities*. This productive occupation was identified by 100% of participants. For some, the will to continue important personal projects or life work drives them to overcome substantial social and health barriers. For example, Johanna (age 73), who now battles ovarian cancer with weekly chemotherapy, still finds a way to continue her elder law practice, in which she sees herself as a helper of mostly older women who face difficult legal situations. Mildred, at age 86, who has multiple sensory and health issues, still writes and revises chapters in textbooks, and volunteers to lead groups of persons with cognitive disabilities, using a technique in which she strongly believes. Pearl (age 79) continues to teach college-level writing courses, despite her balance issues due to Parkinson's. For others, self-care predominates: "living alone, my main role is taking care of myself. I try to remain cheerful and stay busy" (Gerry). "My biggest role is self-management and health maintenance. I must on a daily basis...much time, energy, and attention to medications, changes, and the environment. I can *never* miss a medication, it is part of my routine" (Nancy B.). As a group, the great pride our participants expressed in their very intentionally and skillfully developed self-management truly impressed us.

Reorganizing Life Structure

Part of self-management is choosing meaningful occupations and creating a life structure that supports the most important activities. There is ample evidence from our study that much thought went into constructing a planned lifestyle in retirement that included health maintenance, continuing social connections, and pursuit of self-fulfilling occupations. "An unplanned retirement lifestyle is a recipe for disaster! Yet the execution of a planned retirement lifestyle is clearly an evolutionary process, not always simple in the real, changing world" (Ken). "A planned lifestyle is not automatic; it is developmental and trial and error" (Valnere). "Plan at least 5 years before retirement, not only finances, but also lifestyle. Ask yourself, 'how do I want to spend my days when I am not working?'...Lots of plan-

ning needed...consult others who have retired, what are options?" (Gloria). "I have issues in my life...I could make myself sit home and cry about, but it doesn't do any good. I tell a friend who just wanders around the house, just get out. Seek professional help if needed. You have to take control!" (Mary V.).

In a deliberate and thoughtful way, Pearl describes her intentional planning process: "when I decided to retire in 2009 after 40 years of teaching literature to undergraduates, I began to think about that extra time I would have... free of grading papers and exams and attending meetings. I wanted some of the sense of fulfillment I had as a teacher and learner to continue into my retirement. I wanted the support of an academic community and my own connection to colleagues who had been my friends over the years to continue also. In reviewing what I could do to continue activities and experiences that had provided me with self-fulfillment...I thought first of adjunct teaching, with the idea of scaling back on how much I taught. Going from two courses a semester to one course per year. College teaching has been so much of my identity. It has centered me. It has been a way of defining myself. I had to transform that experience of being a teacher and a learner after I retired. Several colleagues and I began a club to satisfy our social and intellectual needs...we meet at regular times to discuss a novel and a movie based on that novel. The experience is better than reading to teach in a single discipline in the sense that these readers and respondents came from different disciplines and different professional orientations. And best of all, my spouse and I have our 7-month-old grandchild to care for part time. So that could be a continuation of teaching, learning, connection, and self-fulfillment as well."

Clearly there is a sense of *autonomy* and self-determination evident in these statements. Self-management, therefore, implies being in the driver's seat of one's own life. Our participants warn against complacency and dependence, compelling new retirees to take charge of the direction of their lives. *Life management* in retirement includes, but is not limited to, the following,

- Choosing when to retire, and what activities and roles continue thereafter.

- Choosing to stay in one's home or to relocate.

- Finding volunteer roles that satisfy one's needs and wishes.

- Living with others or living alone, continuing or replacing important relationships.

- Deciding to what extent one wishes or feels obligated to provide care to others.

- Finding a second career, or a lower stress/enjoyable way to earn money after retirement.

- Satisfying one's curiosity, traveling, learning new things, keeping informed of news.

- Finding new ways to serve others or to participate more fully in one's community.

- Overcoming barriers to continued engagement in highly valued occupations and relationships.

- Reconnecting with one's lifelong dreams, taking a second chance.

- Nurturing one's own creativity, exploring new parts of the self.

After making these larger decisions, participants need to break down tasks into smaller steps, spreading them out over the course of each day.

Planning Daily Schedules

We asked all of our participants to describe their typical day. Nearly all gave a specific time for getting up in the morning. They depicted specific routines for their morning activities, showering, dressing, eating breakfast, and otherwise getting ready for the day (Figure 6-1). Some used morning time to read a newspaper, while others planned for the rest of their day. Almost without exception, some type of physical exercise figured into their morning routines. At least half of our participants had specific activities scheduled, including part-time paid work, volunteer work, social group meetings, or caregiving obligations, often involving grandchildren. Evening activities included preparing and eating dinner, usually followed by personal time for reading; working on crafts, puzzles or games; and limited TV watching. Specific bedtimes were mostly early (8 to 11 pm), except when an occasional evening event was scheduled (movie, theater, concert, visits).

Skill in managing time and the ability to balance personal tasks with social obligations are needed to successfully manage daily and weekly schedules. *Time management* involves appropriate preparation for the day's activities, planning and sequencing tasks, judgment regarding how long each task will take, and ongoing problem solving when things don't go as planned. A productive self-manager keeps overall goals and priorities in mind as the day unfolds and uses familiar routines whenever possible. *Higher level cognitive functions*, otherwise known as *executive functions*, must be in place to structure a healthy and productive lifestyle in retirement. The OTPF III defines higher level cognitive functions as including "judgment, concept formation, metacognition, executive functions, praxis, cognitive flexibility, (and) insight" (AOTA, 2014, p. S22). "Executive functions are evident anytime multi-tasking is required, when goals need to be formulated to accomplish a task, when tasks have a particular sequence of activities that must be performed for successful completion, when competing stimuli must be ignored to maintain goal-directed activities, or when there is a conflict between what one needs to do and what one would prefer to do" (Connor & Maeir, 2011, p. 53). Most of our participants set

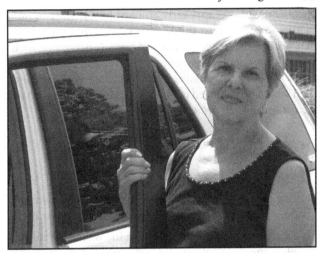

Figure 6-1. Nettie has a busy day planned between errands, volunteering, and social activities. As a good self-manager, she has no trouble managing her time and checking off everything on her list.

goals for themselves and planned activities around those goals. For example, staying informed about local and world news was an important goal for many. Therefore, they found time within each day for reading or watching the news. If service to others was an important priority, they found time each week for volunteering. For example, Betty reads to the blind every Monday afternoon; Mary joins her sister and her family on weekends to volunteer at a local food pantry.

Future Planning

In planning their days participants took into account the need to plan social events with others, or to make appointments and travel plans weeks (or often months) ahead. For example, Peggie and Jack have a goal of keeping in close contact with their family—four sons and a daughter, their spouses, and multiple grandchildren. They set aside a part of each day to e-mail or telephone, search the Internet for interesting things to do together, and make social and travel plans with friends and family members. They also have a routine of family dinners every Sunday, and family vacations every summer.

Some participants expressed unfulfilled plans for the future: "for years I have wanted to move to a new house and get a new car" (Sue S.). Others took steps to plan their own death: "no one wants to talk about it. I've written a letter with all my wishes, along with a living will. I gave it to others upon surgery and they all want to refuse. I have explicit funeral wishes. I want to be cremated and divide my ashes to be with my two husbands. They said they couldn't do it and I told them, 'You can do anything! Figure it out, you can do it!' So the funeral director joked, 'Like Shake 'n Bake?' Yes, I have specific plans for dinner and lunch. Later, I found that earlier letter under a pile of papers that had my second husband's wishes. For me, death has especially been a part of my life because early on I lost people close to me" (Nettie). Mary D. also thinks about "what you want your own death process to be like, not your funeral, but what surroundings, with friends, music? While you are still alive or in the process of passing away. What are your legacies? With whom do you need to make amends? To whom do you entrust unfinished projects you have started?"

Learning Activity 44: Planning Ahead

1. List three ways that you plan ahead in your own life. How does each of these habits contribute to your life?

2. Describe a situation in your own life when you did not plan ahead. What was the outcome? What could you have done differently to produce a better outcome?

3. List three ways that you might challenge your clients to plan ahead in their lives. What might be the benefits of each of suggestion for clients?

Financial Planning and Management

Financial planning is a very important part of managing one's life in retirement. Participants often began saving decades earlier than the anticipated date of retirement, and adequate finances figured strongly into their decision about when to stop working for pay. Malcolm shares one secret of successful aging: "First, eliminate any money concerns by, as soon as you have income, religiously investing a significant portion of that income for your eventual retirement, preferably in tax advantaged vehicles such as 401k plans or IRAs. Those are not, of course, the only investments you should be making. Houses have proven to be good investments with further benefit that you enjoy your home while it (usually) appreciates in value." After 4 years of retirement, Greg has a goal to "never outlive my income…I disciplined myself to save half of my income for many years so I could afford to retire at age 64 with no worries. Now I manage my investments to provide needed income, so I can afford to drive a nice car, go to the city (New York) for dinner and theater, travel and invest in antiques." Ann M. sees a financial advisor: "It was important to save money. We had a retirement person within our school system, and I was able to save in an IRA with help from work." Linval recommends saving as much as you can: "If you are getting ready to retire, save for it." Gloria suggests planning at least 5 years before retirement, "so that your lifestyle won't have to change." Jim M. stated that to "Have money in the bank, it overcomes a lot of the problems of aging."

Saving money was described by several as a *habit* learned early. Bob M. states, "I keep up with the bills. I ask for senior discounts! I learned as a kid I couldn't have it if I couldn't pay for it (no credit card habits)." June states, "You are always trying to overcompensate for what you missed. We

didn't have much money, so I worked to help pay bills from age 16. It is a lesson learned from parents…never stop being productive. I worked very hard to get out of poverty to a more comfortable life. *Self-discipline* is part of who I am."

Learning Activity 45: Financial Management Interview

Identify an older individual whom you believe is a good financial manager. Make sure he or she would be comfortable having a general conversation with you about money management.

1. Investigate the person's lifelong habits and patterns for managing (e.g., income, bills, investments, saving, budgeting, and spending).

2. How is this person planning for retirement, or how has he or she planned for retirement?

3. Inquire about suggestions that he or she would make for your lifetime of money management.

Positive Attitude and Spiritual Beliefs

One of the surprise findings of our study was the unanimous acceptance among participants of the process of aging as a part of life. None focused on aches and pains: "I ignore them. I can figure out what is going on and take steps to correct it. I go to the doctor for my once a year checkup. I thank him, and continue on my merry way for the next year" (Bob M.). "Don't give in to aches and pains. Push through them. You are better off: get up in the morning, limber up and get out and go! You're going to have it [worse] when you are older, so work through it now" (Nettie). Gerry recommends "try to remain cheerful and don't complain all the time. Try to enjoy each day as it comes."

An upbeat attitude predominated most interviews. Ray P. recommends "Take it easy and live every day as it comes. A good attitude is worth its weight in gold." "I want to be like my husband: enjoy every day" (Ann M.). "Keep your spirits up. Tomorrow is going to be a better day.…you need to have a Pollyanna attitude. Try not to be influenced by the negatives of the world—news, other people's down feelings, others who always see the bad side of things" (Nancy B.). Jim M. wears funny t-shirts: "I like to make people smile. I'll never forget what my father taught me, 'It's not the situation but how you deal with it that matters.'" Ellen concurs, "My motto when I worked was 'if you can't laugh every day, don't bother coming to work!' I still try to do that—make others laugh." "Keep a positive outlook and ability to see the humor in various situations" (Jan). June recommends, "Be positive. Expect it to be good. Don't ever give up! Out of all bad things, something good comes. Something unexpected." The positive attitude is not automatic, but intentional, and takes effort. Mildred encourages herself, "Don't judge yourself. Practice being kind. Keep motivated to look ahead, but take small steps. Be more courageous." Participants also suggested using social connections to support their positive attitude, such as "avoiding negative people," "surrounding yourself with others who keep you involved" (Gloria), and "choosing to be with people who understand and support you" (Mary). Some, like Peggie and Margie, turned to their spiritual beliefs and prayer as positive supports, while others suggested ways to deal with the negative: "When faced with distressing situations, remain calm, size up the situation, work at what is needed to relieve stress. Set up steps in sequence, set in motion, avoid panic" (Bob M.). Doing for others helped Sue H. keep things in perspective: "So many people are worse off than me. I am a good listener. I help where I can." Margie recommends: "Go where you are needed, where you can help the most."

Managing One's Own Aging Process (Health Management)

Without exception, participants included taking steps to remain healthy and fit in their planned lifestyles. Health management includes managing one's own health—getting preventive health screenings, making appointments for annual checkups (such as physicals, eye examinations, and dental examinations), and following up on recommendations to prevent illness or injury (such as flu shots, taking dietary supplements, getting enough exercise).

Remaining physically active was a priority for most participants (Figure 6-2). Ken recommends, "take time for exercise—regular exercise to maintain flexibility and tone." Malcolm "maintains a lifetime physical fitness program. Do aerobic exercises for at least 30 minutes at least 5 times a week. Do muscle strengthening exercises with weights at least 30 minutes, at least 3 times a week. Make sure you lose weight as you inevitably lose muscle tone." He continues, "Maintain a lifetime mental fitness program, both in areas where you're already competent and areas you're not. This is not so much from the standpoint of developing erudition as in forcing your brain to continually cope with foreign concepts and ways of attacking problems." This concept is backed up by evidence that engaging in cognitively challenging tasks throughout life can actually prevent dementia later in life (Yang, 2012).

Some participants pointed out the need for *self-discipline* to stick to healthy routines, like daily walks and exercising. Mildred learned self-discipline early: "My ancient parents were role models—just do it, no excuses. If I don't feel like exercising before breakfast, I still hear their voices: '20 minutes won't kill you, Mildred!'...When I feel like taking a nap, I take a walk instead." Gloria concurs, "Discipline yourself to exercise, go for walks." Some participants made exercise a part of their daily routine. *Routines* are "patterns of behavior that are observable, regular, repetitive, and that provide structure for daily life" (AOTA, 2014, p. S27). "Have a daily fitness routine" (Pearl). Bob C., Jack, and

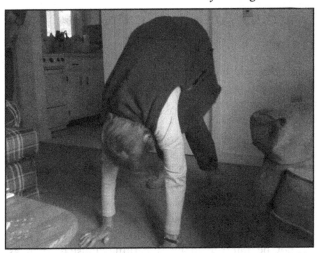

Figure 6-2. Patricia, age 91, demonstrates her flexibility, preserved by her daily practice of yoga stretches.

Peggie exercise daily at a gym. After planning, routines can be helpful for remembering to do things on time, like eating three meals each day, keeping appointments, walking and exercising, and following up with ongoing treatments or medications.

Other parts of *prevention* are also mentioned, like diet and nutrition, a balanced level of activity, and getting enough sleep. Gloria recommends, "Care for your own health. Get enough sleep, food, exercise. Be actively involved in your own health care. I eat earlier, have balanced meals, and exercise early so I can go to bed earlier." Mary likes to "try different recipes for healthy meals." Bob T. suggests eating right, watching Ph balance, and drinking filtered water. "Be informed about your own health. Use the Internet." Peggie "eat[s] healthy and in moderation... exercise, stretch daily, walk, garden, sleep 7 to 8 hours." Bob C. suggests "watch nutrition, exercise to stay fit." "Be mindful of your physical well-being—maintaining your diet and exercising as you are able" (Mary V).

In the opinion of most participants, "keeping tabs on health, regular checkups, and following up on treatments/meds" (Pearl) is only the beginning. It also includes independently gathering information about one's own health through the Internet or other sources and taking steps to correct problems and reduce symptoms that interfere with functioning. For some, this meant regulating their diet, breaking bad habits such as smoking, and stimulating their mind. For others, acute and chronic health conditions challenge their ability to continue life as usual. Some of these include diabetes, high blood pressure, heart disease, stroke, depression, ovarian cancer, fractures, and Parkinson's disease. Many take medications, wear glasses and hearing aids, avoid certain activities such as driving at night or climbing stairs, and make adaptations such as slowing pace, resting more frequently, "pacing self, resting, and taking breaks" (Gloria). Still, an optimistic outlook prevails: "Treat health conditions as problems to solve" (Malcolm).

Learning Activity 46: Breaking Bad Habits

Identify one bad habit you wish to break. Examples might be eating sweets, overeating, procrastinating, smoking, watching too much TV, being late, or playing addictive computer games. Find a partner to work with you, who also has a bad habit to break. You and your partner will need to be in touch daily for 2 weeks or more to complete this activity. (Note: If a partner is not available, you can try this alone, writing the results each day in a journal).

1. Briefly describe the bad habit, how it interferes with your life, and why you wish to break it. Discuss this habit with your partner. Choose 2 weeks that will not be interrupted by something unusual, such as holidays, planned travel, or unavoidable social events or obligations.

2. Write your goal in behavioral terms. For example, "Within 2 weeks, I will limit my intake of sweets to 100 calories per day." Be as specific as possible, but also be realistic.

3. Meet with your partner and both of you create a calendar for the next 2 weeks. For example, create a table on your computer, such as the one below, with days and dates written in. Briefly write your schedule for each day. Enlarge spaces as needed.

SUN	MON	TUES	WED	THURS	FRI	SAT

4. Write one positive action each day to break the bad habit. For example, you might begin by clearing out your room, pantry, or refrigerator of all sweet snacks that might tempt you. You might research alternative healthy snacks and stock up on those. Quitting some things "cold turkey" might have consequences to consider. Looking up relevant information might also become a daily activity. Discuss the feasibility of your plan with your partner.

5. Set a time to contact one another at the end of each day to report the success or failure of your plan. Decide on a reward if you succeeded, and a negative consequence if you failed. Make sure these are also realistic (e.g., one 100-calorie candy bar as a reward). If you failed, you must eat something healthy that you hate or you must go to class or work the next day wearing a big sticker on your chest depicting a frowning face. Choose something appropriate to the goal. Write the rewards and consequences on your calendar. Each of you send a copy of the completed plan to your partner.

6. Carry out the plan for 2 weeks. Afterwards describe the result in a short paragraph. How did your plan work? What about it didn't work? What would you change?

7. What did you learn from trying this exercise?

8. How might you assist a client who wishes to break a bad habit?

Note: Generally, it takes longer than 2 weeks to form a habit and even longer to break one. According to behavioral theory, the key to success is to avoid rewarding a bad habit unintentionally or by repetition of the habit without any negative consequence. A partner helps you by reminding you to stick to the plan, witnessing your successes, and forcing you to face your failures. Encouraging one another gives social support to the effort.

Choosing Occupations and Social Roles That Support One's Individual and Social Identity

It surprised us that so many participants mentioned identity in their answers to questions. For example, Ken states, "You've succeeded if you have made peace with yourself and look forward to defining yourself outside your work identity." Betty identifies herself as a "cultural snob" and a "survivor." She hates ugliness and very much appreciates beauty, especially through the arts. Margie has a strong "Hispanic identity, coming from a large Puerto Rican family." Bob T. mentions a strong identity as ex-military, ex-international pilot for Trans World Airlines, Midwesterner, and conservative Republican. A few mentioned ethnic backgrounds: Gerry is Irish; Sue is an Englishwoman; and June, Betty, and Bob C. identify with the New York City way of life. Some deny a strong identity with religion: Betty is a self-professed "collapsed Jew," meaning she does not practice except for high holy days. Valnere was brought up Anglican but married a Catholic. Mary was formerly a Catholic nun, but now more strongly identifies with her professional identity as an OT educator. Below are some examples of how occupations are viewed as expressions of social identity:

- Planning ahead for travel with friends and family, attending cultural events, getting together with others, participating in organizations.

- Continuing to do what you love (teaching, practicing law, managing finances).

- Serving society, giving back, altruism.

- Creative expression, taking art classes, musical participation.

- Adult learning—Elderhostel, travel tours, book clubs, "stimulating discussions with other mature seekers of wisdom" (Malcolm).

Learning Activity 47: Exploring Social Identities

The participants' comments exemplify some of the reasons why people choose to engage in productive occupations as a way to self-manage by protecting their long-held beliefs about themselves and the image they wish to project to those around them. Review your answers to the social roles questions in Chapter 1 and list five here. What can you say about the way each role contributes to your social identity?

1.

2.

3.

4.

5.

LITERATURE REVIEW

Using the key word *self-management*, two categories currently dominate the literature: business and health care. While these fields define self-management somewhat differently, both resonate with the way our participants viewed their own self-manager role.

Business Literature

Business and education refer to self-management as the skills and strategies by which individuals can effectively direct their own activities toward the achievement of objectives. This includes goal setting, decision making, focusing, planning, scheduling, self-evaluation, and self-development. The way our participants planned and directed their lives in retirement also included these executive processes but aimed them at personal rather than corporate or educational objectives.

The Morning Star Self-Management Institute (2012) describes self-management as "among the most revolutionary organizational models known to modern business." Within this model, employees are "personally responsible for forging their own personal relationships, planning their own work, coordinating their actions with other members, acquiring requisite resources to accomplish their mission, and for taking corrective action with respect to other members when needed" (Morning Star Self-Management Institute, 2012). For example, when Taco Bell created thousands of new locations in the early 1990s, it used self-management training to decrease the number of higher-paid managers necessary for this initiative. Employees were trained and given new technology to enable them to hire, train, and supervise their new colleagues and deal with day-to-day issues under the supervision of a "floating" manager. Teams of workers self-managed each store, result-ing in more highly energized workers, better cost control, higher customer satisfaction, and new ideas for organizing work. Costco and Wal-Mart have adopted similar strategies (O'Toole & Lawler, 2006). From a business perspective, some corporations question the concept of employee or team self-management, citing attitude as equal in importance to skills and abilities (Haskett, 2006). In other words, self-management only works with employees who have the right attitude to begin with and cannot be successful with every worker (Haskett, 2006).

Health Care Literature

In 2004, Albert Bandura used the occasion of his acceptance of the Healthtrac Foundation Award to make some observations about the power of self-management. He stated, "The quality of health is heavily influenced by lifestyle habits. This enables people to exercise some measure of control over their health. By managing their health habits, people can live longer and healthier and retard the process of aging" (Bandura, 2004, p. 143). He predicted that the "days for the supply-side health system are limited," meaning medications and medical-surgical procedures or equipment. "Demand is overwhelming supply…psychosocial factors partly determine whether the extended life is lived efficaciously or with debility, pain, and dependence" (Bandura, 2004, p. 144). Bandura (2004) cites five determinants of health:

1. Knowledge: Knowing the risks and benefits of different health practices.

2. Perceived self-efficacy: The belief that one can control one's own health habits.

3. Outcome expectations: The potential costs and benefits of different actions.

4. Health goals people set for themselves: Concrete plans and strategies for realizing them.

5. Perceived facilitators and impediments: What social and structural conditions help or hinder the changes people seek.

These determinants can also serve as guidelines for OT evaluations and interventions that support the productive occupation of self-management. Bandura (2004) provides some powerful reasons for OTs to place a greater focus on developing and supporting self-management abilities with their older clients.

The health care literature refers to self-management of health risks or conditions, including managing symptoms and taking measures to prevent disability. The Health Council of Canada focuses on self-management of chronic conditions, and defines the critical role of self-management support for health care providers. Self-management support is "interventions to help clients gain the confidence, knowledge, skills, and motivation to manage the physical, social, and emotional impacts of their disease" (Health Council of

Canada, 2012). While patient education lays the foundation for self-management, service providers must follow up with actively shared decision making and empowering clients in assuming personal responsibility. Furthermore, educational interventions should be personalized and individualized to patients, and their follow through with management (of diabetes, in this study) can be tracked, monitored, and reported (Beebe & Schmitt, 2011). In an article discussing self-management of fibromyalgia, Campbell (2012) outlines the skills and challenges of self-management that could apply to any long-term illness. His approach begins with the balancing of acceptance and hope. "Acceptance means that they acknowledged that they had a long-term condition that imposed limits and required that they adapt," but they still retained the confidence that they could do things to improve (Campbell, 2012, p. 1). Four basic skills for self-management are as follows:

1. Learning about the illness.
2. Seeking help from professionals.
3. Experimenting with different strategies to see what works best.
4. Problem solving.

The five challenges are as follows:

1. Managing symptoms.
2. Controlling stress.
3. Getting support.
4. Managing emotions.
5. Adjusting to loss (adapted from Campbell, 2012).

Occupational Therapy Literature

Most OT researchers use the term *self-management* within the context of chronic health conditions. Some authors have differentiated between patient education and self-management: "patient education usually means giving patient(s) information (material and instruction) regarding their condition and possible management… Self-management facilitates problem solving by self: help to define problems, generate possible solutions, implement solutions, evaluate results, based on having enough and appropriate information…Content is based on collaboration between patients and professionals" (Fung & Bobby, 2011, p. 1). These authors suggest a facilitated group format where members can exchange information, both successes and failures, and participate in sharing and discussion. A good self-management program helps patients build the skills necessary for behavior change and fosters "a sense of achievement and self-efficacy" (Fung & Bobby, 2011, p. 2). The distinction between education and self-management is confirmed in a fall self-efficacy study, finding that while education raised awareness of fall risk, it failed to affect self-efficacy or dynamic balance in participants (Garcia, Marciniak, McCune, Smith, & Ramsey, 2012).

In reviewing the literature on diabetes self-management, Pyatak (2011, p. 89) sees OT as a "largely untapped potential to assist individuals who struggle with managing diabetes in the context of everyday life." For self-management of people with migraines, OT practitioners "add a unique dimension to self-management by utilizing it as a means to 1) restore or maintain engagement in valued tasks (or occupations) that have been disrupted by migraine, and 2) achieve a satisfying balance amongst self-care productivity and leisure occupations" (McLean & Coutts, 2011, p. 5). Engagement and balance in occupations have been shown to promote health and well-being (Aegler & Satink, 2009). An OT group intervention for chronic fatigue self-management was converted to an online delivery as a way to increase access by Ghahari and Packer (2011). The content, activities, and discussion topics from a 6-week course for energy conservation reconstructed online were user-friendly for people with basic computer skills and included group blogs for interaction among users. Online facilitators were usually OTs, and authors reported that the most popular part of the program was the group discussions. In a randomized controlled trial of an OT program for early rheumatoid arthritis, self-management significantly increased in the OT group over the control (Hammond, Young, & Kidao, 2004).

For dealing with chronic pain, the International Association for the Study of Pain outlines a proposed OT curriculum, including a section on self-management of chronic pain (Brown et al., 2012). It includes the following:

- Use occupations and activities with meaning to the client.
- Incorporate activity tolerance, energy conservation, pacing, use of pain management strategies, and therapeutic modalities to promote activity, relapse prevention, and management.
- Discuss sleep and sleep hygiene.
- Address intimacy and sexuality.
- Include back care.
- Utilize individual and group approaches for education, support, self-efficacy, and advocacy.
- Provide patient with skills for health system navigation.

This curriculum suggests use of a client-centered approach in which clients collaborate with professionals in creating a daily routine incorporating self-management strategies according to client capacities, goals, and life situation, also involving family members and significant others when appropriate. It further includes developing plans for reintegration into work (productivity) using client goals (Brown et al., 2013).

APPLICATIONS TO CONTINUUM OF CARE

Aging in Place and Community Programs

The best time to develop and support the self-manager role is while retirees continue to live independently in their own homes. In the broader sense, people have always been (to some degree) self-managers, making choices and taking responsibility for those choices over their entire lives to date. Planning for retirement before it occurs, as an individual or group intervention, could be an effective way for OTs to raise awareness of the importance of good self-management as one ages. Targeting community organizations, such as senior centers and other groups whose members might be older (AARP, AAUW, church-related groups, Rotary, Grange), present opportunities to introduce wellness and prevention strategies, such as fall prevention, home safety, medication management, nutrition, and fitness. Models such as the Lifestyle Redesign (Clark et al., 1997, 2011) guide such strategies using a group format, focusing on the importance of occupations in a healthy senior lifestyle.

Primary Care and Home Care

As OTs prepare to expand their roles with older adults, primary care becomes the logical place to support client self-management. According to the interdisciplinary health care literature, the Chronic Care Model, published by Improving Chronic Illness Care (ICIC) (2009), seeks to overcome the fragmentation that now exists in medical service delivery by rethinking public policies and reorganizing the health care system. One of the six main elements of this model is self-management support for an "informed, activated patient" (ICIC, 2009). The model calls for interventions beginning before the occurrence of a health crisis, ideally at the level of primary care. For example, OTs could market their services to primary care physicians, walk-in clinics, or wellness clinics, or they could apply for grants for specific self-management programs, such as those exemplified in the next section. OT practitioners have been encouraged to prepare for interventions at this beginning stage, when a chronic illness is first diagnosed, so that self-management strategies can be put in place to prevent disability. OTs also have the skills to guide clients in adapting ADL and preferred occupations and maintaining or improving desirable levels of physical and mental functioning, so that the older client's quality of life, social identity, and sense of well-being are preserved.

Home care presents another opportunity for OT to support the self-management role, within the context of specific acute or chronic health conditions. During home care visits, OTs can provide education about the condition, teach appropriate skills for self-management, and encourage clients to make choices about adapting their life, as well as managing their illness. Family members, caregivers, and significant others could also be involved. Encouraging, coaching, and otherwise empowering clients to take charge of their own health helps to develop the skill of self-advocacy, enabling them to get their own needs met and to remove barriers preventing them from fully participating in their valued activities, families, and communities.

Because self-management requires maintaining high-level cognitive skills, encouraging clients to continually challenge themselves to learn and problem-solve, and to practice engaging in complex tasks or occupations can help to prevent cognitive decline in older adulthood.

Assisted Living and Retirement Communities

When seniors choose to move into retirement communities, they also need to create their own life structure by choosing activities that help maintain mental and physical fitness, as well as their desired level of social interaction. OTs can assist with the transition of relocation in many ways, such as organizing or downsizing belongings, creating barrier-free environments, and scheduling activities that balance social participation with health-promoting routines and needed rest.

Assisted living centers might represent the next higher level of care. When older adults experience a change in the level of care they need, they continue self-management by choosing their caregivers and supervising and monitoring the care they receive. This type of self-management has also been called "mature dependence" (Soderhamm, Skisland, & Herrman, 2011). When the onset of illness triggers the need for increased care, it might be tempting to allow others to dictate care parameters, which may not consider client choices or occupational priorities. OTs can discuss with clients ways to find or continue meaningful occupations within the new facility, making adaptations or compensating for the limitations caused by illness, without losing valued social and occupational roles. For example, Mildred recently moved into a "congregate housing" facility, which offers multiple levels of care. While the facility requires residents to eat lunch together, Mildred prefers to prepare her own meals. She also continues her own writing projects and prefers outside activities with friends or family to those offered by the facility. She takes charge of her own health with good nutrition and a daily exercise routine, as well as doctor visits. The only service she accepts is a weekly housecleaning. At age 87, she lives with a variety of health risks, but she is determined to make her own choices and remain in control of her own life. As such, she is an excellent self-manager.

Rehabilitation Settings

Clients in rehabilitation facilities have often experienced abrupt changes in health. Concurrently, OT often focuses narrowly on discrete areas of functioning, such as feeding or toileting, as limited by an existing medically oriented reimbursement system. What is the role of client self-management in this environment? In planning for discharge, what might be some ways an OT could think more holistically about what clients need to learn long-term after rehabilitation ends?

Learning Activity 48: Client-Centered Priorities During Inpatient Rehabilitation

Assume that an unmarried older uncle of yours had a stroke and you visit him in an inpatient rehabilitation facility, where he will stay for 90 days. You will be his caregiver when he returns home to his apartment until he achieves a level of independence where he can live alone.

1. Stroke is a layman's term for cerebral vascular accident (CVA). Look this up on the Internet and write a short summary of a typical right-sided CVA, with partial paralysis or weakness on one side of the body.

2. Your uncle has 3 requests of you: a) take care of his dog while he is hospitalized (walked on a leash 3 times a day), b) start up his car and drive it once a week so the battery doesn't run down, and c) bring him his mail and his checkbook so he can pay his bills. Considering each of these activities from an OT perspective, what problems might you anticipate your uncle will have because of the stroke when he returns home?

3. What might an OT do to support self-management in anticipation of the 3 productive occupations your uncle wishes to continue after discharge? For each occupation, describe a skill he will need to strengthen while still in rehabilitation.

   a. Home manager

   b. Caregiver

   c. Driving

Long-Term Care

None of our participants lived in long-term care facilities. However, even there, good self-management remains critical to a resident's quality of life. Clients who retain the ability to bathe, groom, dress, and feed themselves should not be forced to allow others to take over these tasks. Residents in nursing homes can still make choices about how self-care should be done, what clothing to wear, how their hair should be styled, and how they wish to look for their various daily activities. Patricia, one of our participants, had to move to a moderate care setting within her retirement community following a minor stroke that affected her balance. However, she still performed all of her self-care, dressed herself (although she used the laundry service), took daily walks around the halls of the facility in winter, and chose with whom she sat for meals in the dining room, even though she no longer cooked. She enjoyed some of the group activities offered, such as yoga, meditation, and a writer's workshop, which she took turns leading. She cherished her afternoon cup of tea while reading *The Economist* (because it is impartial). Self-management for Patricia was evident in the choices she made and by her continued participation in the occupations she valued most.

IMPLICATIONS FOR OCCUPATIONAL THERAPY PRACTICE

Self-management always means taking control of your own life, even if you choose to give up control of some aspects. For example, in mature dependence an older adult retains autonomy, but delegates assistance with some life tasks to selected others (Soderhamm et al., 2011). One participant, Geno, agrees that "self-management is fulfilling and challenging if one is capable but one must be aware of his/her abilities to do all that is required…whether in full or in part…It doesn't hurt to get help. Why go it alone if you can get help for free or for little money?" Geno's comment brings into focus the concept of self-awareness and the ability to judge when it is no longer safe to participate in certain activities. Geno himself experienced a mini-stroke after our initial interview but before making this follow-up comment. He recognized that a newly emerged impulsivity made it more difficult for him to perform complex tasks, such as meal preparation, baking, or driving to medical appointments, and that his wife now needed to help him with these tasks. OTs need to assess clients' levels of awareness, as well as their other executive functions, to determine the degree of self-management for which they are capable. Families, partners, and friends may provide critical information or offer needed assistance and should be included in any self-management support initiative when client self-awareness and judgment are questioned.

Occupational Therapy Practice Framework (OTPF III)

For the OT profession, the AOTA's (2014) OTPF III defines some aspects of the role of self-manager. *Activities of daily living* (ADL) are defined as "activities that are oriented toward taking care of one's own body…also referred to as basic or personal activities of daily living" (p. S19).

The framework lists these activities as bathing/showering, toileting and toilet hygiene, dressing, swallowing/eating, feeding, functional mobility, personal device care, personal hygiene and grooming, and sexual activity. *Instrumental activities of daily living* (IADL) are defined as "activities to support daily life within the home and community that often require more complex interactions than those used in ADL" (AOTA, 2014, p. S19). The IADLs listed are care of others, care of pets, child rearing, communication management, driving and community mobility, financial management, health management and maintenance, home establishment and management, meal preparation and cleanup, religious and spiritual activities and expression, safety and emergency maintenance, and shopping. IADLs often involve stepping outside oneself and one's home and interacting with others in outside environments. *Rest and sleep* was added in 2008 as a separate area of occupation, which includes "activities related to obtaining restorative rest and sleep to support healthy active engagement in other occupations" (AOTA, 2014, p. S20). The other areas of occupation in the OTPF III document—education, work, play, leisure, and social participation—were all defined as productive occupations by our participants.

The older adults in our study placed emphasis on some of these OTPF III categories, while barely mentioning others. Some areas of IADL fell within the separate productive roles of home manager and caregiver. Participants also added aspects of self-management that are not mentioned in the framework, such as maintaining a positive attitude, nurturing creativity, establishing a life structure (healthy lifestyle), serving others, and pursuing lifelong dreams.

Occupational Therapy Evaluations and Interventions

The first tool available to OTs in supporting the self-manager role for clients is therapeutic use of self. In establishing a foundation for the therapeutic relationship, OT practitioners demonstrate respect for the client's point of view and ask questions that communicate genuine concern for their clients' freedom to make informed choices, set their own goals, plan their own future, and take responsibility for their own aging process.

In thinking about this, it may be useful to consider the possible reasons why older adults might not be good self-managers. Try the learning activity listed below to better understand how potential clients might struggle with self-management.

Learning Activity 49: Barriers to Good Self-Management

Think about people you know whom you do not consider to be good self-managers. List six reasons why they might struggle with this skill. Consider both physical and mental, as well as cultural, issues.

1.

2.

3.

4.

5.

6.

Discuss how these barriers might be removed or these problems overcome.

The OT uses a client-centered approach, allowing the client to choose the direction of intervention, and first supporting strengths while gathering information for the client's occupational profile. While the AOTA (2014) suggests that the initial interview focus on occupational preferences, issues, and goals, the conversation should also allow the OT to determine other self-management prerequisites, such as self-awareness and insight, level of cognitive abilities, belief in self-efficacy, level of self-direction or motivation, future outlook, and existing social connections and relationships that could become supports as the client struggles to overcome barriers to participation. The client cannot choose occupational goals and priorities without basic self-management capabilities in place.

Some basic questions that reveal the client's skills for self-management include the following:

- Describe what you do on a typical day (extent of intentional planning and structuring).
- What habits or routines do you follow to keep yourself healthy and fit?
- What health conditions have challenged your engagement in activities and how did you adapt, overcome, and/or manage them?
- What occupations or activities contribute most to your social identity (i.e., social roles or ways you might describe yourself to others who don't know your occupational history)?
- What activities give you the most pleasure or self-fulfillment?
- To what extent do you continue to participate in self-fulfilling occupations?
- How many social groups do you belong to? What are they, and how often do you attend?
- What are some of your plans, hopes, and dreams for the future?
- What are your current challenges to occupational functioning?
- What are your goals and priorities for OT?

We know from developmental theory that continuity is important for aging successfully, making a good transition to retirement, and staying connected and engaged with others. Therefore, when we work with clients who may not know how to be good self-managers, the more basic skills such as self-awareness, self-identity, and self-efficacy may become a prerequisite to making any well-informed decisions about future occupational engagement. An older adult who has recently encountered an acquired health condition, suffered a significant loss or trauma, or experienced an unwanted and unplanned retirement or an unexpected relocation may need support to pick up the self-manager role again. A starting point might be through reviewing past occupations, roles, identities, and social connections and exploring new ways to put the puzzle that was him- or herself back together within a whole new set of circumstances. This will require the OT to first establish a strong therapeutic relationship through therapeutic use of self to re-engage the client's desire to take charge of his or her own life.

Areas for Occupational Therapy Intervention

OT practitioners and clients need to appreciate the prominence of the self-manager role. Before they take on any other productive roles, they must first take care of themselves. This is especially important for clients who are caregivers because they have a tendency to neglect their own needs and give priority to the needs of care recipients. But this productive occupation is basic to everyone who wants to age successfully, as well as any client struggling to overcome acute or chronic health conditions.

- *Self-Care*: Bathing, dressing, eating nutritious meals, getting rest and sleep.

- *Managing One's Own Aging Process/Health Maintenance*: Taking prescribed medications, getting flu shots, physical check-ups, and dental check-ups, walking and keeping fit, breaking bad habits like smoking, managing chronic health conditions like diabetes and high blood pressure by following medical advice and precautions.

- *Self-Awareness*: Thinking about what you really want to do, finding or continuing the activities that give you the most satisfaction, knowing your own limitations, and asking for help when you need it.

- *Organizing Life Structure*: Choosing and prioritizing the productive roles that mean the most to you, then taking steps to develop or maintain these roles with others, whether working, volunteering, maintaining a home, caring for someone important to you, or learning something new.

- *Structuring Daily Activities*: Whatever the choice, the various tasks that are necessary to perform this occupational role need to become a part of each day's sched-

ule, such as hours for working, caregiving obligations, and social activities. A balance must be found between obligations to others and meeting one's own needs.

- *Financial Planning and Management*: This involves creating and following a budget based on expected income and known expenses. It also includes finding public programs and resources for which you qualify when income is limited, as well as self-discipline in setting spending limits when necessary.

- *Positive Attitude and Spiritual Strength*: Even emotions come under our control. Our participants took intentional actions to remain optimistic, including connecting with others who kept them involved and avoiding negative people. Religious beliefs often supported them in times of trouble, especially when dealing with grief and loss.

- *Setting Priorities*: A higher level function that allows individuals to make decisions based on importance, timing, and situational factors. This includes establishing a balance of occupations and activities that considers one's time, energy, and personal care needs, as well as meaning for oneself.

Self-Management of Basic Activities of Daily Living

A review of the basic self-care might prevent older adults from neglecting something important, such as taking time to bathe and dress appropriately, put on makeup or shave, style their hair, and generally feel good about the way they present themselves to others. Older adults who have scheduled activities that put them in contact with others probably do these things routinely, but those with health challenges may have limited energy or interest in basic self-care tasks. OT evaluation would logically explore any health conditions that might be better managed, freeing up time and energy for engaging in more meaningful, productive occupations. For older adults who take on caregiving roles, it is especially important for the OT to make sure they are also taking care of themselves.

Cognitive Health Self-Management

No one can be a good self-manager without maintaining higher level cognitive abilities. It is necessary to organize and structure one's life, set priorities and future goals, and solve problems that create barriers along the way. With recent advances in research on the prevention of cognitive decline, we can feel confident in advising clients to seek out mental stimulation and challenge themselves with complex tasks and new learning. There are several websites that address this area, but engaging in complex occupations may be more effective when they apply to the client's own life. Please refer to Chapter 11 for more information about maintaining cognitive health.

Self-Management of Chronic Health Conditions

Most studies from the health care disciplines define self-management in terms of managing a health condition, viewing this as a strategy to reduce health care costs for older adults, as well as enhancing their quality of life. Although the participants in our productive aging study revealed a much broader definition, self-management support as an OT intervention has been recommended in the recent literature. "Providing evidence-based interventions that include using self-management support is the key to improving clients' satisfaction with managing their chronic health conditions, thus improving outcomes overall....(It) highlights the pivotal role OT practitioners can play in improving performance outcomes with their clients through the therapeutic use of self and engaging our clients in productive conversations about behavior change" (DeRosa, 2013, p. CE-1). DeRosa (2013) suggests using guidelines from two sources, motivational interviewing (MI) decision support and self-management support techniques, to build partnerships that empower clients to take charge of their own health management. MI, proposed by Miller and Rollinick (2002), prepares clients for change by encouraging internal motivation through three main principles: competence, autonomy, and relatedness/relevance. Home Health Quality National Improvement Campaign (HHQI), (2012) recommends five self-management techniques as follows:

1. *Establish a focus*: The OT fully explores the client's understanding and experience of the chronic health condition, including thoughts, feelings, perceived facilitators and barriers, and strength of self-efficacy and motivation.

2. *Share information*: The OT imparts current evidence about the condition and its treatment, including risk factors, symptom management, and changes to consider.

3. *Develop shared goals*: The OT and client brainstorm together possible tasks leading to controlling the condition, adapting desired activities/occupations, and otherwise making life more manageable in both the short and long term. OTs must lead the client toward self-discovery and active problem solving rather than suggesting solutions prematurely.

4. *Create an action plan*: Based on the client's personal goals, the OT develops a written plan with measurable steps toward achievement.

5. *Use a problem-solving approach*: OTs ask questions that lead the client to an awareness of self-doubting, making poor choices, rejecting needed supports, or otherwise giving up control, allowing these barriers to slow progress toward goals. The OT, through validation of client effort and encouragement of client self-management, enables the client to use feedback, evidence, or other information in ways that help to overcome barriers to goal achievement.

Decision support is the third OT guideline suggested by DeRosa (2013) as a self-management intervention strategy. Decision support is defined as "promoting clinical care guidelines and tools embedded with current evidence-based interventions which will meet the diverse health literacy levels of our patients" (Koh, Brach, Harris, & Parchman, 2013, p. 361). For the skilled OT practitioner, "customizing tools and tailoring information" (DeRosa, 2013, p. CE6) naturally flows with therapeutic use of self, as OTs continually observe clients' responses and check their understanding of each new concept, task, or technique before going further. In "closing the loop," the OT might ask clients to explain, in their own words, their understanding of a new suggestion or strategy (HHQI, 2012).

Self-Management of Lower Back Pain: An Occupational Therapy Intervention Example

Back pain affects up to 80% of adults in the United States (CDC, 2012). In many cases, back pain and associated pain in buttocks, hips, and lower extremities is caused by bulging or herniation of the spinal disks, encapsulated gelatinous substances that cushion the vertebrae of the spinal column. Swelling of the disks often pinches the spinal nerves that exit the spinal column and enervates the lower extremities, causing referred pain such as sciatica. Research has found that one's body position during everyday activities can exacerbate the condition; conversely, correcting one's posture and forming the habit of using good body mechanics can protect one's lower back, alleviating or preventing this condition.

An ongoing research study funded by Quinnipiac University (Cole, 2014) uses the following five principles to educate patients with lumbar lesions in "Protecting Your Back":

1. *Maintain the lumbar curve,* which is the slight arch in the small of your back. Use a lumbar support pillow when working, driving, traveling, or sitting for any length of time. These can be purchased at most drug or surgical supply stores, or online.

2. *Minimize compression* to the lumbar spine by changing the habitual positions in which you perform everyday activities. Sitting in a slouched position and lifting heavy items in a flexed position greatly increase spinal compression and should be avoided. Relaxing in

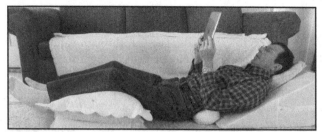

Figure 6-3. The anti-gravity position causes the least amount of spinal compression. This is the best position for relaxing and sleeping to avoid lower back pain.

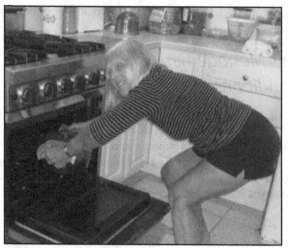

Figure 6-4. Avoid spinal compression and flexion. *Never* lift something heavy while bending over. Adapt by sliding a heavy pot onto a stepstool, then close the oven and lift the pot onto the counter by squatting and keeping back straight. Don't be afraid to ask for help.

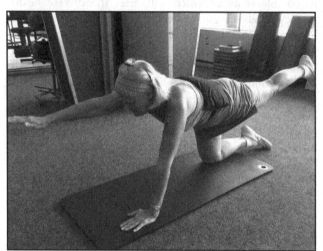

Figure 6-5. Core exercise to strengthen postural muscles to prevent lower back pain/injury.

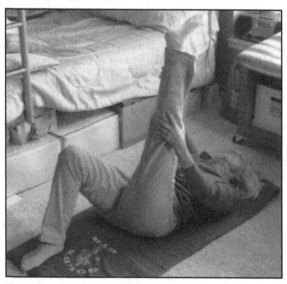

Figure 6-6. Before dressing in the morning, do 10 repetitions for each leg to stretch hamstring muscles. This makes dressing easier when dealing with lower back pain.

an antigravity position represents the least amount of compression (Figure 6-3).

3. *Avoid lumbar flexion.* Flexion is bending forward, which tends to increase the bulging spinal disk, pinching a nerve and causing pain. Always keep your natural lumbar curve (Figure 6-4).

4. *Strengthen the core* muscles that hold your spine upright, so that your muscles help to bear your body weight. Do core exercises, as directed in Figure 6-5, every other day as part of your routine. Three exercises are provided as examples of strengthening the core:

   a. Core Balance Exercise: Position yourself on hands and knees on a cushioned floor. Engage your core by contracting abdominals and squeezing buttocks. Slowly lift opposite arm and leg 10 times, alternating right and left sides. Do three repetitions every other day for a training effect (see Figure 6-5).

   b. Plank exercise: Position yourself prone (on your stomach) on a mat. Raise up on elbows and knees. Lift up to balance on elbows and toes, making your body straight like a plank. Hold for 10 seconds, and work up to holding for 30 seconds. Do three times

every other day for a training effect. This works both abdominals and back extensors.

   c. Hamstring stretch: Stretch hamstrings daily as shown in Figure 6-6. This maintains flexibility to assist in dressing and other self-care activities without having to flex the spine. Additional core exercises may be found on the Internet.

5. *Use good body mechanics* when lifting or performing work activities. Avoid bending from the waist when lifting heavy items off the floor. Squat or kneel to grip items and use leg muscles instead. *Some tips:* keep a chair near your dressing area, keep a step stool near

high or hard-to-reach cabinets, use green shopping bags with handles for groceries, and use a rolling cart to transport heavy items. Don't hesitate to ask for help with lifting when needed.

The OT presents this back pain self-management program in a 1-hour interactive PowerPoint presentation to participants immediately following an epidural steroid injection. The program explains in detail how each of the principles is applied during everyday activities such as grooming and dressing, eating and preparing meals, driving, shopping, working, walking and exercising, using a computer, relaxing, and socializing. Participants are encouraged to ask questions and give examples from their own daily routines.

As the OT member of the research team, I designed a PowerPoint educational program for adults with lower back pain. It shows how clients need to modify their positions in everyday activities in order to apply the previous principles. The following areas are addressed:

- Using a lumbar support pillow to maintain the lumbar curve while sitting; driving; traveling by air, train, or bus; or dining out

- Ergonomic positioning at work or home, positioning for using a computer

- Avoiding spinal flexion and compression by modifying resting and relaxing positions; using an anti-gravity position, with recliners, wedges, and pillows, sleeping positions

- Using good body mechanics when lifting, such as carrying groceries

- Using good body mechanics when dressing, avoiding bending, twisting, and lumbar flexion; avoiding flexing over bathroom counters, adapting ADL tasks (Figure 6-7)

- Rearranging and storing frequently used items at convenient heights to avoid flexion

- Discussion and problem solving for any other activities in clients' everyday lives

This client educational program is currently being researched by an interdisciplinary team with a grant from Quinnipiac University.

Medication Management as an Occupational Therapy Intervention

Older adults in the United States take an average of 3 to 4 prescription medications each day to treat chronic health and age-related conditions (National Center for Health Statistics, 2011). Although medication adherence has been associated with improved health and increased functioning, several studies have found that 50% to 75% of all adults do not take medications as prescribed

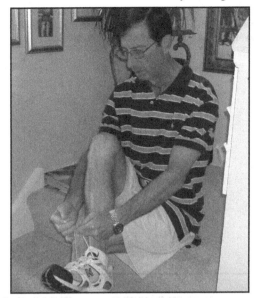

Figure 6-7. Best position for tying shoes without spinal flexion.

(Lococo & Staplin, 2006; Wertheimer & Santella, 2003). According to a recent qualitative study, community dwelling older adults have successfully managed their medications by linking them with other daily routines, such as mealtimes, TV shows, or morning and evening routines (Tordoff, Bagge, Gray, Campbell, & Norris, 2010). Sanders and Van Oss (2013) further investigated the specific medication adherence strategies commonly used by older adults. They found that 91% of their 141 participants embedded medication taking into mealtimes or wake-up and sleep routines. Most used reminders such as keeping their morning pills near the coffee maker and storing evening pills in the medicine cabinet next to the toothpaste. Some used 3- to 4-section pill containers to sort their daily doses, but few used any more complicated or electronic reminders. For example, "Mrs. Smith (age 67) kept her medications in the center of the dining room table since she takes her medications with meals...that way she can see them as a reminder. 'I take out the pills I need for each meal when I set the table...I take the pills right after I finish my meal before clearing the table with a full glass of water'" (Sanders & Van Oss, 2013, p. 96). These results encourage OTs to help clients with multiple medications to form habits for taking them within the context of already established routines (Figure 6-8).

Self-Help Training for Insomnia: A Cognitive Behavioral Intervention for Older Adults

Insomnia is one of the most common complaints of older adults, and this is compounded by the comorbidity

Figure 6-8. Many older adults take multiple prescription drugs as well as supplements. Enabling them to organize and manage medications is a good example of an OT self-management intervention.

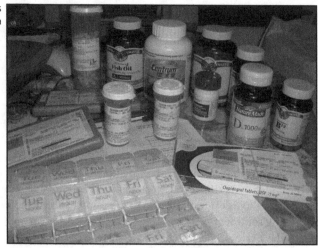

TABLE 6-1		
WEEKLY TOPICS FOR INSOMNIA SELF-HELP		
WEEK	**TOPIC**	**DESCRIPTION**
1	Introduction to Self-Management of Insomnia	Health education on stages of sleep, normal sleep cycles, and the "vicious circle of insomnia" from a cognitive behavioral perspective. Clients set up a sleep diary, kept beside the bed with a pen or pencil, to record times of falling asleep, waking up, use of sleep aides, dreams, and quality of sleep.
2	Sleep Hygiene	Helpful suggestions for optimal sleep, such as keeping a routine, and avoidance of substances such as caffeine that could affect sleeping.
3	Developing Good Sleep Habits	Adjusting bedtimes and wake-up times, controlling environmental influences, and minimizing in bed "awake time" by rising and leaving bedroom after 20 minutes of being awake.
4	Thinking About Sleep	Implementing strategies for "winding down" before bed-time, and de-escalating the anticipated consequences of not sleeping.
5	Sleep Medication	Education about how sleeping pills work, over the counter choices, and issues of dependency and discontinuation.
6	Maintaining Progress	Nurturing good sleep habits for the long term, managing set-backs, and avoiding future problems. Sleep diary.
Adapted from Morgan, K., Gregory, P., Tomeny, M., David, B., & Gascoigne, C. (2012). Self-help treatment for insomnia symptoms associated with chronic conditions in older adults: A randomized controlled trial. *Journal of the American Geriatric Society, 60,* 1803-1810.		

of chronic diseases. However, sleep medications have only modest benefits, but pose a significant risk of harm (Glass, Sproule, & Busto, 2005). Researchers from the United Kingdom report results of a randomized clinical trial for self-management of insomnia for older adults with associated chronic conditions (Morgan, Gregory, Tomeny, David, & Gascoigne, 2012). One of six self-help booklets designed as a structured psycho-educational program was mailed to participants, along with the availability of a telephone helpline to support and clarify the mailed materials. The content of each weekly module is listed in Table 6-1. Results of this study were significant improvements in sleep quality and efficiency, and less severe insomnia severity for the self-help group. These benefits were maintained at 3- and 6-month follow-up. A similar result was independently reported utilizing an 8-week computerized cognitive training program for older adults with insomnia in Brazil (Haimov & Shatil, 2013). The positive results for this good quality evidence suggest that educational programs that support self-management can be highly effective for addressing health issues and overcoming obstacles to productive occupations for older adults.

Journal Entry (M. C.)

Going into the study, I expected self-management to entail mostly self-care, or what OTs call ADL. It is, after all, the most basic of occupational roles enabling a person to function independently. All of our participants checked off this role, which often included the management of a chronic health condition. It included lifestyle choices, too, such as getting enough exercise, sleep, nutrition, and mental stimulation. However, our participants did not emphasize these aspects. What surprised me most is how broadly they did define it.

The most overarching ability connected with self-management was the ability to control their own lives, with descriptors such as self-discipline, self-direction, self-control, and intention. They chose who they connected with socially and intentionally reached out or joined social groups. They structured their days to include the occupational roles with which they most identified, whether working, volunteering, caregiving, home management, or lifelong learning. The older adults who are most happy with their lives have truly taken charge of who they spend time with, what they plan for their future, and even their emotions! People really do have control of their feelings and how their environment influences them. They intentionally plan to nurture optimism, evidenced in statements such as the following, "expect it to be good," "keep doing what you love," "be kind to yourself," "surround yourself with people who are positive," "people who keep you involved," and "avoid negative people!" Wow!

The influence of their personal background—their upbringing—also surprised me. Some participants actually quoted their parents' internalized voices: "Don't just lie there. Get up. Go somewhere. Get out of the house! Call someone! Just do it!" like they were cheering themselves on. Hearing them, I have also internalized their lessons in self-discipline. When it is time to exercise and I don't feel like it, I hear their voices telling me, "When you feel like taking a nap, take a walk instead" and "Twenty minutes [of exercise] won't kill you, Mildred!"

Summary

In Chapter 1, we defined self-management for older adults as the self-directed ability to control and manage their own aging process, to set realistic and meaningful occupational goals, and to structure their lives and daily self-fulfilling activities in ways that continue and reinforce

important social and occupational identities and create and maintain social roles and connections that they find satisfying. Essentially, self-management controls all the other productive occupations in which people choose to engage, the extent and scheduling of involvement, and the balance between self-maintenance and productivity. Therefore, no other productive occupation has greater prominence than this one for determining the health, well-being, and future occupational directions for our older clients. We hope that OTs will take this concept, and the various activities within it, as the focus for individual and group interventions and programming across the continuum of care.

References

Aegler, B., & Satink, T. (2009). Performing occupations under pain: The experience of persons with chronic pain. *Scandinavian Journal of Occupational Therapy, 16*, 49-56.

American Occupational Therapy Association. (2014). Occupational therapy practice framework: Domain and process (3rd ed.). *American Journal of Occupational Therapy, 68*, S1-S48.

Bandura, A. (2004). Health promotion by social cognitive means. *Health Education and Behavior, 31*, 143-164.

Beebe, C., & Schmitt, S. (2011). Engaging patients in education for self-management in an accountable care environment. *Clinical Diabetes, 29*, 123-126.

Brown, C., Engel, J., Holsti, L., Jones, D., Liedberg, G., Martinsson, L., ... Unruh, A. (2012). *IASP curriculum outline on pain for occupational therapy.* Retrieved from http://www.iasp-pain.org/Content/NavigationMenu/GeneralResourceLinks/Curricula/OccupationalTherapy.

Campbell, B. (2012). Living well with long term illness: Role of self-management. MD Junction, Chronic Fatigue Forums. Retrieved from http://www.mdjunction.com/forums/chronic-fatigue-discussions/general-support.

Centers for Disease Control. (2012). Summary of health statistics for US adults national health interview survey, 2010. Series, Number 252. Retrieved from http://www.cdc.gov/nchs/data/series/sr_10/sr10_2!

Clark, F., Azen, S., Carlson, M., Mandel, D., Zemke, R., Hay, J., ... Lipson, L. (1997). Occupational therapy for independent living older adults: A randomized controlled trial. *Journal of the American Medical Association, 278*, 1321-1326.

Clark, F., Jackson, J., Carlson, M., Chou, C., Cherry, B., Jordan-Marsh, M., & Azen, S. (2011). Effectiveness of a lifestyle intervention in promoting the well-being of independently living older people: Results of the Well Elderly 2 Randomized Controlled Trial. *Journal of Epidemiology and Community Health.* Retrieved from http://jech.bmj.com/content/early/2011/06/01/jech.2009.099754.abstract.

Connor, L. T., & Maeir, A. (2011). Putting executive performance in a theoretical context. *OTJR: Occupation, Participation and Health, 31*, 53-57.

DeRosa, J. (2013). Providing self-management support to people living with chronic conditions. *OT Practice, 18*, CE-1-8.

Fung, M., & Bobby, N. G. (2011). A series on self-management of chronic lung diseases – Part 1: Self-management is NOT just patient education. *Occupational Therapy Corner.* Retrieved from http://www.hkresp.com/index.php/administrator/123-copd-and-asthma/1120-2011-may-.

Garcia, A., Marciniak, D., McCune, L., Smith, E., & Ramsey, R. (2012). Promoting fall self-efficacy and fall risk awareness in older adults. *Physical and Occupational Therapy in Geriatrics, 30*, 165-175.

Ghahari, S., & Packer, T. (2011). Occupational therapists online: Equity of access to fatigue self-management. *Occupational Therapy Now, 13.5*, 23-25.

Glass, J., Lanctot, K. L., Herrmann, N., Sproule, B. A., & Busto, U. E. (2005). Sedative hypnotics in older people with insomnia: Meta-analysis of risks and benefits. *British Medical Journal, 331*, 1169-1175.

Haimov, I., & Shatil, E. (2013). Cognitive training improves sleep quality and cognitive function among older adults with insomnia. *PLoS ONE, 8*(4), e61390. Doi:10.1371/journal.pone.0061390.

Hammond, A., Young, A., & Kidao, R. (2004). A randomized controlled trial of occupational therapy for people with early rheumatoid arthritis. *Annals of the Rheumatic Diseases, 63*, 23-30.

Haskett, J. (2006). Are we ready for self-management? Working Knowledge, Harvard Business School. Retrieved from http://hbswk.hbs.edu/item/5507.html.

Health Council of Canada. (2012). Self-management report. Retrieved from http://www.healthcouncilcanada.ca/tree/HCC_SelfManagementReport.CA.pdf.

Home Health Quality National Improvement Campaign. (2012). Focused best practice intervention package: Patient self-management. Retrieved from http://www.homehealthquality.org/getattachment/6a26ad1d-279a-495e-9234-b8d342b16312/Focused-BPIP-Patient-Self-Management.aspx.

Improving Chronic Illness Care. (2009). The chronic care model. Retrieved from http://www.improvingchroniccare.org/index.php?p=The_Chronic_Care_Model&s=2.

Koh, H., Brach, C., Harris, L., & Parchman, M. (2013). A proposed health literate care model would constitute a systems approach to improving patients' engagement in care. *Health Affairs, 32*, 357-367.

Lococo, K., & Staplin, L. (2006). *Literature review of polypharmacy and older drivers: Identifying strategies to correct drug usage and driving functioning among older drivers.* Washington, DC: National Highway Traffic Safety Administration.

McLean, A., & Coutts, K. (2011). Occupational therapy: Self-management for people with migraines. *Occupational Therapy Now, 13.5*, 5-7.

Miller, W., & Rollinick, S. (2002). *Motivational interviewing: Preparing people for change.* New York: Guilford Press.

Morgan, K., Gregory, P., Tomeny, M., David, B., & Gascoigne, C. (2012). Self-help treatment for insomnia symptoms associated with chronic conditions in older adults: A randomized controlled trial. *Journal of the American Geriatric Society, 60*, 1803-1810.

Morning Star Self-Management Institute. (2012). What is self-management? Retrieved from http://self-managementinstitute.org/about_self-management/.

National Center for Health Statistics. (2011). *Health, United States, 2010: With special feature on death and dying.* Hyattsville, MD: Author.

O'Toole, J., & Lawler, E III. (2006). *The new American workplace.* New York: Palgrave Macmillan.

Pyatak, E. A. (2011). The role of occupational therapy in diabetes self-management interventions. *Occupational Therapy Journal of Research, 31*, 89-96.

Sanders, M., & Van Oss, T. (2013). Using daily routines to promote medication adherence in older adults. *American Journal of Occupational Therapy, 67*, 91-99.

Soderhamn, O., Skisland, A., & Herrman, M. (2011). Self-care and anticipated transition into retirement and later life in a Nordic welfare context. *Journal of Multidisciplinary Healthcare, 4*, 273-279.

Tordoff, J. M., Bagge, M. L., Gray, A. R., Campbell, A. J., & Norris, P. T. (2010). Medicine-taking practices in community-dwelling people aged = or > 75 years in New Zealand. *Age and Ageing, 39*, 574-580. .

Wertheimer, A., & Santella, T. (2003). Medication compliance research: Still so far to go. *Journal of Applied Research, 3*, 1-9.

Yang, S. (2012). Lifelong brain-stimulating habits linked to lower Alzheimer's protein levels. Retrieved from http://newscenter.berkeley.edu/2012/01/23/engaged-brain-amyloid-alzheimers/.

Home Manager

Karen C. Macdonald, PhD, OTR/L

"Meaning becomes embedded in place." (Rowles, 2008, p. 130)

Home management has been identified by Knight et al. (2007) as the most frequent productive occupation (89%) of older adults living in the community. According to the PAS, this occupation falls within the guidance of self-management, as older persons make decisions about their own ability or desire to perform the tasks of managing a home. It includes several of the IADLs listed in the AOTA's (2014) OTPF III: home establishment and maintenance, shopping, meal preparation and cleanup, and safety and emergency maintenance. Home maintenance also encompasses outdoor work such as maintenance of yard, driveways, walkways, steps, decks or patios, gardening, and landscaping.

The following are OTPF III (AOTA, 2014) definitions related to the productive role of home management:

- *IADLs*: Activities to support daily life within the home and community that often require more complex interactions than those used in ADL.

- *Home establishment and management*: Obtaining and maintaining personal and household possessions and environment (e.g., home, yard, garden, appliances, vehicles), including maintaining and repairing personal possessions.

- *Meal preparation and cleanup*: Planning, preparing, and serving well-balanced, nutritious meals and cleaning up food and utensils after meals (Figure 7-1).

- *Safety and emergency maintenance*: Knowing and performing preventive procedures to maintain a safe environment; recognizing sudden, unexpected hazardous situations; and initiating emergency action to reduce the threat to health and safety. Examples include ensuring safety when entering and exiting the home, identifying emergency contact numbers, and replacing items such as batteries in smoke alarms and light bulbs.

- *Shopping*: Preparing shopping lists (grocery and other); selecting, purchasing, and transporting items; selecting method of payment; and completing money transactions. Includes Internet shopping and related use of electronic devices such as computers, cell phones, and tablets.

Additionally, because home management also involves making adaptations that allow older adults to age in place, as 88% of all older adults say they wish to do (National Alliance for Caregiving & American Association of Retired Persons, 2009), this chapter also includes a section on OT's role in home modification.

PARTICIPANT PERSPECTIVES

The participants all lived in their own home, a condominium, or an apartment in an independent retirement

Cole MB, Macdonald KC.
Productive Aging: An Occupational Perspective (pp 115-133).
© 2015 Taylor & Francis Group.

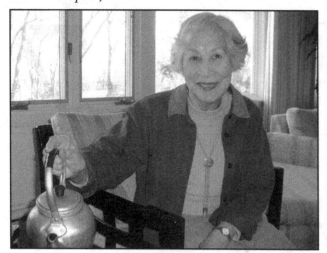

Figure 7-1. Vi pours tea for herself and her guests.

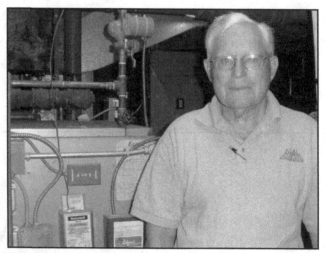

Figure 7-2. Dave periodically changes the filter on the furnace, making sure it is running efficiently.

community, in both urban and suburban settings. Some of the participants owned more than one residence—a primary and a vacation home. We expected that the older homeowners would have mentioned that home and yard care was a challenging or time-consuming task, but it was mentioned with few details. Although all participants had responsibilities for housework, which might be assumed to be increasingly difficult with aging, that was barely mentioned as a topic. Many appeared to enjoy home maintenance and took pride in home ownership and having kept their residence in good repair over a period of years. Condominium or apartment dwellers made little reference to housecleaning or projects. It appeared that home and yard maintenance was a necessary and regularly scheduled responsibility, and did get accomplished, but was not addressed as an interest or important topic for their day-to-day lives.

Home Repair and Safety

Bob M. spoke about owning two homes and maintaining a garden. "I do anything that needs fixing or doing. I keep the cars up, the garden, anything that needs daily attending…cut down dead trees." He commented that "if something seems unsafe, I try to correct it, like steps or the deck, improving possible trouble spots…preventive measures—I hold onto a railing, wear a hard hat in the attic. We have to watch for hazards in the community. Some counters have sharp corners." His mention of daily house or yard upkeep was in the context of timeliness, making sure that it is done as needed and that projects do not accumulate. He mentioned a system of careful awareness of seasonal changes and anticipated whatever preparation might be needed to prepare for the next season.

Mary V. commented that you can't work on your yard in the winter. "I have a ranch house, with one floor. I still have a ramp that we had for my husband. You have to be aware of what is going on in the world, the environment [weather]…the radio had warned of black ice, but I fell, I always thought, 'it won't happen to me!'" Mary had assistance from her sons with needed home repairs and upkeep. She realized what the expenses would be if she did not have family members who were available and capable of offering whatever assistance she might need for the home or yard.

Living alone in a large house, Jan organizes daily home maintenance tasks. The conscious planning, scheduling, and completion of home repair activities requires thought, skill, time, and often purchases. What may seem like a simple repair might turn into a task that could involve driving to the bank, then a store, gathering tools, seeking "how to" advice, or obtaining needed assistance, resulting in hours of time for total completion, even for a simple task (Figure 7-2).

Participants gave attention to safety in several areas such as rugs, lighting, old or poorly positioned cords, and care with heavy or fragile items and hot or sharp items. Adaptations used by some included grab bars, adapted light switches, organizational or enlarged labels, night lights, and carpet texture or stability. When relevant, they were aware of general body mechanics principles pertaining to transfers related to toilet, shower, and bed.

Appropriate storage and use of tools and supplies were described. They often "just knew" to avoid leaving items where they could be lost or damaged by rain. Their lifelong habits of practical skills led to increased safety and competence. For example, even as observers might cringe watching a 90-year-old man move a heavy wheelbarrow, obvious skills would lead to successful performance. At what point does the concerned family member intervene knowing that retained ability and independence are the core of the older person's identity? How can safety be assured without compromising the person's pride in carefully sustained ability?

Joy and Pride in Home Management

Sue S., at 98, happily reported that she likes to clean her house, that it gives her a good feeling, and that the hard work is like exercise but a pleasure. "But now, my place looks like a gypsy camp. It needs a lot of help. But no one will help me. I do things that I have to do, do the laundry. But now, that's all changed, I can't reach the mantle to dust, so now I'll plant things in that dirt [laughing]." Sue had experienced a series of falls and health changes in recent years that influenced her ability to continue with lifelong habits related to home and yard care. She has a small support system, and they do offer help with chores and projects, but she may refuse, saying she would rather find a way to do it herself.

Signian shared that they own an eight-room house, large enough to be comfortable "but it does take time to manage." She stated that neighbors help with lawn care and snow removal. "We love our green spaces and gardens, we like feeding the birds, composting, and enjoying the outdoors." Her comments highlighted the balance that she achieved of responsibilities and work with resulting pleasure and enjoyment.

June takes pride in taking care of her country house. "...[W]hen something is broken, I fix it. I watch workmen very carefully to learn how they do things. I do home projects, redecorating, building additions, subcontracting, and doing it 'hands on.'" She continues that she tries to keep living expenses down and pay down her mortgage.

Living in Seattle, Peggie described how she does laundry the old-fashioned way—by drying everything outside in the sun. She explained that sunshine is sometimes rare in that region. She commented that "...home chores are a given, you must do them every day."

Jack expressed that he does yard work for fun, enjoying the planting of large flower beds, vegetables in a back garden, and landscaping as an annual ritual. He described how "we deck out our yard and house with Christmas decorations each year, they are up by Thanksgiving; it is also a social thing, we are the envy of our neighbors and we come up with a new and lavish décor every year." Jack enjoys his outdoor decorating, knowing that others will enjoy it as well. While some participants spent little in cost or time in their yards, it was a special interest and pleasure for Jack.

Although managed independently, the most demanding chores identified were cleaning, vacuuming, cleaning the tub and toilet, laundry, shopping, and cooking. In relation to these necessary tasks, individuals seemed divided as to whether they were dreaded versus meaningful and enjoyable (Figure 7-3).

Sharing home management responsibilities with her husband, Pearl recalled her Louisiana upbringing. She especially enjoys teaching Cajun cooking of jambalaya, bouillabaisse, and gumbo to her daughters-in-law and grandchildren. Her comments emphasized the nature of

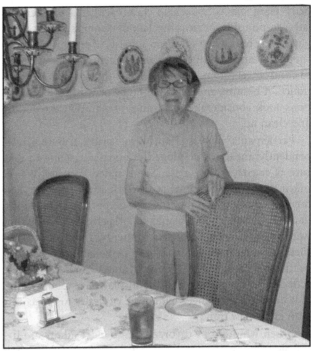

Figure 7-3. Marylyn enjoys maintaining her home and entertaining guests.

cherishing a cultural heritage and the importance of passing down values, skills, and traditions related to home life.

Learning Activity 50: Challenges of Maintaining a Home

1. List your impression of the top five challenges for an older adult to be able to maintain the role of a home manager.

2. What are some community resources to access assistance with home tasks?

Couples Sharing Home Tasks

Finding a way to balance commitments and priorities, Margie shared house chores with her husband, who had recently retired and loves to cook. "I have a fairly large home that demands housekeeping and management—too much cleaning, but great for hosting family and friends. As a full-time caregiver (grandson and granddaughter), I sometimes have conflicts with activities." Margie represents one of the participants who cares for several generations, with pleasure but realized the challenges of balancing her many responsibilities.

Ken stated that his roles include gardening and home upkeep. For the couples interviewed, it appeared that they had a clear division of responsibilities that was acceptable to both. Bob M. shares, "I help my wife with household chores—it's from my Navy training, like how to make a bed." Greg shares household chores with his partner, the latter responsible for cleaning, laundry, computer tasks, and paying the bills. Greg's portion consists of planning menus, shopping, and cooking. He commented that he attempts to control weight and stay healthy. Although seldom mentioned, it became apparent that home or yard care occupations took considerable planning, preparation, execution, and clean up.

Participants expressed an overall pride in living independently and have developed pragmatic systems to take care of needs as they arise. Some stated surprise at how much they could continue to do with advancing age. Few mentioned anything about the large portion of a typical day that these activities would entail, perhaps because they were so routine that not much attention was devoted to them. Home ownership related to personal identity; many participants enjoyed how personal interests and style were reflected in decorating and the display of personal items. However, they no longer felt a need or desire to redecorate with every new trend.

When widowed or divorced, some older adults are living alone for the first time in their lives. Some individuals struggle with this change, while others see it as an exciting new chapter for discovery and growth.

Learning Activity 51: Division of Labor

1. Discuss the issue of sharing chores or division of labor when two individuals share a residence. Many older adults have decades-long routines that are changed when one of the couple has a health change. What are some suggestions for addressing this topic in an open and sensitive way?

2. Identify some likely emotions that would need to be understood and supported.

Learning Activity 52: Pros and Cons of Living Alone

Group activity: With a partner, role play an older individual who appreciates living alone. The other individual is a newly widowed older adult who has never lived alone and is upset.

1. Exchange viewpoints.

2. Share with the larger group (if available). On a whiteboard, record a list of the pros and cons of living alone.

3. When completed, analyze another step by identifying three main themes for each column.

Moving, Downsizing, or Modifying Homes

The generations reflected in the study have typically moved several times—fixing up houses, moving to an "upgrade," and continuing on. At this time of life, they may have been doing the reverse, downsizing and moving to a smaller place of residence, often preferring to give up outdoor responsibilities and moving to a condominium or apartment. Others commented that they knew it was time for them to move or downsize but that the very thought of the moving process was overwhelming, so they remained in their home.

Awareness also focused on effective storage for managing years of accumulated "stuff." Valnere gave herself 2 years after her husband died to clear out her large suburban home. It became her full-time job to find charities, thrift shops, consignment shops, libraries, shelters, antique book dealers, and other appropriate recipients for useful items she no longer needed. She returned photos and letters to relatives or friends who had sent them, sensitive of the feelings they might have about her disposing of them. Now Valnere, the oldest of four siblings, finds herself doing the same at her parents' home after her mother's recent death. Some others spoke of a need for holding a tag sale but hadn't due to anticipation of the massive effort involved.

Participants often expressed awareness that a change in health or ability may prompt a move to a more supportive level of housing. Widows expressed the extensive change in roles and responsibilities and needing to learn new skills or secure assistance. Home modification was seen as a difficult change, often postponed for years, even while recognizing that modifications might raise levels of functioning considerably, such as building an entrance ramp. Lifetime habits of frugality, saving, and investments had provided some financial security to the participants after retirement. However, they commented on the shocking prices of materials for any home repairs or modifications.

Some considered positive new opportunities for housing, including senior housing, assisted living, and gated communities. Several who had moved from private homes to condos described how the decrease in house and yard maintenance responsibilities contributed to overall higher skills and opportunities for social engagement. They mentioned a different lifestyle with condominium and apartment dwelling, in which more frequent contact with other people occurred each day.

Learning Activity 53: Emotions About Moving

Recall older individuals from your own experience who have owned their own home.

1. Discuss the concept of "pride of ownership."

2. Identify the assortment of emotions and reactions that might be typical for an individual who must relocate due to a change in health status.

Learning Activity 54: Task Analysis for the Occupation of Moving

Perform a task analysis on a scenario in which an older adult is moving. Include general considerations, supplies, assistance needed, and timeline.

The participants who lived in a private house often raised the topic of awareness of an eventual need to sell their house. They considered ongoing needs for upkeep and repairs, followed regional real estate trends and noticed the expectations of new buyers (i.e., Do I need to put in granite kitchen countertops to sell my house?). As a result of previous moves, they were well aware of the process of planning, packing, and hiring movers and the process of relocating to another residence and settling in. How would they manage as older adults for the countless issues and steps? What assistance would be possible? What are anticipated needs for future years in selecting the next place to live? Relocation was described by some as a dreaded process, while others saw it as an exciting opportunity for new places and discovery about a community's social, organizational, and cultural and consumer possibilities. (See Chapter 3 for more in-depth discussion of relocation as a transition.)

Accessing Home Maintenance Services

At the mention of home management, Bob C. stated, "I don't cook!...but New York City has great takeout!" For Bob C., home maintenance means mostly keeping his place picked up, paying bills, and using a laundry service. He is most interested in spending time fixing up his car so that he can travel to his girlfriend's vacation home on weekends. Bob's ability to easily benefit from the availability of many services in his urban neighborhood shows a contrast to the suburban participants who had less access.

The location of homes and their access to public transportation, especially taxis and buses, were important. Some relied on others for assistance with rides or used senior van services to get to medical appointments. They described paying attention to calculating distances to drive and with what frequency. Destinations typically included the grocery store, medical appointments, library, bank, shops, pharmacy, family or friends visit, spiritual site, and community activities.

Some expected assistance from family members and community, as well as paid caregivers or workers. Many described the challenges of hiring reliable help. Help was especially needed for painting, moving items, roof repair, and electrical, plumbing, and water issues.

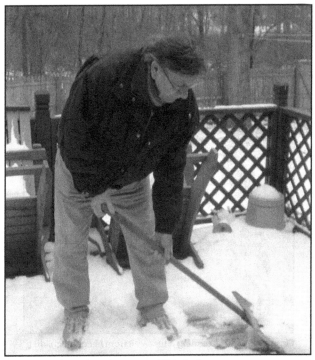

Figure 7-4. Geno shoveling snow off his deck.

Community service projects by teens could assist an elder neighbor with heavy chores, like raking or shoveling snow (Figure 7-4). Also identified as helpful were assistance programs for energy costs, such as senior discounts for oil, gas, electricity, or insulation.

For any home projects requiring the hiring of skilled help, the participants expressed concern about consumer "rip-offs." Locating licensed and certified professionals was often through personal connections and word of mouth. They hoped that quality work would be completed within projected timelines, and that cost estimates would be accurate.

The Meaning of Home

They expressed a consciousness of all that took place in one's home over the years. This included all self- and home-management tasks, as well as hosting family events and holiday celebrations. Entertaining small groups of friends was often mentioned. For example, a "gourmet club" consisted of several couples taking turns entertaining at home over the course of 1 year.

Another "at home" meaningful activity was pet ownership and care. Several described the joys of their relationship with a beloved cat or dog. Caregiving included many responsibilities, such as shopping for food, feeding, play or exercise, attention to a cat litter box or walking a dog, and visits to a veterinarian.

Changing family dynamics also influenced use of home spaces. The participants described scenarios of adult

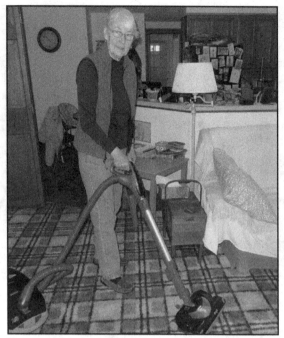

Figure 7-5. Jan vacuuming after a visit from her grandchildren.

children moving back home and/or caregiver roles for grandchildren. With many social changes, such as single parents and economic challenges, some families experienced fluctuations in who was living where and when (Figure 7-5).

Being outdoors in one's own yard offered both a sense of solitary peace and an opportunity for social gatherings. Outdoor seating areas were established for a daily dose of fresh air, a quiet cup of coffee, and a place to sit and enjoy the company of a spouse or partner. Decks, patios, and lawn areas were also structured to allow for visits with neighbors or large gatherings. Cookouts and barbeques were described as eagerly anticipated and special times for family and friends. For these older adults, the family home was still honored and appreciated as the established gathering place for nuclear and extended families. Children and grandchildren had often moved far away or to places that could not accommodate a crowd, or the younger generation was seen as "too busy" with work and family, with the seniors happily continuing in a host/hostess role.

Learning Activity 55: Ideal Housing Situation in Retirement

1. What would you consider to be an ideal housing situation upon your own retirement?

2. How can you plan for this possibility?

The "Business" of Home Management

A considerable amount of "business" took place in the home environment. Sometimes tasks related to paying bills, tax preparation, and correspondence took place at a separate office area or desk. Management of "important papers" included careful organizing, labeling, and filing or storage. They kept an informal inventory of needed materials and supplies. Most of the participants used a computer, some as novices and others as excited experts who welcomed every aspect of new technology, although a few declared they never would use one. Most used it for e-mail, occasional research, online games, or some banking and online shopping. On the whole, they appeared cognizant of mandatory technology changes, such as computer upgrades or changes in television and lighting options. Most had shifted "with the times" to use of CDs for music and DVDs for movies.

They were aware of the need to avoid victimization, such as identity theft or telephone or in-person scams. Several reported a conscious awareness of telemarketers (or whoever the unknown caller was) who were persuasively seeking personal information about identity and existing accounts. Several commented about feeling uncomfortable dealing with solicitors who would come to the door. They expressed anger about the large quantity of "junk mail" that they had to handle. They were being intruded upon by unwanted individuals and promotions. Family members had offered assistance at times to be registered for "no call lists" or with suggestions to screen all phone calls.

In general, the participants identified themselves as having skills in managing the business of daily living effectively and efficiently. They valued their personal space(s) and had an intentional routine of balancing required chores with leisure activities, needed rest, and maintaining healthy lifestyles at home. They organized their kitchens to promote healthy eating, provided for planned rest, established routines for keeping up with chores, and created spaces for entertaining, relaxing, and participating in enjoyable occupations.

Vehicles, Parking, and Maintenance

Living in a private home implied a need for a car and a garage because neighborhoods were a distance from community resources. A garage was another environment for preventing clutter and creating an organized and safe storage system. For example, Jack had a woodworking shop built off the side of his garage and a system for storing his extensive collection of gardening equipment and supplies. For all participants who owned a vehicle, two areas were raised as important. Men willingly took responsibility for the maintenance of their cars, often doing some of the repairs themselves. Women sought professionals to fix their cars and hoped to find a reliable garage or mechanic. All seemed to have an unconscious awareness of "time for a tune-up" or regular maintenance check. If an emergency occurred while on the road, most had cellphones to seek help or had a program for roadside assistance, offering a sense of security.

Automobile owners worried about parking safely. When at home, a garage or driveway hopefully offered easy access to an entry area for unloading numerous heavy grocery bags. Parking in town posed a considerable challenge for many, with confusing parking signs, "new-fangled" parking meters, difficult parallel parking, and poor availability of parking spots near entries. The majority of participants did not have or qualify for a handicapped parking permit. They tended to hope that a parking spot would open up. Most adapted by recognizing times of the day or week that would have less traffic and planned their errands accordingly.

JOURNAL ENTRY (K. M.)

My brother told me a story of an 80-year-old friend who had a lifetime of skilled performance with woodworking, carpentry, and any needed home repair. One time, family members happened to arrive as he was alone atop a ladder and performing a minor repair on his roof. His family was upset, urged him to come down the ladder, and lectured him about never doing that again. The man was never the same again. It was as if they had taken the wind out of his sails, puncturing his pride and capability. For the first time, he felt old.

LITERATURE REVIEW

Owning and maintaining one's private home has been an American ideal for centuries. In past decades, options for owning condominiums or renting apartments have broadened the definition of home. In recent years, the sense of creating a true home-like atmosphere has prevailed for a variety of senior living options, from senior housing to long-term care facilities.

A sense of pride in ownership exists for homeowners who recognize the importance of the value of their property. Renters also experience a deep connection to their own "place." In either environment, home represents comfort, familiarity, and a showcase for one's lifelong possessions. This represents a place where senior individuals do most of their living—self-care, chores, meals, leisure and social activities, and sleep.

Aging in Place

As skills or relationships change with aging, retaining a traditional single family house and yard becomes chal-lenging. Currently, many support services can assist with home and yard maintenance, or caregiving duties. With the increasing percentage of older adults living longer and healthier lives, community services are shifting to allow for a range of life care options. Aging in Place programs have developed that match activity modifications to declin-ing performance skills. Shank and Cutchin (2010) studied older women who sought to negotiate changes in their life. One participant explained that she "...lived by a carefully scripted routine that allowed her to get things done without becoming too exhausted in the course of the day" (Shank & Cutchin, 2010, p. 8). The authors described a process of situ-ational framing, continued negotiation, place integration, and coordinating occupations (Shank & Cutchin, 2010).

Local establishments who traditionally offered extended care facilities have expanded their services to include home care and graduated levels of senior housing. Senior Choice at Home is an example of a spectrum of options offered by Jewish Senior Services. When this author opened their OT department in 1977, they offered intermediate care and a skilled nursing facility, along with a then-innovative adult day care center. Today, they offer home care with many supportive and professional services, as well as assisted liv-ing facilities (Gail Bromer, 2011, personal correspondence). They are envisioning future transitions to new models for life care services, offering individualized health care for higher independent-functioning individuals, which then shifts as residents require more specialized care.

Household Responsibilities in Maintaining a Private Residence

Zur and Rudman (2013) describe an international move-ment characterized by the World Health Organization as "...simultaneous patterns of global aging and urbanization" (p. 370). Shifts from rural farms to suburban neighbor-hoods have matched economic and cultural changes. The expenses of managing and maintaining a private home and property, paying taxes and utilities, and obtaining transpor-tation to shopping or activity areas has promoted attraction to apartment-style living in urban environments. Positive aspects of these changes are described as increased acces-sibility to shopping and services, increased public transpor-tation options, intergenerational contacts, and possibilities for community participation through groups or cultural events. From an occupational science perspective, they viewed these shifts as potentially facilitating many health benefits through increased activity and social participation.

Rowles (2008) explored the role of environmental con-text, stating that "...meaning becomes embedded in place" (p. 130). The essence of home includes "a sense of centering, permanence, ownership, responsibility, control, self-expres-sion, privacy, refuge, belonging, comfort (familiarity) and emotional affiliation" (Rowles, 2008, p. 132). Regardless of location of the home space, deep meaning is associated with one's living environment. Nilsson, Lundgren, and Liliequist (2012) point out that the ability to live at home requires independence and trustworthiness. Perspectives of family, friends, and community create a "surrounding world" with established social norms for ability and health. The ability to live up to shared values implies that the older adult is "keeping up to date." A sense of pride in taking care of the self and home provided important meaning for 90-year-old homeowners in this study.

A striking and poignant example of the importance of personal place is presented in a *Yankee* magazine story of a bachelor farmer in Vermont (Mansfield, 2013). He was the last of a line in his family to own and proudly work a 90-acre farm. At age 64, he was confronted with news that he must move for Interstate 91 to be built through his property. He repeatedly stated, "I will not leave." After much controversy, officials arrived with a court order related to eminent domain. The next night, the house burned down, with the owner inside and doors nailed and locked to prevent being rescued. He sacrificed his life to make a statement that his family's land was sacred.

Household responsibilities are extensive for well older adults and challenging for individuals with health conditions or disability. Stark, Somerville, and Morris (2010) studied how in-home occupations related to priority and life satisfaction. The tasks included ADL performance, reading, writing, meal preparation, bills, household chores, television, pet care, and yard maintenance. They explored the concept of determining a "fit" between the person and the home environment. This resulted in the development of the In-Home Occupational Performance evaluation.

Home Management and Disabilities

With retirement, a recalibration of time used for daily activities often occurs. Performance skills for household occupations were reviewed by Wong and Almeida (2013). Retirement was seen as a time of transition in which there was a decrease in demands and stress and an increase in time for personal pursuits and exercise. It led to a period of uncertainty and transformation as routines shifted to match "multiple domains of responsibilities" (p. 82). If health stressors were present, ability related to personal vulnerability, resiliency, and the availability of resources in the environment. This study highlighted household areas of difficulty for individuals with health challenges, such as lifting, carrying groceries, bathing or dressing, stairs, and mobility.

In a classic analysis, Hossack (1956) offered foundational information concerning home management for disabled individuals. The OT offers varied strategies, including energy-saving methods of work simplification. These included recommendations for assessing the layout of the home, and analyzing roles, abilities, and safety issues. Next, practical approaches were designed to eliminate unnecessary steps or procedures. Scheduling was designed to determine a balance of time and energy, including attention to any shared responsibilities. Body mechanics for posture and positioning are described, with attention to lighting, work height, work pace, and attire. The OT promotes organizational skills with careful planning for sequencing and storage. Clients are encouraged to prevent fatigue, and to acknowledge that methods and habits followed prior to disability will not be feasible. The therapist aids in support for this "shock" as new methods are introduced, rehearsed, and modified for success.

Literature related to home management was reviewed by Tse, Douglas, Lentin, and Carey (2013) through a meta-analysis about participation after a stroke. When focusing on aspects of domestic life, priority topics for publications were acquisition of goods and services, household tasks, meals, housework, caring for household objects, and caregiving for others. They suggested a need for establishing a broader base of evidence pertaining to activities and participation, to aid in understanding chronic illness and disability across cultures.

Learning Activity 56: Work Simplification at Home

Work simplification is an important technique used by OTs related to home management tasks.

1. Consider the occupation of doing the laundry. Identify the steps of the task and considerations for how to simplify.

2. How would this need to be modified for an individual with chronic low back pain?

Maintaining Yard and Property

Occupations pertaining to maintaining yard and property encompass lawn care, raking, snow removal, and tending trees and shrubs. Seasonal changes prompt placement or removal of lawn/patio furniture and outdoor cooking materials. These responsibilities are often of a heavier nature related to performance skills; assistance is often sought through family members or paid workers.

Gardening is one area of outdoor activity enjoyed by many older adults. Along with connecting with nature and enjoying fresh air, gardening promotes physical, mental, and cognitive skills (Wang & Macmillan, 2013). Often described as a way of life, gardens may range from single-pot tomato plants to rows of carefully tended vegetables, fruit, berries, and herbs. Tasks include planning, purchasing materials, planting, watering, weeding, and harvesting.

Learning Activity 57: Safety in the Yard

1. List five hazards for the individual who is independently performing yard maintenance.

2. How could the OT provide information related to preventing hazards and injury? This includes identifying the risk areas and means for offering useful preventative strategies.

Home Modifications

One of the important ways that OTs promote home management skills is to establish systems for safety, ease of functioning, and prevention of injury. Following client education and recommendation for modifications, the client continues with an enhanced self-manager role. Van Oss, Rivers, Heighton, Mocci, and Reid (2012) offer specific suggestions for adaptations and durable medical equipment use in the bathroom. Young (2012) describes considerations of lighting, and the need for OTs to consider a client's full set of daily routines. The OT would assess for changes needed regarding glare and light levels, and background or textural contrasts needed for clients with low vision. Wagenfeld and Buresh (2012) analyzes the task of gardening, a common interest for older adults. They describe seven principles of ergonomics for the OT to evaluate and offer intervention: bending, lifting, kneeling, reaching, turning, standing, and sitting. For each task, recommendations are offered to prevent strain or injury, with examples of optimal techniques. Renda (2012) reviews principles of home modification, and offers information about possible sources for funding for equipment designed to assist older persons in remaining in their home environment. Through attention to all aspects of the home environment and activities that take place in the home and yard, the OT enables clients to engage in a broader scope of self-manager roles.

OTs play an important role in home evaluations to assess the ability of clients to manage in their own home setting. Along with assessing client skills for ADL and IADL performance, the OT determines structural and safety factors that may need attention or adaptation. Woodland and Hobson (2003) identify two categories of risk factors related to potential falls: *intrinsic* includes fear of falling, age, and gender; *extrinsic* refers to environmental factors, such as lighting or slippery surfaces.

Fall prevention is a primary concern in determining at-risk individuals and settings. Arbesman and Lieberman (2012) identify the importance of vision screening and client-centered attention to language and culture. Chase, Mann, Wasek, and Arbesman (2012) further describe a multifactorial perspective, including the assessment of health and safety awareness, the management of medications, visual skills, and gait and balance challenges, and

review the modifications or exercises already in place. Although encouraging the development of further evidence-based practice, their systematic review of 33 articles led to findings that OT home modification and fall prevention programs led to a decrease in the rate of functional decline, decrease in fear of falling, and an increase in balance and strength for older adults (Chase et al., 2012).

Recommendations may be determined and provided by OTs, but connecting with the client's personal goals and preferences influences compliance and satisfaction. Aplin, de Jonge, and Gustafson (2013) explained that one's home is a complex environment with varied meanings. Several dimensions were identified related to a client's decision-making process for modifications:

- Personal: Emotional connections, privacy, safety and security, freedom and independence, and identity and connectedness

- Physical: Structure, materials, services and facilities available, space, location and ambient (light, air, weather)

- Social: Identified as a place to foster relationships, such as family, friends, and neighbors

- Temporal: Issues of past-present-future; cyclical routines or events over the course of a day, week, or year

- Occupational: Home seen as a context for "doing" leisure, rest, ADL, IADL, and work

Respect for individual choice included overall appearance (avoiding a "disabled" look) and led to pleasure in participating in changes that would increase personal functioning. A goal expressed by clients was to avoid disruptiveness and to allow for a sense of choice and control.

Home adaptations are also provided for individuals with psychiatric or mental health conditions. Barrows (2006) relates how clients with a history of mental illness have compounded challenges as they age and experience functional decline in sensory, cognitive, or physical skills. For example, lifelong habits related to low income, poor nutritional status, and heavy smoking contribute to obesity, diabetes, visual decline, and chronic obstructive pulmonary disease. Many may live in older shared-dwelling residences with hazardous steps, poor lighting, or unsafe floor surfaces. Barnes (2006) offers examples of concrete OT recommendations related to lighting, organization, and structural challenges. Suggestions are made for inexpensive and multipurpose adaptations.

The National Organization on Disability was cited by an Information/Education page in the *Archives of Physical Medicine and Rehabilitation* (Morris & Jones, 2013) regarding community-based preparedness for natural disasters or emergencies. Because there may be a decreased access to communication systems and transportation, systems should be in place to ensure safety. They suggest a predetermined plan.

- Check in with personal network.
- Have a known escape route and alternative.
- Have easy access to essential items—medications, assistive devices, special needs.
- Recognize signs of stress—psychological (anxiety, change in sleep), thinking (cognitive change), and physical (headache or digestive problems).
- Emergency kit—food, water, medical equipment, personal information, emergency contacts, copies of important documents, keys, flashlight, cash, soap, warm clothing items, and first aid items. Individuals with special health needs should have a written card explaining their needs in the event communication skills are impaired.

HOME MANAGEMENT ACROSS THE CONTINUUM OF CARE

Primary Care and Aging in Place

OT roles for prevention and wellness ideally occur at this primary level of intervention. Because older adults wish to continue living in their homes, their ability to perform the duties of home management will often be an occupational priority. The older home manager who chooses to age in place also takes on the role of making home modifications that reduce risks and increase safety when adaptations become necessary due to declines in functioning. Making decisions about modifying one's home takes into consideration the financial, physical, and social factors. Can the changes be made at a reasonable cost? Will physical modifications improve functionality given the extent of functional difficulties? How connected is the older person to this neighborhood or community? Is it a safe area for walking? Are needed services located nearby?

OTs work with community dwelling elders to support aspects of self-management that enable the client to gather relevant information, consider all factors realistically, and make good judgments about if and how to modify the home. OTs also perform safety evaluations and assist clients in restructuring home management activities, such as repairs, cleaning, shopping, meal preparation, bill paying, and functional mobility, making necessary adaptations and enlisting the help of others, including community services.

Learning Activity 58: Risk Factors for Falls at Home

1. Brainstorm and create a list that highlights risk factors for falls in a home environment.

2. What would be matching OT recommendations for home safety and prevention of injury?

Home Care

After discharge from a hospital or rehabilitation setting, home care OTs may collaborate with clients and family members to set goals and priorities for home management activities. Together they will determine to what extent the client wishes or is able to resume responsibility for home management, what adaptations will be necessary, and what might be realistic expectations for functional recovery required to perform this productive occupation. The client and OT also must consider other occupations that will be performed at home, such as exercise routines, arts and crafts, entertaining, or gardening, some of which may take priority for the client over housecleaning or doing laundry. OTs must respect the clients' choices and work on those activities that are most meaningful, while letting go of others.

Assisted Living and Retirement Communities

Some of these facilities offer assistance with home management, such as maid services or the provision of meals, often greatly simplifying the client's home management role. The monthly fees in some of these residences are quite high but include various home maintenance services. OTs might consult with clients or do home visits on an individual basis when the client has specified certain home management activities as occupational priorities.

Rehabilitation Settings

OTs in rehabilitation settings often routinely address IADLs, which would typically fall under the home manager role. An example would be health management and maintenance, which includes "developing, managing, and maintaining routines for health and wellness promotion, such as physical fitness, nutrition, decreased health risk behaviors, and medication routines" (AOTA, 2014, p. S19). In addition to ADLs, which typically cover basic self-care, the OT will consider home management activities, such as driving and community mobility, shopping, and home maintenance and safety, as part of discharge planning from a rehabilitation setting.

Long-Term Care

Typically, long-term care settings provide for most of the tasks performed by a home manager: laundry service, meal preparation, housecleaning, and dispensing of medications are among the total care tasks provided as necessary for nursing home residents. However, some attention still needs to be paid to the features of a long-term care facility that provide a more home-like environment. Some personal possessions moved from their previous homes still require residents to perform maintenance tasks, such as remembering to water a houseplant or putting away personal items, such as a book, photograph album, or wristwatch, so that they will not get lost.

The physical environment of a nursing home was identified as an influence on resident behavior and quality of life. Garre-Olmo, López-Pousa, Turon-Estrada, Juvinya, Ballester, and Vilalta-Franch (2012) studied residents of a skilled nursing facility in Spain. Environmental factors of temperature, noise, and heating were determinants of mood and performance in ADL. They identified psychological symptoms of delusions, hallucinations, agitation or aggression, depression, anxiety, euphoria, apathy, disinhibition, irritability, aberrant motor movements, night time behavior difficulties, and changes in appetite or eating. They recommended changes in environmental design to accommodate daily activities, with special attention to eating areas, common shared space, and residents' personal rooms (Garre-Olmo et al., 2012).

IMPLICATIONS FOR OCCUPATIONAL THERAPY PRACTICE

Home management as a productive occupation involves many of the activities OT practitioners have traditionally identified as IADL. The older adults' perspective would be somewhat different, focusing more on the tasks necessary to be able to remain in their homes despite chronic illness or declining function. The OT's role for this productive occupation is to determine which occupations older adults choose to do in their homes and to evaluate those activities. Older clients who are good self-managers will set priorities regarding what needs to be done beyond ordinary maintenance. For example, those who like to entertain will place priorities on cleaning, cooking, and planning seating areas to encourage social interaction among their guests. Additionally, special groups might take place in their home, such as book discussions, card or board games, or viewing movies or sports events together. All of the tasks involved in preparation for one of these home-based events (planning menus, food shopping, vacuuming, dusting, cleaning bathrooms, preparing food items, and providing serving dishes, paper products, receptacles for trash, and parking for guests) fall within the occupation of home manager.

Learning Activity 59: Tasks for the Party Planner

An older client, Ida, with chronic fatigue syndrome wishes to entertain 10 family members for her husband's 70th birthday party. She loves to entertain but does not have the endurance to spend several hours per day preparing the house, cooking, and shopping for decorations, party supplies, and a gift. As her home care OT, how might you assist her in planning 1 week ahead so that she could do a few tasks each day and have enough energy to enjoy the party next Saturday evening? Summarize your plan below:

Sunday
Monday
Tuesday
Wednesday
Thursday
Friday
Saturday

Occupational Therapy Home Assessments

The following is a listing of general considerations when performing an environmental assessment of the home setting. Many therapists create site-specific evaluation forms to represent their typical clientele (e.g., a version for a typical private suburban home vs. an urban high-rise apartment).

The OT may prepare an "OT Tote Bag" containing commonly used supplies for a home visit. This could include pen and paper, clipboard and forms, ruler and tape measure, small flashlight, and small toolkit for minor repairs (tighten bolt on a wheelchair). There are a variety of home safety assessment tools from which to choose. Most include the areas listed in Table 7-1.

Learning Activity 60: Home Safety Internet Research

1. Perform an Internet search on the topic of home and safety checklists. Print three.

2. Compare your findings with the listings found in this chapter.

3. Compile your own one-page home safety checklist that could be used by an OT for evaluating an older adults' home.

Case Example: Jane (Laurie Wallace, OTR/L)

Jane was a 53-year-old right-hand–dominant woman with multiple sclerosis who had been diagnosed 20 years earlier and had several exacerbations and remissions during that time period. She had been living with her mother until about 2 months prior to her referral to OT. Her mother had passed away and the patient subsequently moved in with her brother, sister-in-law, and two nephews. Jane

TABLE 7-1

KEY AREAS OCCUPATIONAL THERAPISTS MAY EVALUATE FOR HOME SAFETY AND ACCESSIBILITY

AREA		
General	Rugs, wood or tile floors Power cords Lights—access, location, night visibility Phone—access, family emergency info Temperature—thermostats, controls Security—locks Access—car, yard, garage, garbage, mail Windows—locks, coverings, shades Furniture—stark vs. clutter Fireplace—use, safety, chimney Calendars and clocks Storage for cleaning—vacuum, dust, mop Heat/AC—space heaters, small fans	Risk for falls Memory problems affecting sequencing and awareness of safety Routine of chores—medications, interaction with others, time out of house (balance and responsibilities) Smoker? Ashtrays, lighters/matches Pests—prevention, poison/toxic items clearly labeled
Entryway	Access to entry, threshold, steps, railings, doormats Security—locks, latches, doorknobs Hang outerwear, umbrellas	View of visitors at door Mud/wet/boots/shoes Bench to put on, take off boots Place for mail, keys, and reminders for self
Kitchen	Storage—medium/low/high, heavy/light Stove—knobs, safety features, potholders Microwave, small appliances Layout—triangle refrigerator/stove/sink Pantry items—storage, often/seldom used Garbage/recycling Clean food preparation areas Floor surface—ability to clean Fridge—freezer, shelves, lighting Rolling cart to load with items Avoid rolling seats and step stools Medications "station," reminders, organize Rubber mat in sink Floor mat—nonskid Fire extinguishers Cleanup area, storage for dishes Pots and pans, can openers, sharp items, utensils	Clear countertops Save steps System for food storage, labels, within reach Organize location in fridge Bend/lift, positioning, body mechanics Pacing—timing: not too rushed, over course of day Avoid "trip" items—pet food, area rug Avoid smoke, burning—timer Avoid distractions—smoke alarm Avoid spills Practice problem solving—What would you do if? Avoid too many plugs in one outlet Have the right tools?

(continued)

TABLE 7-1 (CONTINUED)

KEY AREAS OCCUPATIONAL THERAPISTS MAY EVALUATE FOR HOME SAFETY AND ACCESSIBILITY

AREA		
Hallways	Lighting Floor surface Thresholds, stairs Need for rail/surface to offer support Width to accommodate walker or Wheelchair	Avoid clutter Brighter lighting Exits to outdoors, stairs, basement, garage, locks? Accessibility?
Bathroom	Sharp/hard/slippery surfaces Ability to maneuver, pivot, turn Ability to notify of need for help Supplies and products easily accessed, clearly labeled Razors or other sharps carefully stored Ease in use of faucet	Considerations for modifications—grab bars/raised toilet seat, shower seat, hand-held shower head Safety concerns—type of soap (e.g., slippery if falls on shower floor, may substitute with liquid pump dispenser)
Bedroom	Privacy, covering for windows, door latch Area rugs secure Telephone near bed Lighting—ease in reaching Closets—systems for accessing priority garments Bureaus—sort, organize, label as needed.	Side rail recommended? Chair near bed for support as needed System for hamper/dirty clothing Access to laundry area Area for laying out clothes needed for day
Office area	Computer station, desk, adjustable chair Sort, organize mail, pay bills Safe/lock box—storage of important papers	Electronic safety, Internet safety Budget/finances—utilities, rent, taxes, upkeep
Other areas	Smoke detectors, carbon monoxide detectors Anti-intrusion/security systems Access to basement/attic/yard/garage Television, cable, electronics, games Areas to relax and socialize Specialized areas for hobbies Clear areas for exercising, equipment	Avoid strain for opening and closing windows All precautions related to electricity and water Medical alert systems Attention to hazardous waste materials (e.g., old paint)
Yard	Outdoor activities, gardening Level versus slope or hill Condition changes due to weather/seasons Storage of tools for fixing things Decks, patios, grills, fire pits	Ability to access help when out of doors Safety of steps and railings Sidewalk condition Storage of garden items, shovels
	What other ideas would you add to this list?	
Created by K. C. Macdonald, 2015.		

could ambulate short distances with a quad cane, but her proximal leg and arm strength were rated only fair-minus to fair. She had great difficulty with overhead reaching and stair climbing due to significant quad weakness. She had significant fine motor deficits as well but had been compensating for many years and was able to bathe, dress, toilet, and groom herself independently with increased time. Jane already had traditional adaptive equipment such as a reacher, sock aid, long-handled shoe horn and bath sponge, handheld shower, and bath bench that she had acquired over the years. Her primary concern with this recent move was accessibility of her brother's home. She needed help determining simple changes that could be made to help her function in his home without incurring renovations that would be expensive or disruptive to the household.

Her brother lived in a multilevel home set into a hillside, which had four steps to enter through the front door, four steps to enter through the garage entrance, and a one-step entry through the backyard. The front steps would have necessitated her negotiating an uneven flagstone pathway, so that access point was not feasible. The backyard was a grassy area that was not level, so that was not an option either. That left the garage entrance as her best option. However, the one-car garage could not accommodate a wheelchair ramp. The steps were particularly steep and her quad weakness did not allow her to lift her legs high enough to negotiate the steps without great effort and difficulty on her part. We were able to find a "half step" cane online that was basically a quad cane with a lightweight plastic platform attached to the base that reduced the step height by half so she could climb up the steep steps with ease.

The other major problem area was grooming and hair care because the narrow bathroom could not accommodate a chair for her to be able to sit at the sink to brush her teeth, dry her hair, or perform other grooming tasks. The simple structural change of removing the two doors and low threshold under the sink were recommended to allow her to fit a chair under the sink when not in use, leaving the path open past the sink to the tub and toilet beyond. A gooseneck clamp was also mounted on the sink to hold her hair dryer overhead, leaving her hands free to prop her elbows on the edge of the counter so she could style her hair while seated at the sink. She also used this propping technique for applying makeup, donning jewelry, and performing oral care. These simple changes allowed her to conserve energy and maximized her independence without disrupting the household. It only required a few sessions to resolve problems that had seemed insurmountable to her at the initial evaluation.

Adapted Gardening

Gardens may be adapted for size, accessibility, and social contact. Raised garden beds are designed for indi-

viduals in wheelchairs. Hanging planters may be used in an enclosed sunroom for an individual who should not leave the house unescorted.

Garden groups or clubs cater to individuals who enjoy plant care, whether in the community or within an adult day care center. Intergenerational projects are possible with shared responsibilities for researching and planting seeds or propagating from cuttings.

As a health promotion activity, the harvested results of a "crop" may lead to cooking and eating, enjoying them raw, or drying or preserving them through canning or freezing. Other items may be transformed into decorative or craft projects. Examples include use of pressed flowers for stationery cards or dried herbs and flower petals blended for a potpourri.

Occupational Therapist's Roles in Relocation Decisions and Adjustment

When managing a home becomes unrealistic, many options are now available. Downsizing, relocating, and adjusting to a new living situation and neighborhood are challenging. This can potentially lead to decreased participation or can open new avenues for positive possibilities. Throughout the process of home evaluation and promoting independent skills in any living environment, OTs have important responsibilities.

OTs may have assorted roles relating to varied definitions of home. Many clients in adult day care have recently relocated to a family member's home, usually a daughter or son. The home visit in this setting includes attention to some additional factors, especially of a social-emotional nature. A new family system has to be developed, with changes in roles and routines. The OT would determine the context of the client within the new living situation, addressing role expectations, acceptance, and coping with change.

The new residence may need significant modification depending on the health condition of the client. Observations should include safety risks, including symptoms of neglect or abuse by caregivers. This could be manifested in several ways, including physically, emotionally, or financially.

If the client has a cognitive impairment, adjustment to a new setting may be difficult. Attention may be focused on locking and disguising stairs, or adding large-print calendars and labels. The family member may be in a new role as a caregiver. The OT would offer suggestions related to scheduling, toileting, medication management, storage systems for easy access, and adherence to therapy recommendations from other professionals, such as exercise and dietary protocols.

Occupational Therapist's Roles in Long-Term Care

In a long-term care facility, it is important for health professionals to respect that even a shared room is perceived as home. Encouraging residents to bring some items that offer a sense of familiarity may ease the transition when first arriving. Pictures, pillows, and small decorative items help to identify a new area as "their" space. OTs may make helpful recommendations for 24/7 issues for awareness in the long-term care facility to offer a sense of respectful consideration of resident's basic needs. Examples include the following:

- Pleasing appearance in all areas, attractive colors and homelike atmosphere, aesthetics, not childlike
- Cleanliness
- Avoidance of clutter and fire hazards
- Practicality of all items—how to clean, store when not in use, durability, ergonomics, comfort
- Chairs, clocks, sound levels, traffic flow near nursing station
- Access to telephone, television
- Areas for privacy, small family/social gatherings
- Accessibility to common areas for recreation/dining
- Protected/supervised access to outdoor walking areas
- Decorative items as potential hazards (plants)
- Rapid attention and response by staff to spills, call buttons, or residents with calling-out behaviors
- No access to medicine/cleaning supplies/sharp items
- Options for personal control—lighting, temperature, scheduling of care activities, bedtime hours
- Durable medical equipment, adaptive equipment, restricted access to stairs, elevators, balconies, and assistive devices.; a careful system of inventory, labeling, and storage is necessary with a shared home setting

The OT may participate in general team discussions on these important topics. In other settings, the OT may be a consultant hired to determine needs for environmental changes. The OT might work closely with architects, subcontractors, or interior designers to determine practical yet pleasant living spaces.

Therapeutic Use of Self

Entering an individual's place of residence for the first time is a significant event. He or she is allowing the OT to witness and evaluate a private domain. In some cases, the client will be known from a previous rehabilitation setting. In many instances, the OT will be a stranger arriving for a home visit.

A client may be proud to invite you into his or her well-kept household. Another client may feel ashamed that due to recent changes in ability, he or she has not been able to "keep up" with usual standards for cleanliness and order. It will be apparent with some clients that housekeeping has never been a priority. Finally, some individuals may be collectors or borderline hoarders and may live in unsafe conditions representing years of that lifestyle.

The client or family may have spent significant time, energy, and even expense in preparing for the therapist's home visit. They may be fatigued from a flurry of cleaning to "make the house presentable" and to make a positive impression. In an example of poor therapeutic use of self, I will describe one of my few professional regrets at the end of this chapter.

Occupation-Based Activities—Occupational Therapy Group Example

An example follows of an OT group "going home again" in a subacute inpatient rehabilitation setting. Participants represent acute conditions, such as fracture, stroke, and cardiac, with members anticipating discharge to home within weeks. The group would be held 3 times weekly with an average of 4 to 6 participants. A module would contain 6 sessions, each 45 minutes, held in the OT clinic with the following themes:

- Session 1: *Introductions. Safety and hazards at home*: Discussion, identify risks and solutions, demonstrate examples in clinic.
- Session 2: *Helping yourself heal through doing*: Clinical instruction about importance of returning to familiar IADL activities.
  - Members share experiences of how they were recently performing household care. What may be different? Ideas for strategies and challenges.
  - Group is seated in chairs near clinic's bathroom setting. How would cleaning of the bathroom be different while healing?
  - Review restorative nature of performance of actual activities pertaining to usual habits and routines.
- Session 3: *How do you move?* Introduction to body mechanics and modification for positioning and transfers. Meet in clinic with chairs near bed setting. OT will offer follow-up consultation with professional and family caregivers to reinforce teaching and promote consistency.
- Session 4: *Asking for help:* Seated at table with paper and pens. Supportive session acknowledging need for some changes in methods and standards of home management, such as frequency of dusting.

○ Discuss assertiveness technique for self-advocacy in requesting assistance.

○ Review of community resources for temporary or permanent help with home and yard care. OT may contact local agencies and advocate for senior discounts for individuals who need short-term home management assistance.

○ Describe community programs and health services that may be available to match current and future needs, such as Meals on Wheels and home care rehabilitation, respectively.

- Session 5: *Maintaining financial health*: Seated at table with paper and pens.

  ○ Discuss how some medical conditions may have a cognitive component, and that an unexpected role as a patient may disrupt prior money management systems.

  ○ Review of budget, new expenses related to medication or durable medical equipment, scheduling bill paying, online possibilities for direct payment.

  ○ Review precautions about protecting financial information.

- Session 6: *Am I ready to go home?* Circle of chairs at table.

  ○ Supportive final group discussion to review principles of home management prior to discharge.

  ○ Acknowledge feelings that may range from anxiety to excitement.

The OT may photocopy a congratulations theme "cover" for a card; on the inside is printed Good Luck to ____. Each person writes his or her own name, then passes to the left. As cards are passed, one by one members write well wishes to the person whose name is printed on that card. When the card is returned to the original member, he or she reads the comments and then offers a verbal reaction and final remark to the group members.

  ○ Structure graduation-style festivities.

A group of this nature meets many goals with supplemental concurrent individual sessions. The group members can identify with others "in the same boat," compare progress, express emotions in a supportive setting, and participate in group problem-solving. Identifying with peers is a powerful therapeutic connection. The OT is skilled in designing group goals, structuring thematic sessions, guiding for group development, and addressing group dynamics issues.

Purposeful Activities

A patient with an anxiety disorder attends a day treatment program specializing in geropsychiatry. He experiences difficulties in focusing his thoughts, planning, sequencing, and task completion. He states that he is overwhelmed when he thinks about caring for his beloved vegetable garden. His wife depends on his produce for cooking and canning.

In individual sessions, the OTA sets goals with him to list the steps of his gardening tasks. Together, they sequence them for a daily, weekly, and seasonal "to do" list on an enlarged calendar. She engages him to participate in watering and weeding/trimming for houseplants in the day treatment center. A personalized garden journal is created with images of his favorite plants that are downloaded and printed. Together, they list notes about special care. For homework, he records one entry per day about a task completed, even if limited to a walk to look at the garden. In a subsequent session, the OTA inquires about the latest entries and discusses progress and obstacles.

Learning Activity 61: Cookbook Project

Diana is a homemaker who loves cooking. She has some residuals from a recent mild stroke and wishes to find simpler recipes. The OT suggests a homework project in which Diana will create a cookbook for her own use.

1. What would be the criteria for inclusion, such as: simple, no more than five ingredients, no bake, microwave only, and serve cold?

2. How will Diana locate recipes? Cookbooks? Internet?

3. How will Diana record, organize, and store, to create a hard copy "cookbook"?

Case Example: Ann and Catherine (Dr. Mary Ellen Johnson, OTD, MHS, OTR/L)

Catherine and Ann are mother and daughter clients, with home management to be shared between them. Ann is a busy professional, married with no children. She and her husband own a single story, 4 bedroom, 2.5 bath home in a suburban area in the Northeast. Ann's mother Catherine, who recently moved in with them, has a diagnosis of Alzheimer's disease evaluated at stage 3 (mild) on the Global Deterioration Scale. Catherine previously lived alone in another state, where she and her late husband both retired 14 years ago at age 65; that home is now listed for sale. Ann has one younger brother, but he works in Tokyo and is not available for caregiving.

Ann works in health care and is familiar with a local company specializing in aging in place run by two OTs. She contacted them and explained that she would like them to evaluate her mother's needs in relation to her new living environment. Safety is a primary concern but so is making accommodations for her mother's osteoarthritis in her hips and knees. Ann also wanted to plan ahead because she knew her mother's cognition would deteriorate over time.

The OT practitioners came to Ann's home, where Catherine was agreeable to being evaluated. They assessed her cognitive level at 4.6 using Allen's Cognitive Disabilities frame of reference (Allen, Earhart, & Blue, 1992), the lowest level required for living alone, according to this theory (Toglia, Golisz, & Goverover, 2014). They evaluated her ADL performance and found that although she was able to independently stand up from a chair, bed, and toilet and ambulate, she was unsteady when she first stood up secondary to hip and knee stiffness and pain (3 on a scale of 1 to 10). She uses a cane.

The OT discussed with Catherine and Ann the home management occupations they wished to do. Ann expressed she would appreciate having her mother's help with cleaning and dusting, laundry, and meal preparation and cleanup because she would continue to work full time. Catherine asked the OTs if she would be able to garden. She has won awards for her gardening, both indoor and outdoor, and her flower arrangements. Last year, she let her garden go because it was too difficult to bend down with her arthritis.

The OTs also evaluated the home using the SAFER-HOME v.3 (Chiu et al., 2006). Several areas of concern were identified:

- Catherine was at risk of falls getting in and out of the tub to shower (her preference) and in standing unsupported to take a shower. There were no grab bars and the shower head was fixed.

- The toilet seats in her bathroom and the half bath are 16 inches high and make it difficult for 5'9" Catherine to stand up easily.

- The door to the stairs leading to the basement was right next to the door to the half bath, and looked the same. It did not have a lock.

- The bathroom in the guest room (Catherine's room) was not accessible from the hallway and, with the bathroom and bedroom doors closed, it would be difficult to hear Catherine call for help, especially at night.

- The one concrete step leading into the house did not have a handrail.

- The kitchen was safe with supervision. Ann reported that Catherine has, on occasion, left the stove on when she boiled water for tea.

- There is a flight of six steps from the back deck to the yard and the steps are not gated. The deck is off the kitchen and accessible through french doors without any step.

- Catherine's medications were in a bag in her bedroom and she is still self-administering them.

Ann and her husband are willing to make modifications to the home as long as they don't involve major construc-

tion. Catherine has given durable power of attorney to her daughter and they have discussed using the funds from the sale of her home to retain a companion to be with Catherine while Ann and her husband are at work.

The OTs made the following recommendations:

- *Bedroom and bathroom:* Put night lights in the outlets near the bathroom to illuminate the floor between the bed and bathroom, a night light in the bathroom, leave the bathroom door open so that Catherine can find it when she awakens during the night. For the bed, insert a 12" width bed rail to assist rising and standing. Place a two-way baby monitor in Catherine's room and in Ann and her husband's bedroom.

- *Shower and toilet:* Install a shower chair that extends over the side of the tub so transfers can be done while a sitting position, a handheld shower, grab bars in the shower (vertical and horizontal) for rising and standing, comfortable height toilets in Catherine's bathroom, and, in the half bath, grab bars next to both toilets.

- *Kitchen:* Leave a covered plastic pitcher with ice water and cups on the island to encourage hydration; leave prepared snacks on the island or in the refrigerator to eliminate the need to use knives. Supervise any hot beverages or foods or when assisting family in food preparation.

- *Deck:* Add a locked gate to block the steps. Add raised planters around the deck for gardening.

- *Basement stairs:* Put a combination lock on the door.

- *Front step:* Install a handrail or landscape and pave a walkway that rises equal to the door sill in the event that stairs become too difficult or a wheelchair is needed.

- *Medications:* Use a pill box and assistance to help Catherine to set up her daily medications. Monitor that they are correctly taken.

The OTs discussed occupational goals with Ann and Catherine. Ann realized that shopping and storing food, as well as tending to her mother's medications, would have to be her responsibility. Catherine could do some familiar homemaking tasks by herself when Ann set out the needed items, such as a dust cloth and spray cleaner for the wood furniture or a laundry basket full of dry clothes to be folded on the bed. It is not recommended that Catherine use any electric appliances without supervision. However, Catherine could put a salad together if ingredients are left out on the kitchen counter and could set the table for the evening meal without assistance. She and Ann would need to do meal preparation together, so that the use of appliances could be supervised. With the above-mentioned home modifications in place, Catherine could plant and maintain a patio garden with tools for the task set out in plain view.

The OTs discussed with both women how Ann could assist Catherine in maintaining her familiar self-care routines by placing all of the needed items for a task in plain sight. Applying Allen's Cognitive Disabilities Theory, individuals at Level 4.6 only attend to items they can see; they can perform multistep tasks only when everything they need is clearly visible, and items they should not use are put out of sight. For example, items for bathing and grooming need to be laid out in the bathroom so that Catherine can perform these activities independently. Likewise, she can dress herself if clean clothes are laid out for her, but dirty clothes should be stowed out of sight. Ann needs to take extra care to sort and store household items, keeping her mother's living areas as clutter free as possible. Following this principle, Ann can assist her mother in remaining independent in ADLs for as long as possible.

Journal Entry (K. M.)

I arrived at the home of a woman with multiple sclerosis. This visit was my first session with her. She had agreed to be interviewed for my doctoral study on women adapting to physical disability. Her husband and a morning aide had provided very challenging morning care. When I arrived at 9-o'clock in the morning, I could tell they had already experienced several hours of difficult tasks, paced to allow my client time to rest before my arrival.

When I was settled into a chair, the home health aide immediately appeared with a plate of homemade cookies, proudly offering them to me. She stated that she had made them from scratch at 6-o'clock that morning in the midst of all the morning care. I thanked her and smiled and said, "No, thank you" and switched to beginning my information gathering. But I knew at that moment, when I looked at the three of them, that I had broken my opportunity for a certain level of respect and rapport. They had envisioned "getting acquainted" in a normal social manner: offer a guest a little something. I, in hindsight, could have certainly enjoyed a cookie at the same time as beginning some questions and note taking. I consider myself a very polite person. Why didn't I know how to side step from "being a professional" and "getting down to business" and simply add empathy and acknowledgment?

In mentioning the experience to other home care therapists over the years, all expressed similar experiences in which clients have prepared full meals and expect a very lengthy visit... chatting... showing cherished possessions... "But I have to be across town for my next appointment in 30 minutes, and it's a 20-minute drive!" was a shared sentiment. How can we best develop a sense of trust and rapport, while at the same time setting some boundaries for time and establishing a professional relationship, which is different from visiting a personal acquaintance? How do I separate out my perceptions and findings from knowing that they "prepared for company" versus their usual patterns of home management?

Therapeutic use of self is especially vital in home care service provision. Careful attention is important related to respecting individual values and standards for housekeeping. The therapist has limited time for each session and a large overall number of sessions each workday, requiring exceptional skills in identifying priority areas for concern. Careful instruction and communication become the basis of shared problem solving, with proposed interventions reviewed and adapted until they are realistic. The therapist needs to consider past, present, and future needs, which are often in a state of transition. For example, a fall leading to a fractured dominant shoulder would result in many changes in ability for many weeks and possibly months of healing. This could lead to modified techniques or shifts in role responsibility, where a spouse might need to take responsibility for laundry or vacuuming.

Summary

The sense of home, representing comfort and family memories, is viewed through realistic eyes. Older adults have typically experienced many moves for many reasons, such as employment, family locale, retirement, finances, and changes in ability. Having seen their parents and many peers shift in home management abilities, most participants seemed to have the perspective of, "I'll manage the best I can for as long as I can, and then I'll have to think about moving." Several participants moved to a condo after widowhood or change in health status.

Another motivation to change from a place of residence was to seek companionship. Many older adults, when widowed, state that they have never eaten alone in their lives or find it gloomy to cook for one. Developments of senior and congregate housing offer options for shared meals, as well as a vast reduction in home and yard tasks.

Some seniors have difficulty adjusting to a new living situation, while others are excited about the possibilities of a new community. This generation of seniors, who have witnessed radical social changes and lived through life's personal transitions, are familiar with coping and adjusting. The OT may play an important role in assessing factors of safety and function to any living environment. Equal consideration may be given to how the individual is managing responsibilities or adjusting to change.

References

Allen, C. K., Earhart, C. A., & Blue, T. (1992). *Occupational therapy treatment goals for the physically and cognitively disabled.* Bethesda, MD: American Occupational Therapy Association.

American Occupational Therapy Association. (2014). *Occupational therapy practice framework: Domain and Process.* (3rd ed.). Bethesda, MD: Author.

Aplin, T., de Jonge, D., & Gustafsson, C. (2013). Understanding the dimensions of home that impact on home modification decision making. *Australian Occupational Therapy Study, 60,* 101-109.

Arbesman, M., & Lieberman, D. (2012). Methodology for the systematic review on occupation-end activity-based intervention related to productive aging. *American Journal of Occupational Therapy, 66,* 271-283.

Barrows, C. (2006). Home adaptations: Creating safe environments for individuals with psychiatric disabilities. *OT Practice, October 9,* 12-16.

Chase, C. A., Mann, K., Wasek, S., & Arbesman, M. (2012). Systematic review of the effect of home modification and fall prevention programs on falls and the performance of community-dwelling in older adults. *American Journal of Occupational Therapy, 66,* 284-291.

Chiu, T., Oliver, R., Ascott, P., Choo, L. C., Davis, T., Gaya, A., ... Letts, L. (2006). *Safety Assessment of Function and the Environment for Rehabilitation: Health Outcome Measurement and Evaluation (SAFER-HOME) Version 3 Manual.* Toronto: COTA Health.

Garre-Olmo, J., López-Pousa, S., Turon-Estrada, A., Juvinyá, D., Ballester, D., & Vilalta-Franch, J. (2012). Environmental determinants of quality of life in nursing home residents with severe dementia. *Journal of American Geriatric Society, 60,* 1230-1236.

Hossack, J. R. (1956). Home management for the disabled. *American Journal of Occupational Therapy, 10,* 143-149.

Morris, J. T., & Jones, M. L. (2013). Emergency preparedness for people with disabilities: Guide and checklist. *Archives of Physical Medicine and Rehabilitation, 94,* 219-220.

Knight, J., Ball, V., Corr, S., Turner, A., Lewis, M., & Ekberg, M. (2007). An empirical study to identify older adults' engagement in productivity occupations. *Journal of Occupational Science, 4,* 145-153.

Mansfield, H. (2013). Romaine Tenney loved his farm to death. *Yankee, 77,* 102-110.

National Alliance for Caregiving & American Association of Retired Persons. (2009). *Caregiving in the U.S.* Retrieved from http://www.nationalallianceforcaregiving.org.

Nilsson, J., Lundgren, A. S., & Liliequist, M. (2012). Occupational well-being among the very old. *Journal of Occupational Science, 19,* 115-126.

Renda, M. (2012). Home modifications: An introduction to practice considerations. *OT Practice, 17,* 1-7.

Rowles, G. D. (2008). Place in occupational science: A life course perspective on the role of environmental context in the quest for meaning. *Journal of Occupational Science, 15,* 127-135.

Shank, K. H., & Cutchin, M. P. (2010). Transactional occupations of older women: Aging-in-place: Negotiating change in meaning. *Journal of Occupational Science, 17,* 4-13.

Stark, S. L., Somerville, E. K., & Morris, J. C. (2010). In-home occupational performance evaluation. *American Journal of Occupational Therapy, 64,* 580-595.

Toglia, J. P., Golisz, K. M., & Goverover, Y. (2014). Cognition, perception, and occupational performance. In B. A. Boyt Schell., G. Gillen, & M. E. Scaffa (Eds.) *Willard & Spackman's Occupational Therapy* (12th ed.); (pp. 779-815). Philadelphia: Lippincott Williams & Wilkins.

Tse, T., Douglas, J., Lentin, P., & Carey, L. (2013). Measuring participations after stroke: A review of frequently used tools. *Archives of Physical Medicine and Rehabilitation, 94,* 177-192.

Van Oss, T., Rivers, M., Heighton, B., Mocci, C., & Reid, B. (2012). Bathroom safety: Environmental modifications to enhance bathing and aging in place in the elderly. *OT Practice, 17,* 14-19.

Wagenfeld, A., & Buresh, B. (2012). Ergonomic gardening: Teaching safe movement patterns. *OT Practice, 17,* 14-19.

Wang, D., & Macmillan, T. (2013). The benefits of gardening for older adults: A systematic review of literature. *Activities, Adaptation & Aging, 37,* 153-181.

Wong, J. D., & Almeida, D. M. (2013). The effects of employment status and daily stressors on time spent on daily household chores in middle-ages and older adults. *The Gerontologist, 53,* 81-91.

Woodland, J. E., & Hobson, S. J. (2003). An occupational therapy perspective on falls prevention among community-dwelling older adults. *Canadian Journal of Occupational Therapy, 70,* 174-182.

Young, D. (2012). Light the way: Providing effective home modification for clients with low vision. *OT Practice, 17,* 8-12.

Zur, B., & Rudman, D. L. (2013). WHO age friendly cities: Enacting societal transformation through enabling occupation. *Occupational Science, 4,* 370-381.

8

Caregiver

Marilyn B. Cole, MS, OTR/L, FAOTA

"Caregiving's value can't be overstated." (Appleby, 2012)

Usually, one thinks of older adults as recipients rather than providers of care. Caregiving ranks third (30%) of 5 productive roles identified by older adults in the United Kingdom (UK) (Knight et al., 2007). Caregiving in older adulthood occurs in a variety of contexts. While younger mothers and fathers bear the full responsibility for raising their children, older adults mostly take on caregiving roles by choice and according to their own conditions and limitations. When a spouse or elderly parent, sibling, or close relative becomes disabled, older adults often feel a sense of obligation to provide care. However, there are other acceptable options, such as home care workers paid by Medicare or out of pocket, adult day care, or escalating levels of long-term care. Older adults in the PAS chose to take care of adult children or grandchildren more often than expected, with mutual benefits to both. In more than one instance, PAS participants provided both emotional and financial support to their returning adult children.

A caregiver, quite simply, provides for the personal needs for survival, health, and well-being of another living being. The terms *caregiver*, *care giver*, and *carer* have equivalent meanings, although *caregiver* is standard terminology in the United States, Canada, and China, while *carer* is more common for the UK, New Zealand, and Australia. Carer and caregiver generally refer to unpaid help of a relative, friend, or child with a disability (National Alliance for Caregiving & American Association of Retired Persons, 2009). More

formal caregiving may fall into various categories of service providers, such as home health aides or health care workers, as well as a host of medical personnel. The AOTA's (2014) OT Practice Framework III includes "care of others, care of pets, and child rearing" within the broader category of instrumental activities of daily living (IADL) (p. S19). *Care of others* is defined as "(including selecting and supervising caregivers)—Arranging, supervising, or providing care for others" (AOTA, 2014, p. S19). Care of pets is defined as "Arranging, supervising, or providing the care for pets and service animals." *Child rearing* is defined as "Providing the care and supervision to support the developmental needs of a child" (AOTA, 2014, p. S19).

There is a distinction between being in a grandparent role and custodial grandparenting. Grandparents laugh about "spoiling" their grandchildren and visiting while having the option of going back home. Grandparents enjoy teaching their grandchildren about their ancestry, culture, or traditions and providing or sharing pleasurable experiences with them as part of the grandparent role. *Custodial grandparenting* means taking on the primary responsibility of child rearing in lieu of parents, not just occasional visits, fun activities, or babysitting on weekends.

Caregiving, as a productive role, usually refers to providing unpaid care for someone close, such as a family member, and involves a personal commitment to another person's well-being. In a national study, 89% of

Cole MB, Macdonald KC.
Productive Aging: An Occupational Perspective (pp 135-153).
© 2015 Taylor & Francis Group.

spousal caregivers were over age 65 and 53% were over age 75 (Spillman & Black, 2005).

PARTICIPANT PERSPECTIVES

Caring for Aging Parents and Spouses

Caregivers in our study reported most often caring for spouses or relatives who became ill or disabled. Valnere cared for her 90-year-old mother long distance by visiting her for about one week each month at her retirement community. During these visits, she managed her mother's finances, took her shopping and to medical appointments, and met with service providers to review her mother's care. They spoke by telephone every evening between visits. Earlier in her life, Valnere reported caring for her husband, who suffered from Parkinson's and a stroke, as well as her father and her adult daughter who died of cancer at age 26. At one point, she felt an obligation to quit work so that she could spend more time in caregiving. "I fell into retirement instead of planning it. Really, caregiving duties dictated what happened. I stopped working at age 58 when my husband became ill. But caregiving began many years before that. I took care of my mother-in-law, who lived with us until she died in 1979…I had to set certain limits as to how much time I could devote because I was still working and caring for a teenage daughter then. Nicole was sick for 2 years before she died in 1995 at age 26. Father became disabled, and I adapted our home so he could live with me, while also caring for a disabled husband. I could only work a few hours a week to keep up my certifications." In contrast, Bob C. cares for his mother long distance, mainly by managing her finances on his computer from his apartment and one or two weekend visits each year. She resides in an assisted living facility. He and his younger brother take turns calling her occasionally.

When Betty's first husband had multiple sclerosis, she cared for him while raising their two sons until he died at age 49 after 20 years of marriage. Her second husband was an established New York artist, and Betty worked at his gallery. After 15 years, "He had a stroke and turned nasty—I dreaded coming home after work." After her divorce, "my friends try to fix me up. I tell them I don't need another old man to take care of!"

Sue feels the burden of caregiving at home for her husband who had a stroke, "He used to be violent but is now fairly docile." She also provides care for her mother-in-law, who has her own apartment in Sue's home: "She's now showing signs of dementia, and health workers come in while I'm working." Sue begins each day caring for her four dogs, who also have special needs. "One has diabetes and I give him a shot of insulin before breakfast. They all get fed and walked before I have my morning tea." She finds herself in the role of advocate for the health care needs of her husband and mother-in-law: "advocating is part of the caregiving role." Sue's daughter lives nearby and comes over daily to help with dinner because Sue has difficulty carrying trays of food because of her own balance and mobility issues. Her divorced son has recently moved back home, but he works full-time, contributes to expenses, and is more a support than a burden.

Bob M. reports providing care for "my wife who fractured her shoulder—helping her with dressing, meals, dishes, and driving." Ellen assists her partner who has multiple sclerosis, "with tasks like shopping, laundry, and meal preparation…[B]eing a caregiver gives me great satisfaction [her family appreciates it], if not for me, she'd be in one of those places." Alice provided care for her husband at home for his last 6 months. A health worker "would come in from 8 to 4, then I cared for him in the evening. Then he needed a wheelchair. To get him into bed, we got a hospital bed and the aide would get him into bed before she left. Then he kept changing and declining. Thank goodness I was working or I would have lost my mind. He went to adult day care and ended up enjoying all the programs. He went through depression in his life when he lost his job. Later, he was delusional, [and] we weren't sure if it was post-traumatic stress disorder or Alzheimer's or Parkinson's. He would say things in the middle of the night. He would get angry or frightened. After, it took me 6 months to get back on track. It was very hard for me."

Caring for Adult Children and Grandchildren

Adult children represent another category of care recipients. June's older sons are both married and raising families of their own. Her youngest son, however, has a chronic mental illness. "For him, I'll always be a mother, a caregiver. I drive to get him every weekend and he comes with me to my apartment [in New York] or my house in the Berkshires. I'm always making sure he's taken care of, finding a place for him to live that's decent and safe (subsidized apartment near a mental health clinic). I'm interfacing with his doctors and other caregivers, advocating for him, making sure no one takes advantage of him. I feel I must be there to see who takes care of him. So many unqualified helpers are cheap, but not equipped to handle severe mental illness."

Malcolm reports caring for wife with multiple sclerosis for 10 years (died several years ago); he now shares his home with his adult son and cares for two grandchildren on weekdays while his son works. "My 50-year-old son has had some great jobs in the past—his best yearly income was about $125,000. Since his divorce 10 years ago, his combined income might not equal that. I have kept him afloat while he has sought several new careers. He has soaked up most of the money I could have invested more productively. He has done an outstanding job as a Mr. Mom, but a terrible job as an income provider."

Those who reported caring for grandchildren by choice almost always found the experience emotionally rewarding. Sue tells us, "I love being number one Nanna for my baby granddaughter," who visits each day for dinner. Malcolm reports "my grandchildren are a powerful source of joy to me. They are exceptionally well mannered. They do well in school in spite of having outside activities. My grandson is following up his black belt in Tae Kwando with an intense interest in Aikido. My granddaughter spends more than 12 hours a week figure skating under the tutelage of a man recognized as one of the world's best coaches."

Margie, another full-time Nanna, takes care of her two grandchildren, ages 1 and 4, every weekday while her daughter works. They get dropped off at her home at 6:45 a.m. and are picked up around 5:00 p.m. each evening (Figure 8-1). Nanna's duties include dressing and bathing them, fixing breakfast and lunch, changing diapers and potty training, providing learning experiences for them during play time, and driving her grandson to and from preschool. Margie reports having some difficulty balancing caregiving with getting her own needs met. Being naturally nurturing, she sometimes feels she does too much, and she would like her daughter and son-in-law to take on more of the primary parenting responsibilities. Pearl and her husband also take care of their grandson 2 days each week while their son and his wife work. They cherish the time spent with him even though it is a challenge for Pearl to run after an active 18-month-old toddler.

Mildred enjoys having her 8-year-old grandson "sleep over" on weekends. They do crafts together, and she cooks his favorite dishes. She has voluntarily taken over his religious education—she takes him to synagogue and is teaching him Hebrew (as her father did for her at the same age). Jan does some long-distance babysitting when her Texas son and his wife go on vacation. With her nearby son, Jan cares for grandchildren as needed and goes to all of their school events. Peggie identifies herself as a caregiver by nature. Peggie and Jack often travel long distances to attend the sports events of their grandchildren. They plan family vacations each year, and spend time every summer with each of their five children's families at Peggie's sister's home at the New Jersey shore. Their adult daughter is struggling financially; she is divorced, working daytimes, and going to school at night. Peggie often takes her daughter's kids shopping for things they need to get them ready for a new school year or for sports equipment. Recently, they bought their daughter's house so the bank wouldn't foreclose and she wouldn't have to move her kids out of school. She pays them rent by working part-time.

Signian and Ken, also long-distance grandparents, see the grandkids on almost every holiday. Nettie often babysits her grandchildren: "I take my 4-year-old to the playground and I go on the slide with him! I go hiking with my granddaughter even though it's a challenge."

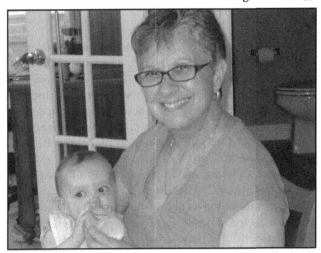

Figure 8-1. Margie cares for granddaughter Emma (age 1) every weekday from 6:45 a.m. to 5:00 p.m.

Grandparenting isn't always easy. Betty went on a cruise with her daughter, son-in-law, and their two children. As a captive grandma (staying in close quarters for the duration of the cruise), she had major problems with their parenting style, and felt deeply embarrassed by her grandchildren's undisciplined misbehavior during their vacation. Afterward, Betty got depressed and didn't speak to any of them for 1 year. She has since sought some counseling, and now visits her daughter's family, but she chooses not to be their caregiver.

LITERATURE REVIEW

Caregiving as an occupational role in older adulthood has not been widely researched. Existing studies tend to cluster around specific issues, such as caregiver strain, end-of-life family caregiving, spousal caregiving, and grandparents raising grandchildren. Specific issues around caregiving for a relative with dementia have recently received widespread attention.

In a qualitative study of productive occupations of older adults, Knight et al. (2007) report carer (caregiver) as one of the five most common productive occupational roles. Carer ranked as the third most often identified role (27%), after homemaker (89%) and volunteer (30%) (Knight et al., 2007). The recipients of care included not only family members, but also pets, neighbors, and friends. Women held caregiving roles more frequently than men. These researchers cited altruism (doing something for others, making them happy) and pleasure (feeling useful, sense of satisfaction, love and companionship) as the most common motivators for engaging in productive occupations generally, as well as caring in particular (Knight et al., 2007).

Caregiving Statistics

Most statistics on caregiving in the United States do not distinguish caregivers by age. The gender statistics, however, still apply: of unpaid family caregivers, 66% are women, and their average age, now 48 years, is increasing. Male caregivers spend 17.4 hours per week in caring, while women average 21.9 hours (National Alliance for Caregiving & American Association of Retired Persons, 2009). However, the provision of care for a spouse over age 75 is about equal for men and women (Family Caregiver Alliance [FCA], 2012). Of those caring for someone over age 50, the average caregiver age is between 50 and 64 years. Of those caring for someone over 65, caregivers average age is 63, with one third of these in fair to poor health themselves (FCA, 2012).

National surveys also summarize caregiver time spent in various caregiving tasks. In a Gallup survey, caregivers spent approximately 13 days per month doing IADL such as meal preparation, housekeeping, laundry, transportation, and giving medication. Personal care ADL, such as feeding, dressing, walking, bathing, and assistance with toileting, accounted for about 6 days per month (Gallup Healthways Wellbeing Survey, 2011).

In the Home Alone study of family caregivers who provide complex chronic care, nearly half (46%) also performed medical and nursing tasks such as handling incontinence supplies, administering enemas, providing wound care, and giving intravenous medications or injections (Moorman & Macdonald, 2013). Furthermore, for older family caregivers, the average number of hours dedicated to caregiving increases with age (FCA, 2012):

- Caregivers ages 55 to 64 provide an average of 25.3 hours per week.

- Caregivers ages 65 to 74 provide an average of 30.7 hours per week. (FCA, 2012)

- Caregivers over age 75 provide an average of 34.5 hours per week

A Gallup survey reports that 72% of caregivers cared for a parent, step-parent, or mother/father-in-law, and 67% of care recipients were over age 75 (FCA, 2012). Approximately 20% of caregivers live with their care recipients, while 74% live less than 20 minutes away (National Alliance for Caregiving & American Association of Retired Persons, 2009).

Other activities included in caregiving are transportation (83%), housework (75%), grocery shopping (75%), meal preparation (65%), managing finances (64%), and arranging or supervising outside services (34%). Advocating for care recipients with paid service providers, government agencies, or schools and researching health conditions through the Internet are cited as important supportive activities of the caregiving role (National Alliance for Caregiving & American Association of Retired Persons, 2009).

Transition to Caregiving

Some studies report that as older relatives need more care, adding new caregiving responsibilities for the younger or healthier family member can have unanticipated emotional consequences (Cress, 2001; Knotts, 2008). Certainly, when thrust into caregiving for a spouse who has unexpectedly experienced a disabling illness, such as a broken hip, a heart attack, or stroke, the well partner's life may change substantially as traditional roles are reversed. A caregiving wife may find herself driving, mowing the lawn, and managing the family finances; a caregiving husband may need to learn his way around the kitchen, handle laundry and house chores, and do the grocery shopping. Thus, in transitioning to care giving and receiving, the older couple finds their relationship itself has changed. This is especially true when one's spouse suffers from dementia. In caring for a spouse or any relative with dementia, the caregiver must find the right balance between doing things for the person and providing autonomy with oversight (Knotts, 2008). Tasks for this situation include safety-proofing the house and assisting with bathing, grooming, and toileting, while also creating meaning, life quality, and dignity. The caregiver concurrently must cope with his or her own stress, fatigue, and, often, profound sadness and loss (Gitlin & Corcoran, 2005).

Five PAS participants described caregiving for spouses, parents, or partners. Sue has major caregiving responsibilities for her spouse, a stroke survivor, and her live-in mother-in-law, who has dementia. Valnere currently performs IADL for her 91-year-old mother, who lives in a retirement community, and describes formerly caring for her spouse (stroke, Parkinson's), her father, and mother-in-law in her home. Ellen cares for her partner with MS, and Alice provided end-of-life care for her husband with dementia and other complications. Their experiences mostly concur with recent studies, except for Bob C., who provides only long-distance care for his elderly mother.

Grandparents Raising Grandchildren

From a developmental perspective, a grandparent's role coincides with Erikson's generativity stage of life, making sharing one's wisdom and life experience with younger generations a priority. Grandparents whose adult children have primary child rearing responsibility can enjoy periodic visits and share leisure activities with their grandkids, such as taking them to parks and playgrounds, teaching them to fish or bake cookies, and even taking them on camping trips or excursions to Disney World. As most of our participants reported, such occasional shared experiences provided a great source of joy for grandparents.

However, custodial grandparenting or taking on primary responsibility for raising grandchildren under age 18, a rapidly rising trend in the United States, implies a very different caregiving role for older adults. A U.S. Census Bureau (2010) report stated that 39% of grandparent caregivers had cared for their grandchildren for more than 5 years, and 1 in 10 grandparents in the United States will be a primary caregiver for a grandchild for at least 6 months. Five percent of all children are currently living in grandparent-headed households (U.S. Census Bureau, 2010). With this role comes increased stress associated with parenting at an unexpected life stage, including financial burden, worry, health issues, and freedom restriction (Williams, 2011). Research cites several reasons for the recent increase in custodial grandparenting (which may or may not involve actual legal custody), including birth parent substance abuse or incarceration, teen pregnancy, emotional problems, untimely parental death, and, more recently, financial burden and military deployment of the birth parent (Bunch, Eastman, & Moore, 2007; Butler & Zakari, 2005). When grandparents have physical custody but lack legal custody, many complications arise, such as difficulty obtaining child health insurance, obtaining medical and dental care, and enrolling children in school, day care, or sports activities. Additionally, there is a gap in qualification for income assistance from government programs for grandparents without legal custody of their grandchildren (Bunch et al., 2007; Williams, 2011).

According to Butler and Zakari (2005), most grandparents assume caregiving responsibilities because of a crisis situation, having no prior plans to raise their grandchildren. In their study, 17 mostly lower-income grandmothers raised an average of 2 grandchildren with up to 8 other grandchildren, and sometimes great grandchildren, living in the home. Within this sample, 87% reported at least moderately impaired physical health, and half indicated high anxiety, moderate depression, and inadequate social relationships. They depended mainly upon their extended families and the church for needed social support. Only 3 of the 17 reported having adequate financial resources—the remainder were still in need of child support, clothing, transportation to clinics and special schools, and medical benefits (Butler & Zakari, 2005). Additional negative outcomes for older grandparents include decreased peer network interaction, social isolation, depression, and lowered life satisfaction; custodial grandparents lack the freedom to participate in recreational or leisure activities that could provide self-fulfillment for people at their age (Williams, 2011).

Two PAS participants performed the productive role of custodial grandparents, although neither had legal custody. Malcolm's son and two children live with him, and he takes primary care of his preteen grandchildren on weekdays. His schedule is full, but he makes the most of his remaining free time and considers his grandchildren sources of pride and joy. Margie feels privileged to care for 2 grandchildren, ages 1 and 5, every weekday while her daughter works. Although she has help from her husband who recently retired, she often feels the need for more freedom to do things for herself and struggles with balancing her multiple roles.

Caregiver Strain

Caregiver strain is defined as "caregivers' perceptions of negative physical, psychological, social, economic, or spiritual effects from providing care to a terminally ill relative" (Townsend, Ishler, Shapiro, Pitorak, & Matthews, 2010, p. 52). This definition comes from a hospice perspective, which estimates that 25% of all family caregivers are age 65 or older (FCA, 2012). In a national survey, caregivers report poorer health (17% fair or poor) on average than the general population (13%), with those providing care over 5 years being twice as likely to report poorer health as a result of caregiving (FCA, 2012). Emotional situations, such as caring for someone with cognitive or behavioral challenges, tends to increase stress, with co-residence and burden of care significantly contributing to caregiver strain. Financial challenge is highly correlated with greater caregiving burden (longer hours, more difficult tasks) and is a source of increased caregiver stress (National Alliance for Caregiving & American Association of Retired Persons, 2009).

From a professional perspective, McGhan, Loeb, Baney, and Penrod (2013) studied older women caring for their spouses using 3 health care models: (1) cooperative network model, in which care is directed at disease progression and symptom management, which may or may not involve the family caregiver; (2) interdisciplinary teams, in which the caregiver is considered a corecipient of care; and (3) provider dominant model, in which a medical specialist retains sole responsibility for the patient and considers the spousal caregiver a coprovider of care with no consideration for the caregiver's own needs. This qualitative study identified five dominant themes of older caregivers (ages 71 to 80):

1. Balancing multiple morbidities: "I don't know how this treatment is affecting his other problems."

2. Feeling overwhelmed and exhausted: "I can't do what I did when I was 50."

3. Dealing with personal health issues: "I've come up against my own mortality."

4. Feeling isolated: "I'm not a gad-about, but I do need social interaction."

5. Coordinating care for patient and caregiver: "They said they'd call, but they haven't yet."

This study concluded that the caregivers felt most supported and helped by members of an interdisciplinary team. This was the only approach that provided assistance with coordination of care and considered both patient and caregiver needs; the other two models required the caregiver to "navigate uncoordinated services, which contributed to their distress" (McGhan et al., 2013, p. 54). Another study looking at transitions in care for older adults in long-term care facilities comes to similar conclusions that the family caregivers "do not receive needed information about the reasons for their transfers to hospitals, medical diagnosis, and planned treatments to address acute changes in health" (Toles, Abbott, Hirschman, & Naylor, 2011, p. 40). These authors identify an "urgent need for ... health care team members to talk with ... family caregivers [to] ensure that they are engaged and informed participants in care" (p. 40).

A study by Townsend et al. (2010) sought to identify predictors of caregiver strain, as well as protective factors. They found that predictors varied according to the type of strain. Younger end-of-life caregivers had higher levels of psychological strain; protective factors were being able to plan ahead, having good intrapsychic resources, and the availability of caregiving help from others. Caregivers of patients with cancer reported lower psychological strain. These same protective factors applied to social strain. Caregivers in poorer health and in unpredictable caregiving situations reported the highest physical strain. Higher economic strain was found by caregivers with diabetes, and those with lower incomes and poorer physical health. Higher spiritual strain was reported by White caregivers, those with fewer intrapsychic resources, and those in poorer physical health. No differences were found by caregiver gender or the length of caregiving. Surprisingly, in this study of 162 family caregivers, older caregivers reported lower levels of strain, with caregiver health having the strongest relationship to cumulative strain.

Learning Activity 62: Caregiver Stress

1. Many resources for caregivers may be found on the Internet. Locate 3 assessments of caregiver stress and print them, with reference(s).

2. Explain why managing stress is important for both caregiver and recipient of care.

3. How can occupations help caregivers manage their stress?

4. Write a summary of how you, as an OT practitioner, might incorporate a caregiver stress quiz as a basis for supporting caregiver self-management.

Respite Utilization

Caregiver respite refers to temporary relief from caregiving duties to allow the caregiver to tend to his or her own needs and to restore energy and a sense of well-being. For the most part, studies of caregiving tend to portray caregivers as needing more respite, but often putting the needs of the care recipient above their own. One recent study comparing the experiences of spousal caregivers with adult child caregivers of older adults with physical and cognitive impairments concluded that respite utilization varied according to their own grief responses during caregiving

(DeCaporale, Mensie, & Steffen, 2013). Among caregivers with a mean age of 69, they found that grief reactions made adult child caregivers more likely to use respite, but grief had no effect on spousal caregiver use of respite resources.

Caring for Pets

Pets often provide valued companionship to older adults and have also been shown to improve health status (Gulick & Krause-Parello, 2012). A study of women who live alone revealed that 40.8% had companion cats and 34.3% had companion dogs (Krause-Parello, 2008). Dogs and cats can meet relational needs for consistent, reliable bonds and can facilitate transitions through disruptive changes (Walsh, 2009). Research shows that pet ownership can improve social, emotional, and physical well-being by providing:

- A sense of security and safety.
- Social integration with other pet owners.
- Reassurance of self-worth.
- Opportunities for nurturance (Krause-Parello, 2008).

Dogs, in particular, contribute to physical fitness because of their need for frequent walking. Research shows that companion dogs are stronger facilitators of recovery from illness than companion cats (Wells, 2007).

While pets provide comfort and companionship to elders, the animals themselves also need adequate care. Regular feeding, fresh water, and a warm and clean sleeping area are minimum requirements, along with outdoor walking for dogs and regularly refreshed litter boxes for cats. Pets also need medical check-ups, vaccinations against diseases, treatment to ward off fleas and ticks, toenail clipping, and occasional bathing and grooming. Elderly pet owners need to be physically able to care for a pet or need to arrange for someone else to do so. Individuals with mild to moderate dementia may not be capable of remembering to do needed pet care and should be supervised in this role so that the animal is not abused or neglected. For example, one client with moderate dementia forgot to walk her pet Chihuahua before she took her to bed; therefore, she would wet the bed every night, making additional work for morning caregivers. When family caregivers investigated, they also found the dog could not chew her dry food because of loose teeth, and that she was surviving by eating her elderly owner's own lunch, fed to her piece by piece from the table.

APPLICATIONS TO CONTINUUM OF CARE

Community and Aging in Place

Most family caregiving takes place at home—whether the home of the caregiver or care recipient. Although medical services focus mostly on the recipients of care, family members taking on the role of caregiver could benefit from education regarding the health risks so that they can take preventive measures. Much of the evidence mentioned earlier shows that older caregivers often feel overwhelmed and socially isolated and lack respite or other types of support. For older caregivers living in the community, several studies have suggested that health professionals should provide more information about resources available to them in their caregiving role. For example, Williams (2011) suggests creating caregiver support groups for custodial grandparents, who have a stated need for more peer interaction and decreased isolation. Similarly, caregivers of loved ones with terminal illnesses have indicated their need for more social interaction (McGhan et al., 2013). For every client attending an adult day care center, there is likely a family caregiver who transports him or her there, but otherwise bears the burden alone, and could benefit from the support of others in similar roles.

Another need in the community might be helping caregivers navigate the complexities of the health care system, which usually falls on their shoulders (McGhan et al., 2013). OT practitioners might, as part of their advocacy role, become better informed about community services available to caregivers. They could become more knowledgeable about how the current health care system works, so that they might better guide caregivers in getting help for complex medical problems.

Supporting Caregivers in Primary Care

The family caregiver often accompanies the recipient of care to medical appointments, either to follow up on chronic conditions or to address emerging health issues. This would be an ideal opportunity for OT practitioners to provide caregiver education and support, either individually or in groups. With primary care physicians increasingly under stress to spend less time with patients, OTs might seize the opportunity to provide additional guidance both in self-management for the patient or client and in wellness and prevention strategies for the caregiver. Offering supportive group interventions might be the most cost-effective way to meet this growing need, perhaps organized by specific health condition populations, such as dementia, stroke, or bone fractures that interfere with functional mobility. Some niches for OT have been suggested by AOTA, including low vision, driver safety, fall prevention, and home modification and safety for aging in place (Yamkovenko, 2014).

Learning Activity 63: Primary Care Physician's Office Interview

OT students and new graduates might become advocates for the profession by laying the groundwork for OT entry into this important area of productive aging practice.

Find a primary care physician's office or clinic where older adults are frequently treated. Often such offices are very busy, but hopefully they are willing to spare 30 minutes (or less) to help a student with a learning assignment. Be sure to identify yourself as an OT and remember to thank them afterward.

1. Make an appointment for an interview regarding the needs of their older clients who have family caregivers. (If this is not possible, create a survey for their staff to fill out within 1 week—give due date).

2. Find out the following:

   a. What percentage of their patients are Medicare recipients (over 66 years of age)?

   b. About how many are living independently in the community?

   c. If cared for at home, about how many have a full-time family caregiver?

   d. To what extent do primary care staff work specifically with caregivers who accompany patients to appointments?

   e. Does the MD (physician's assistant or nurse practitioner) see a need to spend more time educating and supporting caregivers?

   f. To what extent do patients rely on caregivers to carry out recommendations, facilitate medication compliance, and/or follow up with this office?

   g. If funding were available, would this office support OT individual or group interventions to promote self-management, wellness, and prevention for patients/clients and their caregivers?

Home Care

OTs may encounter older caregivers during home care visits, where both client and caregiver may be considered recipients of care. For example, when a client returns home after a total hip replacement, the family caregiver needs to be aware of certain procedures and precautions, such as a safe way to assist the client with transfers from wheelchair to toilet or shower chair, sitting to standing, wheelchair to bed, and the reverse. At a minimum, the home needs to be adapted to accommodate the wheelchair, at least temporarily: furniture cleared, throw rugs removed, doorways decluttered, and, sometimes, doors to bedrooms, bathrooms, and closets removed to provide enough space for the wheelchair to navigate. Other options, such as rolling walkers, may make mobility throughout the house easier when the client's strength and balance improve. Basics of care need to be discussed, because the client's limitations do not allow him or her to do everyday tasks the same way as before surgery. There will likely be a home exercise program that the caregiver will need to supervise.

TABLE 8-1	
INTERNET RESOURCES FOR CAREGIVERS	
http://www.caregiver.com/articles	For caregivers of individuals with Alzheimer's and related disorders
http://homecare.com/hiring-home-health-care-worker-without-agency	Guidelines for hiring and managing home care aides
http://www.aoa.gov/aoa_programs/hcltc/caregiver/index.aspx	US Administration on Aging (2010): caregiver support and resources
http://www.caregiver.org	Family Caregiver Alliance, National Center on Caregiving (2012)
http://www.aarp.org/(home-family/caregiving)	American Association of Retired Persons
http://www.caregiveraction.org	US National Alliance for Caregiving
Compiled by M. B. Cole, 2015.	

With earlier discharge from hospitals and rehabilitation centers becoming more common, many semi-medical tasks now fall to the family caregiver. As described in the caregiving statistics, it is not uncommon for the caregiver to insert or remove urinary catheters, change wound dressings, or administer injections in addition to assisting with daily hygiene such as bathing and maintaining clean surroundings. Although training the caregiver to do these medical tasks usually falls to a home care nurse or nurse practitioner, other aspects of caregiver education will be an important role for the OT. An OT home care visit should include helping the client and caregiver set priorities and schedule caregiving tasks at a pace that is acceptable to both the giver and recipient of care. The unique focus of the OT will be to rearrange belongings so that things needed by the client are easily accessible. Ideally, the client should be able to occupy him- or herself doing something meaningful for extended periods throughout the day without constant attention from the caregiver. Both time and stress management could be included in this process. A list of online resources for caregivers may be found in Table 8-1.

Obtaining In-Home Assistance

Sooner or later, most family caregivers reach a point where they realize they cannot provide all of the care needed by a care recipient. When that occurs, several options should be considered: (1) finding a volunteer helper (neighbor, friend, fellow church member, extended family); (2) hiring an aide directly; or (3) hiring an aide through a home care agency. Although finding a volunteer saves costs, this type of assistance is often temporary because others do not share the same level of commitment to caregiving as the primary family caregiver. Family caregivers may need guidance in acquiring a paid home care worker to take over some of the caregiving tasks. When cost is an issue, Medicare or Medicaid may cover some of the expense of a home care aide but within specific guidelines, including acquiring the worker through an approved agency. This does not necessarily mean that the worker comes with any experience or training—many agencies do not even require a high school education (DeGraff, 2013). Furthermore, if medical insurance does not cover the cost, aides from agencies cost 2 to 3 times more than hiring an aide directly. The average cost of an aide is $19 per hour, with a range of $9 to $30 per hour (Genworth, 2011).

With or without an agency, the home care aide will be trained and supervised by the family caregiver. The caregiver and care recipient need to give a paid helper specific tasks and a specific schedule; it falls to the family member to recruit, interview, hire (either aide or agency), train, and then supervise and manage aides onsite on a daily basis (DeGraff, 2013). An agency does provide screening (such as drug screenings and criminal background checks) but provides only telephone supervision. Some agencies limit what an aide is allowed to do, usually for liability reasons. If control is important, or the caregiver wants the aide to do certain things (such as giving medications or transporting the recipient of care in his or her own vehicle to appointments), these arrangements are more easily accomplished with a non-agency aide. Additionally, hiring directly offers greater choice, an option of setting house rules (no smoking, no personal phone calls), and the authority to replace undesirable aides when necessary. The downside of hiring directly is having to maintain financial records, pay salaries, and, when appropriate, pay taxes and file required government employment documents. At this writing, paying an aide who is not self-employed more than $1500 per calendar year requires reporting that person's income to the Internal Revenue Service, and withholding Social Security and Medicare Taxes (Care.com, 2013).

When hiring a home care aide, guidelines recommend that a caregiver communicate clear expectations from the outset of the relationship, including a list of tasks, a written

TABLE 8-2
TYPICAL TASKS FOR A HOME HEALTH AIDE/HOUSEKEEPER

- Cooking, serving, cleanup
- Cleaning house, sweeping, vacuuming, dusting
- Doing laundry
- Changing bed linens
- Helping with toileting and lifting
- Planning meals, planning schedule as needed
- Assisting with medications
- Caring for wounds and bandaging
- Helping with showering and dressing, hair and nail care
- Driving and transportation assistance
- Shopping and running errands
- Providing companionship, engaging in leisure activities

Adapted from Friedland, R. The Home Care Guide: Home Care Aide Options. Retrieved from http://www.care.com/senior-care-home-care-aide-options-p1145-q7415.html

schedule, and emergency contact information, with time set aside for communication at the end of each session. A list of functions typically performed by home health aides is outlined in Table 8-2. A list of things the family caregiver should discuss during an interview with a home health aide candidate may be found in Table 8-3.

The *Occupational Outlook Handbook 2012-2013* (U.S. Census Bureau, 2013) distinguishes between a home care aide and a home health aide. Home care aides provide personal care to a client and the client's home but do not provide medically based services. Home health aides usually work for certified health or hospice agencies under the direct supervision of a medical professional, usually a nurse. Health aides keep records on the client's condition, report changes to case managers, and work with therapists and other medical staff to carry out home medical regimens, such as therapeutic exercise, massage, use of special equipment (e.g., braces, ventilators), changing wound dressings, and administering medications. Some home health aides also provide personal care and light housekeeping, within the limitations of the supervising agency (U.S. Census Bureau, 2013).

Rehabilitation Facilities

Older caregivers who are adult children or spouses of those receiving rehabilitation services often go unnoticed or are not given due recognition, guidance, and support. However, upon discharge, patients and clients depend on these caregivers to continue meeting their complex and ever-changing medical and functional needs. Because care-

giving has been called a *co-occupation*, OTs might work with both the client and caregiver as collaborators in setting goals for discharge or for creating a home program for outpatients. Again, this might be a good opportunity to offer caregiver education and support groups within the rehabilitation setting, especially because funding from the Affordable Care Act (PPACA, 2010) may become available for such pilot programs (prevention, self-management).

Assisted Living and Long-Term Care

A family caregiver's job does not end when the recipient of care moves to a residential facility, but it does change considerably. The decision to institutionalize has recently been the subject of much public policy research because of the high cost of residential care and the likelihood of increased numbers of the aging population needing care in next few decades. Because of greater Medicare flexibility in paying for more health care services in one's home, elders have been able to age in place much longer than they have in previous years, therefore entering long-term care in a more severely disabled state.

When an elderly parent or spouse enters a long-term care facility, the caregiver usually helps to orchestrate the move. Decisions must be made about what to bring to a single room or apartment from a much larger space. The new residence usually accommodates framed photos or artwork on the walls, quilts or blankets, a TV or radio, and perhaps a small table, bookshelf, or rocking chair but not much else. Clothing is limited to one closet and one chest of drawers. Just as with children going to summer camp, all clothing

TABLE 8-3
HOME HEALTH AIDE INTERVIEW—THINGS TO DISCUSS WHEN HIRING DIRECTLY

- Setting work hours and schedule, variability, and prior notice
- Terms of payment, amount, frequency, and method (cash, check, etc.)
- What the care provider is expected to do—specific and in writing
- Openly discuss personal preferences, candidate's strengths and weaknesses
- Ask questions about candidate's personal situation, career goals, and attitudes
- Discuss house rules about smoking, TV watching, personal phone calls
- Provisions for sick days, vacation days, taxes, and health benefits if applicable
- Cancellation procedures and terms for rescheduling missed days
- Clearly communicate level of supervision needed and what client can do for self
- Other benefits, such as eating lunch with the client, gas money when using own car
- Candidate should provide at least three references from prior clients—call them all!
- Expectations of communication, daily in-person, evenings by telephone, in writing
- A regular schedule for discussions about quality of care and problem solving
- Terms for ending the contract. What are the deal breakers for both parties?
- Make sure recipient of care and other family caregivers have input to the interview
- Discuss emergency procedures for various scenarios and provide contact information

items must be labeled with the resident's name so they will not be lost in the laundry. Some values regarding care of one's belongings have to be compromised. Of course, family caregivers may volunteer to have certain clothing items dry cleaned, but at the facility, everything goes into a washing machine and a dryer with no special care. Furthermore, security for any good jewelry or other valuable personal items is usually not guaranteed. An in-house resident account often takes the place of checks and credit cards, and there is no longer need for cash. The resident might spend some money (from the account) at a beauty parlor, barber, or gift shop, but otherwise, all meals and personal care needs are provided by the facility. When clothes wear out, family caregivers might be asked to provide new ones, as well as clearing out unused items to make room for new purchases. Residents who are still able might enjoy a trip to their old hairdresser or shopping for clothes in a familiar department store. Such outings usually need to be pre-arranged with the staff and should consider safety precautions while traveling and navigating in public. The family caregiver is then responsible for returning the resident after the allotted amount of time.

Upon the admission of an ill relative, the family caregiver's role changes to that of team member and advocate, with a long-term continuing commitment to attending periodic meetings with nursing staff; dietitians; recreation, physical, and occupational therapists; social workers; and sometimes pastoral caregivers and others who, together, review and revise the plan of care for the resident. Because the family member knows a new resident better than anyone else on the team, he or she may be called upon to provide historical or background information. For example, "the best way to get my husband to open his eyes for eye drops is to hand him the dropper and let him do it himself," or "the reason my mother has that rash on her arm might be that you are giving her strawberry milkshakes and she has always been allergic to strawberries."

Former family caregivers still need to visit regularly, advocate for their loved one, and help solve problems experienced by a resident within the long-term care setting.

IMPLICATIONS FOR OCCUPATIONAL THERAPY PRACTICE

Some research on caregiving occupations is embedded in studies of older adults with specific disabilities, such as stroke, spinal cord injury, and dementia. Previously, research has noted that the maintenance of stroke survivors' occupations outside the home was dependent on caregiver problem-solving skills and resourcefulness (Jongbloed, Stanton, & Fousek, 1993). Caregivers who take on additional roles during the initial phases of their spouses' stroke recovery report reduced social and leisure activities and often experience a disruption in social life, isolation, and physical exhaustion (Anderson, Linto, & Stewart Wynne, 1995). Rudman, Hebert, and Reid (2006) looked at the impact of wheelchair use on the occupations of older stroke survivors and their caregivers. They identified two main themes: living in a restricted occupational world and challenges to participation in occupation. Of the 15 caregiver informants in this study, 13 were spouses. Spousal caregivers reported a "spill-over effect," in that their "spouses' restrictions also meant that their own occupational worlds had narrowed." For example, "We used to go down south in the winter and play golf and have fun...can't do that sort of thing anymore," or after attending church "we usually had coffee downstairs after the service, and we can't now because the church doesn't have an elevator" (Rudman et al., p. 146). Some caregiver restrictions were also self-imposed, "If I go out and he did have to use the urinal, he would possibly fall," or when paid homemakers come in "I have to be there to supervise, to make sure that what is to be done is done" (Rudman et al., p. 146). Some caregivers felt reluctant to even attempt community outings; "there's just no spontaneity left...by the time you go through all the rigamarole of getting him ready, you don't care whether you do it or not" (Rudman et al., p. 146).

In reporting challenges to participation in occupations in the community, caregivers noted the following barriers to wheelchair use: inclines, poorly repaired sidewalks, stairs into buildings, small washrooms and close aisles in stores, curbs, revolving doors, gravel or bumpy terrain, lack of handicapped parking, bad weather, heavy traffic, and short green signal time to cross streets. Therefore access to community events for the couple was restricted to buildings with street-level entries without stairs, and those with wide or automatic doors, wide hallways, and elevators. Fatigue was also a factor for both stroke survivor and spousal caregiver: "It's...get him down the stairs, put him in his wheelchair. [Push] him to the car. Take him out. Put him in the car. Put the wheelchair in the car...bring him home. Go through it all again. It kills me...I'm lugging a wheelchair all the time" (Rudman et al., 2006, p. 147).

Another study looked at health-related quality of life (HRQOL) for stroke survivors and their spousal caregivers beyond 2 years post stroke (Godwin, Ostwald, Cron, & Wasserman, 2013). HRQOL refers to physical, functional, psychological, and social dimensions of health. Not surprisingly, caregivers experienced higher levels of depression and more frequent physical illness when their physical, social, and psychological quality of life scores were low and this negative trend worsened over time. This study recommends that mental and physical evaluation of stroke survivors and their caregivers be extended beyond 2 years to meet the needs of long-term caregivers.

On the positive side, *mutuality* refers to the shared pleasures for both the giver and receiver of care resulting

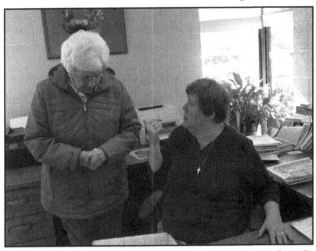

Figure 8-2. Sue (seated) and Gerry confide in each other, informally providing one another emotional support. The church office where Sue works provides her needed respite from multiple caregiving duties at home.

from the caregiving relationship, which is associated with greater positive outcomes for both (Lyons, Sayer, Archbold, Hornbrook, & Stewart, 2007). In a study of persons with Parkinson's disease, mutuality between patient and caregiver is associated with a higher mental health quality of life, but had no association with physical quality of life (Tanji et al., 2008). Mutuality also increased life satisfaction for both stroke survivors and their spousal caregivers (Ostwald, Godwin, & Cron, 2009).

As an example, Sue takes care of her husband who had a stroke several years ago. She works part-time as a church administrator, with a flexible schedule and lots of opportunities for social interaction. She confides in Gerry, her mentor and former coworker, and the two provide social support for each other (Figure 8-2). Sue has multiple caregiving duties and has also obtained hired help for her live-in mother-in-law who has mild dementia. She needs this time away from recipients of care to refresh herself mentally and spiritually and is fortunate that she also provides a service and earns an income to help with the costs of caregiving.

OTs may encounter older caregivers when providing home care for clients or when treating them in an outpatient rehabilitation facility. When working with elderly clients, family caregivers are also recipients of service. Caregiving is considered a "co-occupation that involves active participation on the part of both caregiver and recipient of care" (AOTA, 2014, p. S6). Clearly, caregivers need the support, guidance, and respect of OT professionals when attending to family members facing difficult health challenges. OTs *listen to caregivers* while evaluating the client's concerns, problems, and occupational goals as part of the collaborative, client-centered approach. During interventions, OTs often provide *caregiver education*, especially when home adaptations are necessary or for client safety considerations when engaging in desired activities. When the client needs to work on occupational goals between treatment sessions, it is often the caregiver who initiates practice sessions and convinces the client of the importance of following through.

While much has been written about how caregivers can best help clients, little has been written about helping clients for whom caregiving is identified as a preferred occupation. In *supporting the occupation of caregiving* itself, OT might have an occupation-based focus, using the tasks of caregiving as interventions. As the literature tells us, caregivers who are themselves older adults also need to take better care of themselves, pay attention to their own health issues and lifestyle factors, and intentionally nurture and develop their own social connections. Therefore, an important new role for OT with older caregivers should be *supporting caregiver self-management*. For example, caregivers must get adequate rest and sleep to competently perform the tasks of this productive role. Balancing their own need for rest and sleep with those for whom they provide care falls within the occupation of caregiver self-management. Emerging data illustrate the heavy toll caregiving can have on sleep. Peng and Chang (2013) found that 92% of caregivers for persons with dementia experienced poor sleep quality. Fredman, Gordon, Heeren, and Stuver (2013) found that depressive symptoms were associated with increased sleep problems; some studies report 40% to 70% of family caregivers have clinically significant symptoms of depression. Conversely, caregivers with positive attitudes (affect) had fewer sleep problems (Fredman et al., 2013). These findings provide clear evidence to support OT interventions with caregivers, to assist them in exploring ways to reduce stress, develop and nurture positive attitudes, or engage in activities that promote relaxation, and to improve the quality of their rest and sleep.

Listening and Developing Therapeutic Relationships With Older Caregivers

OTs begin to develop rapport with caregivers from their first meeting, mostly by listening carefully and communicating support and empathy. In therapeutic use of self, the OT does the following:

- Includes both the client and caregiver when evaluating client strengths and concerns.

- Asks open questions about relevant issues to fully understand both client and caregiver perspectives relative to occupational concerns. "What makes it difficult for you to continue to play cards with your friends?" "How could (caregiver) make participation easier for you?"

- Communicates empathy through accurately reflecting the emotions both client and caregiver express and their context. For example, "You seem frustrated because you still can't dress yourself without pain," or

"You sound angry because (care recipient) keeps asking the same questions over and over."

- Avoids premature problem solving and advice giving. Facilitating collaborative problem solving will lead to greater motivation and more meaningful outcomes with the added advantage of empowering both client and caregiver.

- Suggests some concrete ways to further explore the problems expressed with roles for each. For example, the client might keep a journal each day noting the tasks that bring on pain; the caregiver might search the Internet for information about the specific condition (such as lower back pain); and the OT might gather current evidence on possible approaches, techniques, and interventions.

When the OT takes time to ask probing questions and to listen carefully to the answers, the most pressing concerns of client and caregiver in all their nuances and complexities become better defined.

Within the initial session, the OT also needs to clarify which issues of concern to the client and caregiver fall within the domain of OT. Despite illness or disability, clients still need to engage in meaningful occupations to feel happy and satisfied with their lives. OTs may need to summarize the evidence for this reality in everyday language, so clients and caregivers understand the importance of productive occupations in protecting and enhancing health and well-being.

The next step for the OT, client, and caregiver will be to identify the facilitators and barriers to occupational engagement and participation in productive occupations. Interventions are designed to increase facilitators such as enhanced or adapted environments and to overcome barriers such as poor endurance or lack of transportation to a desired activity. Therapeutic use of self continues with the OT facilitating ongoing collaboration throughout the intervention.

Learning Activity 64: Interview an Older Caregiver

Find an older adult who spends at least 20 hours per week caring for a relative with an illness or disability who lives with him or her.

1. Focus your interview on the following: how she first became a caregiver, how long has she performed this role, what are her caregiving tasks, how does she feel about being a caregiver, how has caregiving affected her relationship with her disabled relative, how has caregiving affected her own quality of life.

2. Write a short case study, summarizing her answers.

3. Design one individual OT intervention for the caregiver with the goal of preventing risk factors

enhancing quality of caregiving, and/or improving the well-being of the caregiver. Explain your reasoning and give specifics.

Family Caregiver Education

The OT educator role is defined as "imparting knowledge and information about occupation, health, well-being, and participation that enables the client to acquire helpful behaviors, habits, and routines that may or may not require application at the time of the intervention session" (AOTA, 2014, p. S30). When educating caregivers, this may involve many things, including facts about the specific illness or disability and its management, the current evidence regarding interventions that have worked, and the interdisciplinary evidence about wellness and prevention in relation to productive aging.

At an organization or population level, an OT might address a group of caregivers, such as those caring for individuals with dementia, spouses of stroke survivors, or grandparents raising grandchildren. Each of these situations requires careful planning, including gaining an understanding of the needs and concerns of group members beforehand, and providing information directly addressing those concerns. In a formal presentation, sometimes group participation is limited, but with smaller support groups, the OT can invite discussion, provide examples of problems and solutions, and ask questions for the whole group to problem solve. OTs have excellent training in group leadership, which can easily be applied in organizational and community group settings to facilitate learning.

In designing group interventions for caregiver education, many good resources are available in the OT literature. For example, caregivers of individuals with dementia are especially vulnerable to emotional and behavioral aspects of this health condition. An OT might use the evidence from the Cognitive Disabilities Reconsidered model by Levy and Burns (2011) to promote greater understanding of the thinking process of persons with dementia that might cause their emotional or behavioral reactions, and offer some helpful suggestions for managing their daily occupations. Table 8-4 shows Levy and Burns' (2011) caregiver education guidelines, which are based on the original Allen Cognitive Levels (Allen, Blue, & Earhart, 1995).

This author was recently invited to share the findings of the PAS with a group of inner city grandparents raising grandchildren. After explaining the three main themes—prominence of self-management, social connections, and self-fulfilling occupations—the focus quickly turned to the actual tasks involved in their role as grandparents and how they felt about them. Many concerns had to do with inadequate finances and lack of time to socialize with their peers. Being older, they found it difficult to relate to the younger parents they met at school functions, and the only connection with others for most was the support group facilitated by a part-time OT one evening each week which was paid for by the area Agency on Aging. We discussed how they could make caregiving more of a social activity and what self-fulfilling activities might be shared with their grandchildren. Some ideas include the following: organizing play groups; meeting other grandparents at a local park or playground; organizing a monthly clothing, book, and toy swap; or eating at McDonald's with grandparents of other similar-aged grandkids. Activities might be baking or cooking together getting hairstyles and manicures, or playing cards, board games, or electronic games.

Supporting the Occupations of Caregiving

When the client is an older caregiver who may have difficulty with some of the tasks of caregiving, an OT can provide both training and guidance. For example, when the recipient of care is unable to use a shower or bathtub, the OT can help the older caregiver to sequence the steps of giving a sponge bath and changing the sheets while the recipient of care remains in bed. Likewise, when the patient gains strength, the older caregiver might need training and practice in assisting with transfers from a bed to a wheelchair, a wheelchair to a toilet or shower seat, and back. OTs need to teach caregivers the principles of good body mechanics when lifting or supporting during transfers and positioning (James, 2014). In lifting, it is usually best to keep one's back straight, to use leg muscles to support a heavy weight, and to keep the load close to the chest. Safe transfers depend on the strength and balance of the care recipient, with the caregiver supporting the weaker side, preventing the knee from buckling. The reader is referred to Focht's (2009) analysis of lifting to prevent lumbar back injury.

Supporting Caregiver Self-Management

This OT role may begin with some educational components, but quickly becomes much more complex. The main difference between educating and supporting is the self-direction of the recipient. Self-management requires a person to take charge and, ultimately, responsibility for his or her own life, from daily personal care and structuring daily activities to choosing and enacting occupational and social roles that have meaning, joining and participating in social groups or networks, and setting future goals for him- or herself. For older adult caregivers, self-management involves providing good care for someone else, while also balancing the care of their own health and meeting the other needs that are consistent with the caregivers' own life stage.

In supporting caregiver self-management, the OT should address the following:

- What are the caregivers' reasons for performing this role? Some adult children feel obligated to care for

		TABLE 8-4		
		CAREGIVER EDUCATION CHART		
CPT LEVEL	**GDS/ FAST STAGE**	**NORMAL FUNCTION (FOR CLIENT AT DECLINING ALLEN COGNITIVE LEVELS)**	**CLIENT DIFFICULTIES**	**CAREGIVER ASSISTANCE**
5.6	1	Plans actions; anticipates effects; uses symbols and abstract ideas	Independent	None
5	2-3	Has poor short-term memory and problems with planning and judgment; may be hesitant or impulsive; may be anxious or depressed	Difficulty with complex tasks, abstract thoughts, and seeing the whole picture	Encourage independence; watch for anxiety; simplify tasks; provide printed information; help plan ahead; point out consequences; help family to understand and support the person
4	4-5	Shows decline in many areas of thinking (orientation, perception, attention, concentration, language, coordination); is goal directed for familiar activity; needs visual cues; uses trial and error	Increasing confusion and errors; inability to perform complex tasks accurately or safely; may have delusions and catastrophic reactions; needs supervision for hazardous activities; needs assistance with ADLs	Set up items for each task; remove extra items from sight; give simple and concrete directions; maintain simple daily routines; remind and help person to keep on track; monitor for safety and errors
3	6	Demonstrates generalized confusion; manual actions only (needs tactile cues); grasps and uses objects but is not aware of the goal; may perseverate or misuse; often enjoys 1-to-1 social contact as a means to focus attention	Profound confusion: may have restlessness, sleep disruption, psychotic ideation, agitation, and aggression in response to stress; reacts to many stresses; balance may show decline and increased risk for falls	Simplify environment, approaches, and interactions; give step-by-step help for basic tasks; hand items to the person (demonstrate; use simple nouns and verbs; remind when to go and stop); keep dangerous objects out of reach; provide object-centered repetitive leisure activity; monitor all activity
2	7	Exhibits postural actions only (little use of objects); slow reflexes; focuses attention on touch, movement, and sound, and things that come in contact with the body; may cooperate with or resist care	Needs total care; there is a risk for falls; may exhibit repetitive verbalization, grasping, pinching, or hitting others	Learn efficient total care techniques for all ADLs, including dressing, bathing, toileting; may offer one food item and utensil at a time or finger foods; monitor for swallowing difficulties; provide stimuli in the environment (comforting textures, massage, range of motion, colorful or moving objects, music)
1	7	Shows continual decline; uses reflex actions only (responds to internal stimuli); may respond to touch or being moved	Needs total care, monitoring, and comfort; increased risk of skin breakdown, aspiration, and infections; needs late-stage decisions regarding life-sustaining measures	Comfort care; family support

CPT = Cognitive Performance Test; GDS = Global Dementia Stages; FAST = Functional Assessment Staging Instrument; ADLs = activities of daily living.
Reprinted with permission from Levy, L., & Burns, T. (2011). The cognitive disabilities reconsidered model: Rehabilitation of adults with dementia. In N. Katz (Ed.), *Cognition, occupation, and participation across the life span* (3rd ed., pp. 407-442). Bethesda, MD: AOTA Press.

their elderly parents, even when the role is unfulfilling for them. Span (2013) called these "reluctant caregivers" (p. 2). Others care for their family members out of love rather than obligation and feel a satisfaction from being needed and appreciated in return.

- What is the caregivers' state of health? Much can be done to monitor and manage chronic conditions, including taking time for exercise and good nutrition and designing a health-promoting lifestyle. Chronic health conditions require treatment and follow-up.

- Monitor the emotional and mental status of caregivers, watching for signs of mental fatigue or strain, and address their needs for emotional support.

- How does the caregiver cope when the health status of the recipient of care is unstable or constantly changing? How can the OT help to problem solve and to establish routines that consider the need for ongoing adaptation?

- What is the extent of social participation for the caregiver apart from the care recipient? One of the greatest risks for a family caregiver is social isolation, especially when the care recipient requires 24-hour supervision. The caregivers' resources for social support are critical to their own health and should not, under any circumstances, be neglected. The OT might need to identify community resources to provide respite while caregivers have lunch or dinner with a friend.

- What other occupational goals does the caregiver have for the future? Good self-managers do not sacrifice their own development while caring for a loved one, but they are able to develop a life plan that includes both. For example, some caregivers work part-time for pay at a job they love, and they can then afford to hire home health aides to cover their caregiving duties while working.

- What self-fulfilling activities can be shared between caregiver and care recipient? Caregivers might take classes to learn a craft, such as quilting or woodworking, that they can then teach their loved one. Or both might develop skills in baking, gourmet cooking, or gardening—things they can learn from books or the Internet.

- Under what circumstances would the caregiver be willing to ask for help? Family caregivers notoriously neglect their own needs to always meet the needs of their care recipient. The OT might help an older caregiver to better define when help is needed and how often. Then, a list of resources might be developed with people he or she can call or consult about various kinds of issues, such as other family members, religious leaders, medical professionals, trusted neighbors and friends, or people willing to perform needed services, such as housecleaning, yard work, or shoveling snow.

- How does the caregiver advocate for him- or herself? Self-advocacy is an important self-management skill that usually comes into play when encountering environmental barriers, such as dealing with the health care system (doctors, insurance companies, or pharmacies), gaining access to community or financial resources, or public policy issues generally. What are the external barriers to providing both good caregiving and good self-management? To whom should an appeal be made and what needs to change?

When the family caregiver is one of several family members who could perform this role for a relative, the OT might help the caregiver to call on others to help or coordinate caregiving tasks and roles, with consideration of long-standing family dynamics.

Learning Activity 65: Occupational Therapy for the Caregiver

Choose one of these as a focus for this exercise: Alzheimer's, Parkinson's, stroke, hip replacement, or diabetes/obesity. Imagine you are an OT working with a client with one of these disorders and his or her family caregiver.

1. Find out the basics of the disorder, using textbooks or the Internet, and write a short summary.

2. Write another paragraph explaining the expected stages of decline or recovery to a potential caregiver. With which occupations will the recipient of care need assistance?

3. Summarize the main safety concerns for the client when participating in a social activity (specify one, such as going to a dinner party, attending a senior line dancing class, playing poker at a friend's home).

4. What adaptations might be necessary to facilitate the client's activity engagement? What actions should the caregiver take to ensure both safety and successful participation?

5. Focusing on the caregiver, what OT interventions might you design to support caregiver self-management? Describe two specific interventions.

Occupational Therapy Group Interventions for Caregivers

In my *Group Dynamics in Occupational Therapy* textbook (Cole, 2012), I give an example of six weekly sessions with a family in which the grandmother has been diagnosed with Alzheimer's disease. In this hypothetical family, the parents are part of the sandwich generation, caring for an elderly parent while still raising three school-age children. If the family wants to keep grandma in their home, education and cooperation are necessary for all family

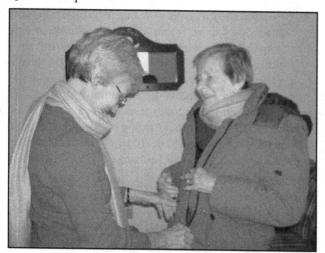

Figure 8-3. Valnere helps mother Pat (age 91) to zip her winter coat. She will take Pat out for a haircut on a snowy February day.

members in dealing with the ever-present need to balance grandma's autonomy with the safety and well-being of the whole family. These family sessions were based on Schutz's group theory of inclusion, control, and affection.

Of all the possible disabilities, caregivers of someone with Alzheimer's have the most psychological stress. This results from the unpredictable behaviors, illogical emotions, and personality changes that typically occur as the disease progresses. An OT intervention can explain the typical progression of the disease to caregivers, making some behaviors more understandable. Additionally, there is much that OTs can teach caregivers about facilitating the highest level of functioning for the care recipient and providing cues that will make ordinary tasks go more smoothly.

Because much recent attention has been given to this growing, but thus far incurable, disease of older adulthood, this might be a good topic for a learning activity. A caregivers group could use Levy and Burns' (2011) Caregiver Education Chart, based on Allen's Cognitive Disabilities Reconsidered model, which gives concrete suggestions and strategies for caregiver assistance at each progressive level of dementia.

Planning Occupational Therapy Groups for Caregivers of Individuals With Dementia

The purpose of these groups is to educate and support caregivers of loved ones with dementia, using everyday activities to measure and maintain cognitive functioning. Because caregivers often don't feel they have the time to attend a support group, the OT might set up a program in conjunction with an adult day care center, so that their recipients of care will also be occupied during the meeting time. Suggested themes for the group might be one of the following: getting through the day, understanding the stages

of Alzheimer's, communication strategies, safety-proofing the home, promoting independence through routines, and meeting social needs through reminiscence.

Learning Activity 66: Using Internet Resources for Caregiver Groups

Plan three group sessions for caregivers of family members with Alzheimer's dementia who are living in their own homes. Choose three themes and search the Internet for resources. Create a group activity around each theme, followed by a list of open questions for group discussion.

1. Theme 1:
    a. Activity Description
    b. Discussion Questions
2. Theme 2:
    a. Activity Description
    b. Discussion Questions
3. Theme 3:
    a. Activity Description
    b. Discussion Questions

Case Example: Valnere

"[In] one way and another, I had a caregiving role from 1993 until 2012. I came into it gradually with my daughter, Nicole, being the first to become ill. Consciously, I never defined the caregiving role. I found I responded to a need or crisis as it occurred. My first experience came as a shock when my daughter (at age 26) was diagnosed with cancer. Initially, we both needed emotional support from each other; it was gradually that physical and other needs defined both our roles. In caregiving, there is so much interchange. I found in all my family members to whom I was caregiver, I got so much support from them in return, too. Their need for my help was genuine and I was rewarded by being able to help and I needed their support, too. We all were tired at times, but I don't remember feelings of resentment or being overburdened (Figure 8-3).

"In finding a balance, I feel with each family member we supported one another. I was always able to work, attend conferences, participate in a group activity, or take a trip that was beneficial to me. And, in reverse, I could help my family member do what he or she wanted to do. To do these things, we sometimes needed to enlist extra help. This help wasn't always close by, but we could plan on it.

"Coping after my family member died took time. So many family and friends were supportive and spiritual belief in an 'afterlife' and a comfort in 'knowing' that we are all spiritual beings sustained me and still does to this day. I do not feel I have lost someone, I feel I have a different connection and that the family member can be very 'present.'

"Afterwards, there were the practical tasks of taking care of their possessions and their estates. But I am lucky, I have always felt resourceful. Yes, holidays are a time of memories and reflection, but I have never felt alone. For example, if no plans for the holidays are materializing, I make plans. I invite people to come to me. I enjoy entertaining" (V. McLean, personal communication, 2013).

Learning Activity 67: Lessons From Valnere

Assume you are an OT assigned to home care for Valnere's daughter, Nicole (age 26), shortly after she is given a terminal cancer diagnosis. Nicole is currently experiencing an especially difficult episode of cancer treatment (chemotherapy), during which there is a significant decline in her ability to perform everyday activities due to pain and fatigue. Search the Internet to more fully understand the effects of chemotherapy treatments and their expected effects. Although Nicole is your primary client, Valnere as her family caregiver will be the focus of this learning activity.

1. How might you evaluate Valnere's caregiving role? Explain what Nicole can expect from the chemotherapy, using your research. How she might best help her daughter through this crisis?

2. What questions might you ask Valnere to determine the extent of her physical and emotional distress?

3. Based on the case description, what are three strengths Valnere brings to her role as caregiver? What are three areas of possible vulnerability?

4. How might Valnere use occupations in her home to meaningfully engage with her daughter to help her cope with her current situation?

5. Locate three resources Valnere might use to obtain social support (both in the community and Internet). Briefly describe each, and explain why you chose them.

JOURNAL ENTRY (M. C.)

Caregiving for elderly parents is an occupation with which I have considerable experience. This role was thrust upon me in 1991 when I became aware that my own aging parents, who lived about a mile from my husband and me, were about to have their power shut off. I was at their back door, picking up my dog, who usually spent the day with them while I worked, when the postman delivered the certified letter and asked my mother to sign for it. At first, I thought it must be a mistake, my father always paid the bills on time. But we scrutinized the check register and it was true; there were no checks to the power company recorded

for the previous 3 months. My father kept all the financial records neatly stacked inside his desk. In it, I found several recent bills with due dates later that month. The paid bills were marked as such, and stored in a folder—I found the power bills under the section labeled "utilities," and the most recent of these, for service ending 3 months earlier, was marked paid with no outstanding balance. Of course I helped them call the power company right away, and I was able to pay the balance over the phone with my credit card. But the mystery remained: where were the past 3 monthly invoices?

My father was 91 at the time, had survived two strokes and took medication for Parkinson's, was hard of hearing, blind in one eye, and could barely see out of the other because of macular degeneration. Still, his mind was sharp. He could balance his checkbook in his head, and he knew almost to the dollar how much cash was in his wallet. He instructed my mother, 11 years younger than he, with excellent vision and hearing and no physical health conditions, to read him the mail, physically write the checks with his guidance, put stamps on the envelopes, and mail the payments at the post office. They did this together at least once a week. My mother drove them both to the nearby town almost every day, where they ate lunch at a local diner, shopped at the grocery store, and visited the post office, the dry cleaners, the barber, or the bank as needed, all in the same small complex.

"What happened to the bills?" I asked my father the next day.

"I don't know for sure," he answered, "but lately your mother has been confused about what to do with all the junk mail that comes. I think she's been stashing it under the bed." I found a treasure trove under there! Everything mixed together—personal letters, bank statements, credit card statements, and other bills in among magazines, newspapers, and advertisements. Now I was worried. I began searching the rest of the house, finding it more cluttered and disorganized than I remembered. I found sour milk in the refrigerator, moldy bread on the counter, and rotting tomatoes in one of the kitchen cabinets. In the bedroom, soiled clothes lined the closet floor, and still others, soiled and foul smelling, hung on hangers in the closet. The bathroom hamper contained only my father's soiled pajamas and underwear. My mother followed me as I searched, making excuses, and ultimately accusing me of interfering and meddling. This was not unusual because she was always a very private person, never revealed the details of their lives or finances, and mostly ignored my offers of help or well-meaning advice.

But now I had no choice. I had to "interfere" because they both needed help. Later that month, their family doctor confirmed my suspicions: my mother had entered the beginning stages of Alzheimer's disease. So for the next 8 years or so, I was a reluctant caregiver for my mother, who more or less resented my presence most of the time. And I was also a joyful caregiver for my father, who always valued my advice and appreciated my help.

My father had one bottom line request—that neither of them would enter a nursing home no matter what. That was a hard one for me because it meant I'd have to be there every day to arrange for housekeepers and health aides as needed and to modify the house dramatically to accommodate both their needs and mine. Eventually, my husband and I sold our large home, which, with our five children grown, we no longer needed, and moved into an addition (in-law apartment) we had built atop my parents' ranch-style home. I did all the cooking and shopping, helped my father with the bills, and hired various helpers to clean, do laundry, serve meals while I was teaching, and eventually assist both of them with bathing, dressing, and other ADLs. My mother did her best to obstruct. When a new washing machine was needed, my mother stood in front of the old one, refusing to allow the workmen to remove it. She left me scathing messages at work, accusing the health care worker who helped my father shower (after he broke his hip and could no longer walk), with "seeing him naked" and "taking advantage of him behind the closed bathroom door!" She "put away" the health worker's purse, and they couldn't find it anywhere when it was time to leave.

In her later stages, my mother walked out the door at 6 a.m. to walk the dog, wearing only a cardigan over her underwear in the middle of winter. Once, a frantic health care aide called me at work. While she was assisting my father, my mother had walked out the front door, leaving it wide open, and disappeared. Luckily, I'd had an ID necklace made for my mother that she couldn't easily remove, with her name and address, and my telephone number. A policeman eventually found her walking down Main Street and brought her home. It became necessary for me to be there whenever health workers came in, so with my husband still working full-time, I had to take an unpaid leave of absence.

We eventually did some modifications to make life easier. We disconnected the stove and refrigerator, using only the in-law apartment to cook and store food. We bolted the front door at night and fenced in the backyard, so neither the dog nor my mother could leave the property without our knowledge.

We'd go out to lunch or for outings when my mother eventually calmed down. We invited longtime friends of my father's to visit and a few of my mother's cousins too. Children home from college would stay in the single guest room or sleep on the sofa bed, and we'd have Thanksgiving and Christmas dinners all together. My mother liked these, and she could still help by setting the table, slicing tomatoes and cucumbers for a salad, or peeling apples for pie. She could empty the dishwasher, dry the drips, and stack dishes on the counter for me. She would say grace and tap her feet when we played familiar music. Seven years after her diagnosis, she had become almost childlike again and accepted the care she had previously refused.

At age 97, my father died at home. He was sitting at the breakfast table and I was feeding him applesauce, when the doorbell rang. The visiting nurse came in for her weekly visit, and by the time I returned to my father's side, he had stopped breathing. At first I panicked, but the nurse took his vitals and said to me calmly: "This is why we have a DNR [do not resuscitate], this is how he wanted it, to die peacefully at home." Thank goodness she was there. She was right, of course.

SUMMARY

Caregiving in older adulthood has not been as well defined in the literature or studied as extensively as caregiving or parenting for children. It is not defined as a separate occupation by AOTA's (2014) OTPF III. However, whether it is defined as an IADL or one of many social roles, caregiving represents a major commitment for the older adult. Caregiving as a productive occupation requires extensive scheduling, planning, and skill and often expands the role of self-manager, not only for oneself, but also for the recipient of care. Furthermore, as evidenced in the literature, older adult caregivers have a strong tendency to neglect their own self-management to meet the needs of a loved one, placing them at risk for both physical and mental decline. For this reason, OTs need to recognize the full impact of caregiving as a productive occupation and to better define the tasks involved in the role of a caregiver.

REFERENCES

Allen, C., Blue, T., & Earhart, C. (1995). *Understanding cognitive performance modes.* Ormond Beach, FL: Allen Conferences.

American Occupational Therapy Association. (2014). Occupational therapy practice framework: Domain and process (3rd ed.). *American Journal of Occupational Therapy, 68,* S1-S48.

Anderson, C. S., Linto, J., & Stewart Wynne, E. G. (1995). A population-based assessment of the impact and burden of caregiving for long-term stroke survivors. *Stroke, 26,* 843-849.

Appleby, J. (2012). From the executive director: Caregiving's value can't be overstated. *Gerontology News, 40*(12), 2.

Bunch, S. G., Eastman, B. J., & Moore, R. R. (2007). A profile of grandparents raising grandchildren as a result of parental military deployment. *Journal of Human Behavior in the Social Environment, 15*(4), 1-12.

Butler, F. R., & Zakari, N. (2005). Grandparents parenting grandchildren: Assessing health status, parental stress, and social supports. *Journal of Gerontological Nursing , 30*(10), 43-54.

Care.com. (2013). *The home care guide: Home care aide cost.* Retrieved from http://www.care.com/senior-care-home-care-aide-cost-p1145-q212516.html.

Cole, M. (2012). *Group dynamics in occupational therapy* (4th ed.). Thorofare, NJ: SLACK Incorporated.

Cress, C. (2001). *Handbook of geriatric care management.* Gaithersburg, MD: Aspen.

DeCaporale, L., Mensie, L., & Steffen, A. (2013). Respite utilization and responses to loss among family caregivers: Relationship matters. *Death Studies, 37*, 483-492.

DeGraff, A. H. (2013). *Paid aides—an agency's or your own?* Retrieved from http://www.caregiver.com/articles/print/paid-aides.htm.

Family Caregiver Alliance. (2011). *Fact sheet: Selected caregiver statistics.* Retrieved from http://www.circlecenterads.info/documents/FCAPrint_SelectedCaregiv...pdf.

Focht, D. (2009). Lifting analysis. In K. Jacobs (Ed.). *Ergonomics for therapists* (3rd ed., pp. 173-190). St. Louis, MO: Mosby.

Fredman, L., Gordon, S., Heeren, T., & Stuver, S. (2013). *Positive affect is associated with fewer sleep problems in older caregivers but not non-caregivers.* Presented at The Gerontological Society of America, 66th Annual Scientific Meeting, Nov. 20-24, New Orleans, LA.

Gallup Healthways Wellbeing Survey (2011). *Most caregivers look after elderly parent: Invest a lot of time.* Retrieved from http://www.caregiver.org/caregiver/jsp/print_friendly.jsp?nodeid=439.

Genworth (2011). Cost of care survey. Retrieved from http://www.care.com/senior-care-aide-cost-p1145-q212516.html.

Gitlin, L. N., & Corcoran, M. A. (2005). *Occupational therapy and dementia care: The home environmental skill-building program for individuals and families.* Bethesda, MD: AOTA Press.

Godwin, K., Ostwald, S., Cron, S., & Wasserman, J. (2013). Long-term health-related quality of life of stroke survivors and their spousal caregivers. *Journal of Neuroscience Nursing, 45*, 147.

Gulick, E., & Krause-Parello, C. A. (2012). Factors related to type of companion pet owned by older women. *Journal of Psychosocial Nursing, 50*, 30-37.

James, A. (2014). Activities of daily living and instrumental activities of daily living. In B. Schell, G. Gillen, & M. Scaffa (Eds.), *Willard & Spackman's Occupational Therapy* (12th ed., pp. 610-652). Philadelphia, PA: Lippincott Williams & Wilkins.

Jongbloed, L., Stanton, S., & Fousek, B. (1993). Family adaptation to altered roles following a stroke. *Canadian Journal of Occupational Therapy, 60*, 70-77.

Knight, J., Ball, V., Corr, S., Turner, A., Lowis, M., & Ekberg, M. (2007). An empirical study to identify older adults' engagement in productivity occupations. *Journal of Occupational Science, 14*, 145-153.

Knotts, V. J. (2008). Transitions for older adults. In S. Coppola, S. Elliott, & P. Toto (Eds.), *Strategies to advance gerontology excellence: Promoting best practice in occupational therapy* (pp. 109-134). Bethesda, MD: American Occupational Therapy Association.

Krause-Parello, C. A. (2008). The mediating effect of pet attachment support between loneliness and general health in older females living in the community. *Journal of Community Health Nursing, 25*, 1-14.

Levy, L., & Burns, T. (2011). The cognitive disabilities reconsidered model: Rehabilitation of adults with dementia. In N. Katz (Ed.), *Cognition, occupation, and participation across the life span* (3rd ed., pp. 407-442). Bethesda, MD: AOTA Press.

Lyons, K. S., Sayer, A. G., Archbold, E. G., Hornbrook, M. C., & Stewart, B. J. (2007). The enduring and contextual effects of physical health and depression on care-dyad mutuality. *Research in Nursing and Health, 30*, 84-98.

McGhan, G., Loeb, S. J., Baney, B., & Penrod, J. (2013). End-of-life caregiving: Challenges faced by older adult women. *Journal of Gerontological Nursing, 36*, 45-54.

Moorman, S., & Macdonald, C. (2013). Medically complex home care and caregiver strain. *The Gerontologist, 53*, 407-417.

National Alliance for Caregiving & American Association of Retired Persons. (2009). *Caregiving in the U.S.* Retrieved from http://www.nationalallianceforcaregiving.org.

Ostwald, S. K., Godwin, K. M., & Cron, S. (2009). Predictors of life satisfaction in stroke survivors and spousal caregivers twelve to twenty-four months post discharge from inpatient rehabilitation. *Rehabilitation Nursing, 34*, 160-167.

Patient Protection and Affordable Care Act. (2010). Pub. Law 111-148, #3502, 124 Stat. 119, 124.

Peng, H., & Chang, Y. (2013). *Predictors of sleep in family caregivers of individuals with dementia.* Presented at The Gerontological Society of America, 66th Annual Scientific Meeting, Nov. 20-24, New Orleans, LA.

Rudman, D., Hebert, D., & Reid, D. (2006). Living in a restricted occupational world: The occupational experiences of stroke survivors who are wheelchair users and their caregivers. *Canadian Journal of Occupational Therapy, 73*, 141-152.

Span, P. (2013, February 20). The reluctant caregiver. *The New York Times.* Retrieved from http://newoldage.blogs.nytimes.com/2013/02/20/the-reluctant-caregiver/.

Spillman, B. C., & Black, K. J. (2005). Staying on course: Trends in family caregiving. *AARP Public Policy Institute*: Issue Paper #17. Retrieved from http://assets.aarp.org/rgcenter/il/2005_17_caregiving.pdf.

Tanji, H., Anderson, K. E., Gruber-Baldini, A. L., Fishman, P. S., Reich, S. G., Weiner, W. J., & Shulman, L. M. (2008). Mutuality of the marital relationship in Parkinson's disease. *Movement Disorders, 23*, 1843-1849.

Toles, M., Abbott, K., Hirschman, K., & Naylor, M. (2011). Transitions in care among older adults receiving long-term services and supports. *Journal of Gerontological Nursing, 38*, 40-47.

Townsend, A., Ishler, K., Shapiro, B., Pitorak, E. F., & Matthews, C. (2010). Levels, types, and predictors of family caregiver strain during Hospice home care for an older adult. *Journal of Social Work in End-of-Life & Palliative Care, 6*, 51-71.

U.S. Census Bureau (2010). *People and households.* Retrieved from http://www.census.gov/population/www.socdemo/grandparents.html.

U.S. Census Bureau (2013). *Occupational outlook handbook 2012-13 edition, home health and personal care aides.* Retrieved from http://www.bls.gov/ooh/healthcare/home-health-and-personal-care-aides.htm

Walsh, F. (2009). Human-animal bonds I: The relational significance of companion animals. *Family Process, 48*, 462-480.

Wells, D. L. (2007). Domestic dogs and human health: An overview. *British Journal of Health Psychology, 12*, 145-156.

Williams, M. (2011). The changing roles of grandparents raising grandchildren. *Journal of Human Behavior in the Social Environment, 21*, 948-962.

Yamkovenko, S. (2014). *Emerging niche in productive aging.* Retrieved from http://www.aota.org/en/Practice/Productive-Aging/Emerging-Niche.aspx#sthash.pajVEFbo.dpuf.

9

Volunteer

Karen C. Macdonald, PhD, OTR/L

"A sense of accomplishment, positive energy gained, and a joy in being out in the world and making a difference."
(K. C. Macdonald)

Volunteering is unpaid work. The types of tasks are endless, ranging from driving an elderly neighbor to the grocery store to serving on a national advisory committee. Formal volunteering, usually for charitable or service organizations, requires specific schedules, duties, and expectations. Informal volunteering includes occasional helping and/or ongoing support for others, such as serving as executor of a friend's will or supplying chicken soup for a neighbor who is sick. However, the activities of caregiving for family members are not considered volunteering.

Volunteer tasks often would be paid work in a different environment. For example, the demands of working in a church thrift store would be paid work in a comparable privately owned consignment shop or retail store. People who volunteer often are devoting their time and energy to benefit a cause for an organization or event. The time frame ranges from a single day, such as a fundraising event, to an ongoing weekly or monthly schedule, such as mentoring students or reading to the blind.

Older adults may approach volunteering from several perspectives. Some have had a lifetime of volunteering. Some may have looked forward to beginning a volunteer role upon retirement. The latter group may wish to continue in a related field or may wish to embark on a totally different type of occupation. Some people may wish to design and initiate their own volunteer experience based on an unmet

need they have discovered. Other volunteers are recruited based on their personal expertise. In either case, volunteers bring a unique set of personal interests, qualities, and skills that reflect their previous activities. The skills required for each job vary, creating an important opportunity for OTs to assist in finding ways to match ability to activity.

In a study of older adults in the United Kingdom, 30% of participants said they volunteered both for enjoyment and altruism (Knight et al., 2007). In the United States, volunteers are a significant resource for the unpaid work provided. For example, volunteers who assist in clean-up efforts after storm damage yield an important savings to the Federal budget. One of the major motivators for this age group is altruism, accompanied by the need to feel useful and productive (Brown et al., 2011). In considering both formal and informal roles, 26% of older adults volunteer for organizations, 29% informally help the sick or disabled, and 33% help to care for their grandchildren (Caro & Morris, 2001). For many older adults, volunteering replaces the lost worker role, fills gaps in increased leisure time, and provides meaning or purpose in daily activities (Mutchler, Burr, & Caro, 2003).

Volunteering has a unique meaning to each individual, from physical and mental health benefits to connecting with others to "give back to the community." Settings may vary from "at home" projects, such as knitting prayer

Cole MB, Macdonald KC.
Productive Aging: An Occupational Perspective (pp 155–169).
© 2015 Taylor & Francis Group.

shawls for a cancer center, to service projects in which the volunteer travels to another country to offer training for sustainable farming. Whatever the task, time commitment, or location, volunteering provides a chance to give of one-self for the benefit of others, with no expectation of reward.

The Domain of the OTPF III identifies volunteering within the occupation of work (AOTA, 2014). Volunteering is defined in terms of volunteer exploration and volunteer participation:

- Volunteer exploration: Determining community causes, organizations, or opportunities for unpaid work in relationship to personal skills, interests, and time available.

- Volunteer participation: Performing unpaid work activities for the benefit of selected causes, organizations, or facilities (AOTA, 2014, p. S21).

Exploration refers to the process of searching for volunteer opportunities and may include visiting agencies, networking with personal contacts, performing online research, and posting offers of assistance for public viewing (Cole & Macdonald, 2011). Volunteer *participation* encompasses the experience of securing a volunteer position, training, performing required tasks, and terminating the experience, as appropriate.

OTs as a group are known for their volunteering, with many "above and beyond" activities beyond employment. These include state and national committee work, research and writing, advocacy and activism, and participation in community and organizational fundraising for health care concerns. "I have known so many OTs, and they never go home; their work doesn't end at 5:00. They are forever going to meetings or working on another project. They don't get paid for that. It's not like that in other fields" (S. Brooks, personal communication, May 2011).

As our population ages and embraces community-based interventions, volunteering is viewed as a way to promote health and prevent deterioration related to chronic conditions. Volunteering is activity based, and promotes feeling of self-worth, accomplishment, and altruism. It provides concrete results that benefit individuals, agencies, and communities. OTs, often personally familiar with a lifetime of volunteering, have a unique expertise to assess the skills and needs of prospective volunteers, and match them to a setting or project in need of volunteer workers.

Learning Activity 68: Exploring Your Own Volunteer Experience

Identify a volunteer experience in which you personally participated.

1. Briefly describe the experience. How did you hear about it? How did it begin?

2. What did you do? Who benefitted from your work?

3. Who accompanied you? To what extent was this an experience shared with other volunteers?

4. What did you most enjoy about it?

5. How did it end? Review the process of the volunteer experience from beginning to end.

PARTICIPANT PERSPECTIVES

The participants explained several motivations for volunteering. These included learning new activities, helping others, being around other people, believing that activity is important for mental and physical well-being, and having an overall sense of "giving back to the community." From their life experiences, participants were confident that they had much to offer and appreciated the variety of volunteer opportunities that existed in their communities. Most connected with community-based organizations, such as churches, schools, and cultural agencies.

Feeling Needed

When discussing volunteer experiences, the participants expressed a feeling of deep personal meaning, for their own satisfaction and also for the sense of being helpful to others. Judi H. stated that her reason for volunteering comes "from my own personal need to be helpful. Doing things with other people, being a team player. When I volunteer, I am helping others and they appreciate that I am there... Sometimes it feels like that's all I do; I have to stand back and realize I do have free time of my own."

Ray offers other examples of types of volunteering. He is proud to have earned a Mason's 50-year pin. "I have been a blood donor; I am more proud of that than anything. At 100 pints you get honored. I had donated 27 gallons until I had surgery and developed anemia. I also volunteer at a thrift shop. All the customers seem to like me and ask about my health. They appreciate my service and help. It's been 17 years now."

Continuing Prior Work Skills

Many of the participants have had years of experience with volunteer activities prior to retirement. Others had looked forward to retirement as a time of life when they could pursue interests in volunteering. Some continued in volunteer work related to their paid career.

Margie continues to apply her expertise with preschool education through a volunteer role. She maintains a strong identity as a college graduate and teacher. Phyllis explained that after she retired from teaching, she remained actively involved in a mentor program, such that she witnessed the graduation of a young woman from a junior college after working with her beginning in third grade. She stated that she had volunteered her entire life and "had been president of a national cancer research organization." She now serves on her condominium board. Many active seniors find varied ways to be involved within their immediate community, and to be influences for positive change.

Betty, 89, felt that volunteering gave her a certain status, and that "doing something meaningful" gave her a sense of fulfillment and made her feel whole. She had been involved with voluntary backstage activities on Broadway when her first husband was a theatrical producer and worked in her second husband's art gallery (Figure 9-1). Most of the participants had been paid workers for a significant portion of their adult lives. Volunteering represented a continuation of some of those skills. For most, a full day of some type of purposeful activity had been the norm for decades of life and volunteering served as a means to preserve that routine.

Also offering church-based volunteer services, Jan serves on the Board for a Birth to Three program (early detection of special needs children), defined as a public service program for the State of Connecticut. Many of these volunteers called upon a lifetime of experience to offer contributions toward important program planning and organizational systems management.

June works directly with teens with brain damage, helping them to shop and cook for themselves. This stems from her experiences in successfully assisting her special needs son to manage more independently. There was a common theme of teaching others from their own life's learning, as if consciously helping others to avoid "reinventing the wheel." They knew that many things were not available for learning through education or research, but rather were best shared by an individual who had lived through a similar circumstance.

Utilizing her professional expertise, June also offers pro bono work in her former paid career of professional recruiting. She helps friends through job searches, making recommendations for interviews and real estate ventures. Several participants viewed occupations as volunteer work because they knew in other circumstances, someone would be paid for the same activity. They appeared to be able to offer it as a sort of service to others.

Raising Awareness for a Cause

Margie serves as a volunteer in her church, advocating for the Spanish sector at several levels of responsibility. She is a church ministry coordinator and a Hispanic leader and translator. She sets up and monitors altar schedules, is a youth group organizer and a lay Eucharistic leader, and helps publish a newsletter for a Spanish congregation. She also leads two weekly Bible studies—a ladies group and a Spanish group. Along with those commitments, she also is a site and program coordinator for a reading tutorial program at a local school. She coordinates a paper recycling program. It became evident that some of the participants

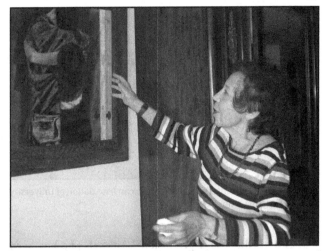

Figure 9-1. Betty, age 90, is a docent at the Metropolitan Museum of Art in New York City.

would need several paid workers to do an equivalent amount of work! However, the participants felt strongly that this was personal service and for many, like Margie, it held a spiritual meaning.

Vi demonstrated how one person can make a difference as a volunteer, influencing many through teaching about her personal life experiences. In this case, she is autonomous, designing her talks and arranging for speaking opportunities independent of any supervisor or organizational system. Vi gives talks in the community about American history in the era of Japanese internment camps. "It is an opportunity for people to find out about one of the most egregious periods in our history. It's not in textbooks. I usually speak to high school students after they have a segment on World War II history. I also speak to senior citizen groups, assisted living…they are particularly interested, they lived through it…I'm one of the younger ones left, I feel I should do it while I can. My father was arrested the night of Pearl Harbor; he was not allowed to be an American citizen. The whole west coast became a military zone. We took the last train out of Seattle to Texas, with 3 days' notice. I was 1 of 2,000 to leave without going to a camp. My husband spent 2.5 years in a camp. When I went to Texas, it was a whole different world—Dr. Pepper, tacos, 2-inch scorpions. Everyone thought we were Chinese. I was sent to a Catholic school." The opportunity for Vi to share her story as a volunteer has offered deep meaning in her life, expressing perspectives through her shared oral history that make a deep impression on her audiences.

Social advocacy was another area described within a volunteer role. Mary stated that "currently I am bringing petitions for a constitutional amendment to prevent corporate control of elections" to clubs and organizations of which she is a member. She partakes in a national walk related to mental illness awareness, as well as rallies and a walk across the Brooklyn Bridge. She serves on professional committees

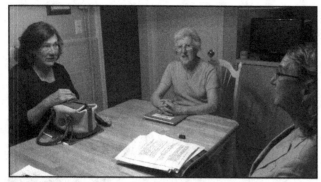

Figure 9-2. Gloria (center) chairs the American Association of University Women finance committee.

and is a coeditor of a professional journal. She has been mentoring others to take on some of these roles, which she wishes to cut back on or relinquish, but it is difficult to find replacements.

Seeking Social Interaction Through Volunteering

Along with stimulating physical and intellectual skills, the social component of volunteering was clearly very important to the participants. Some preferred to seek leadership roles, while others purposely avoided leadership responsibilities. The camaraderie of the volunteer colleagues was consistently noted as important. Individuals looked forward to the day(s) of the week in which they were scheduled for work. Other volunteers were sole volunteers in a setting, felt much appreciated for their efforts, and enjoyed being treated as a part of the paid worker team when sharing important responsibilities. As the years passed after retirement, many of the participants lost friends through death or relocation or experienced their own moving to a new locale. Volunteering often served as a means to meet new people who shared similar interests.

Mary balances profession-related duties with social participation through a sailing club, for which she has served on the Board several times. She coordinates speakers for educational programs, and connects this to local seashore venues for dinner meetings. Volunteer responsibilities at this level involve a tremendous amount of time, scheduling, and personal and social skills. Several of the participants engaged in high-level leadership positions in the role of a volunteer. Gloria volunteers in her church on many levels—visiting members in the hospital and nursing home, giving communion, and serving on the altar guild and in prayer groups. She also holds leadership positions in several organizations (Figure 9-2). All of these require a great deal of time, travel, and personal engagement with individuals, groups, and church leadership.

Learning Something New Through Volunteering

Ellen, who retired at a younger age, moved to a new city and volunteered at a zoo. Her responsibilities are entirely different from her former career in a health care profession. Working at a zoo matched with her lifelong love of animals. She has a variety of important responsibilities, including many data entry projects. She appreciated the opportunity to be helpful at needed work, and to learn about the zoo and special projects for animals, continuing a lifelong pattern of enjoying being involved in a project, and for new learning. She especially emphasized that she appreciated the new friends that she made in the volunteer setting after moving to a new city. "I find it is personally fulfilling and have made lots of new friends after moving to a new state."

Giving Structure to the Day (With Perks)

Some participants appeared to parallel the schedule of a very busy full-time employee, with many hours per week devoted to volunteering. At age 89, Betty shared that she goes to a different charity nearly every day. On Mondays, she reads to the blind. Two days a week she serves as a docent, leading tours in a historic theater. On another day, she teaches English to immigrants, which she states makes her feel useful. She also serves as a docent for a nationally renowned art museum and critiques newly trained tour guide leaders at a large library. She has a goal to volunteer at the United Nations in the future. She expresses a sense of deep fulfillment as a result of how these involvements have enriched her life. She also mentioned certain perks as a volunteer, such as free admission or tickets to events. Volunteer tasks at this level require a strong commitment, extensive training, and many skill demands during the course of any session of work. Rather than reporting the actual fatigue that might result from lengthy standing, talking, or hands-on work to complete a detailed task, the participants reported a sense of accomplishment, positive energy gained, and a joy in being out in the world and making a difference as a direct result of their involvement.

Some volunteers had trade-off programs; for example, Patricia's husband had worked for Exxon. In a matching program, they contribute money to a charity for specified blocks of volunteer work. She stated that "it is easy work, like stuffing envelopes," which she does for 21 hours per quarter. For some individuals, a simple project is welcome, while others seek very challenging activities. Volunteering is so varied that there is something for everyone.

Informal Volunteering

Examples of informal helping take many forms—some of them unexpected. Patricia lives in an assisted living setting and now helps less able-bodied neighbors, taking them to church services. She recommends taking time to help people: "many people need help in a place like this need something fixed help them fill out a form for maintenance to do it, even if they dropped something and can't bend down to pick it up." Although simple caregiving or assistance to others may not fit into strict definitions of volunteering, this type of service to others was an intentional way of life and, therefore, a type of informal volunteering, as defined by some participants.

Ray states, "I often write to the editor of my newspaper with comments and corrections." Although the latter may not seem a volunteer role, he takes it very seriously, as if he is an assistant to the editor, with whom he has established a nice relationship. He is doing it on his own time and enjoys the feeling of making a difference.

Sue expressed that her way of volunteering is by helping other people who are worse off than herself. She is a church administrator; troubled people often land in her office on church business, and she lends a compassionate ear. She states that she is a good listener and helps where she can. Some might question how this is distinguished from being a good friend? These participants distinguished volunteer activities as stemming from identifying a need not met by others and finding a means to offer assistance personally. This was seen in the context of preventing a need for formal or professional help in which fees would be involved.

Gloria also described another volunteer role, that of an executor of a will. She described how after a friend died 2 years ago, she is still working on that task. She plays a role in determining what happens to the property and personal possessions of a person who was a collector: "Who are the beneficiaries, who should get what? All must be evaluated and sold...work with a lawyer to do everything correctly. People should understand what to do before they die, to downsize and consolidate assets and keep a well-documented, up-to-date will to lessen the burden on the executor." This served as an example of a volunteer role that was a heavy responsibility, extended over a long period of time, and involved complex problem solving.

Most of the participants, as active and healthy retirees, made helping others a priority. Peggie related how she empathizes with those less fortunate by contributing to charities. She also described participation in informal volunteering through helping older neighbors or church members, by running errands such as filling prescriptions, by advising or giving medications, and by communicating and "checking in." This type of sensitive involvement addressed important needs to enable others to function at home with minimal but necessary assistance.

Over-Commitment in Volunteering

A comment from Marilyn highlighted the "lifespan" of a volunteer commitment. She stated, "I retired from volunteering at a thrift store after more than 20 years. I should have done that much sooner." She continued working even though it was very taxing on her and she felt that what she was contributing was decreasing. Volunteer roles often have no end point, and some older adults may need assessments as to whether it is still meaningful or safe to continue. Because they represent a generation who took work very seriously, it may be difficult for them to retire from volunteering. Volunteering becomes an important part of their identity, and leaving that position may be a welcome relief or an unwelcome signal that their abilities are changing. It would be helpful for volunteer supervisors to be sensitive to recognizing when volunteers need to discontinue their services and offer support for that transition.

Judi H. reports, "I volunteer at the senior center, my church thrift shop, the choir at church...and at the community theater, I assist with the costume department—now they store their things in my attic." Judi raised an interesting concept of a need to set boundaries on her involvement. This was also expressed by some others because they knew the need for volunteer participation was great and knew that a skilled and committed volunteer is an important resource to the operations of many groups.

Although a volunteer is generally expected to make a commitment to match scheduling needs and stay for some length of time after being oriented, the participants appreciated knowing that they could leave if their needs were not being met and transfer to some other type of volunteer situation. Some became so devoted to their volunteer responsibilities and network of peers that they found it difficult to retire from volunteering. They often would experience a series of efforts to modify and grade activities to continue to participate and would often only discontinue involvement when health or driving abilities decreased to the extent that they could not continue.

Learning Activity 69: When Is It Time to "Retire" From Volunteering?

1. Some older volunteers are so dedicated that they wish to continue beyond what is safe or beneficial. Identify five possible areas of difficulty or challenge for an older volunteer.

2. If a community center hired you as a consultant to determine "retirement" criteria for when an older adult

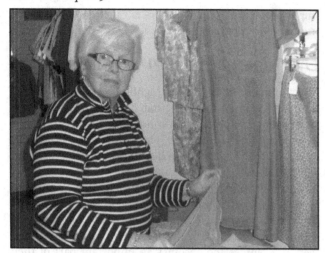

Figure 9-3. Mary V. volunteers at a church thrift shop.

is no longer capable of engaging in volunteer activities, list five factors that you would include.

Importance of Volunteering

Although often working in large and small groups, Phyllis stated how meaningful it was to have an individual connection with one student over many years. In a long-term role, a volunteer may see progress and change and feel accomplishment in making a deep difference in one person's life. Phyllis had been serving in volunteer capacities her whole life, enjoying different types of opportunities. She believed it had been a very important part of her life and hoped that others would start young in a volunteer role because it enriched her life in many ways.

Through several venues, Ray demonstrated his concern for others, involvement in his community, and knowledge that he has made a difference. Many of the participants believed that volunteer activities led to self growth and an important role in meeting community needs (Figure 9-3).

The participants all wished to serve, be involved, and contribute. Through the productive occupation of volunteering, we began to see their connections to all ages in their communities. Their services offered the recipients a perspective of intergenerational connecting and an appreciation for all that seniors are capable of contributing, even in their most elder years.

Learning Activity 70: Finding Volunteer Opportunities for Older Adults

1. Over the next week, collect information about volunteer opportunities for older adults in your community from senior centers, library, newspaper, or the Internet.

List and describe three different volunteer jobs, giving sponsoring organization and references.

a.

b.

2. List specifics such as hours, how often, tasks involved, and skills required.

3. For each volunteer role, give your reasons for choosing it for an older adult.

LITERATURE REVIEW

Volunteering is a vast topic for older adults. What opportunities are available? Who is best qualified to do what? How do volunteer sites recruit and accommodate for seniors? What are the motivations for participating in often challenging work? What is the connection to OT?

Benefits for Health and Well-Being

The OT literature is limited in explaining this rich and meaningful occupation for older adults (Cole, 2007). Literature from other disciplines portrays many issues related to personal and social needs for volunteers and attention to boundaries and challenges. Health benefits range from physical to emotional, cognitive, and social (O'Reilly & Caro, 1994; Tomas Sancho, Kennedy, Colomer, & Revuelta, 1998). Studies have revealed important benefits, such as lowering risk for depression (Hawkley & Cacioppo, 2004), increasing immune function (Hawkley, Masi, Berry, & Cacioppo, 2006), and increasing longevity (Musick, Herzog, & House, 1999). Volunteering provides a sense of well-being (Wheeler, Gorey, & Greenblatt, 1998), social integration (Backes, 1993; Okun & Schultz, 2003), and increased integrity and self-esteem (Ruler, 1998). Tavares, Burr, and Mutchler (2013) reinforced that volunteering promotes personal health and contributes to life satisfaction and a sense of enhancing programs in their community.

These benefits are in proportion to the number of hours spent participating in volunteer work. The number of hours per week increases health and influences and strengthens a sense of identified role and social involvement (Morrow-Howell, Hinterlong, Rozario, & Tang, 2003; Van Willigen, 2000). Quantified by Fried (2005), 15 hours minimum per week is related to promoting influences in health. Ongoing connection to a particular organization also increases personal benefits (Musick et al., 1999).

Increased Socialization

In older years, individuals appreciated opportunities for new or increased social roles, including volunteering (Cornwell, Laumann, & Schumm, 2008). Following retirement or decreased family responsibilities, older adults sought to increase their interpersonal social network. Specifically, they found this effective when sharing common work activities. Rook and Soskin (2003) provided an example of a foster grandparenting program in which the workers formed friendships with their peers, which led to the establishment of meaningful social ties.

Informal volunteering is tasks provided for non-family members, such as assisting with household or yard chores, driving to appointments or grocery shopping, or emotional support (Johnson, 2003) provided on an as-needed basis. *Formal volunteering* is regularly scheduled, often for ongoing projects, including fundraising, teaching, labor or piece work, or assisting professionals (U.S. Bureau of Labor Statistics, 2004). Connotations of volunteering have evolved from rather negative stereotypes such as stuffing envelopes (Tanz & Spencer, 2000). In recent years, identification as civic engagement or community involvement has emerged (Cavanaugh, 2005). These labels imply skilled participation with increased responsibility, reflecting years of experience in a professional career. Examples could include serving on a state board, consulting, or advocacy.

With the increasing percentage of retired elder adults and economic changes leading to downsizing and the consolidation of work positions, a connection between the two could have significant benefits for all. Seniors often have experience, "people skills," and a strong work ethic, making them reliable workers who wish to contribute as well as benefit from personal rewards of satisfaction and wellness promotion.

Volunteer Choices, Motivation, and Incentives

Volunteering is defined as giving time without being paid and is one's own choice (Tavares et al., 2013). It is considered a productive role, whether full- or part-time, with a commitment to a schedule and expectations of supervised compliance with established roles and procedures (Cole & Macdonald, 2011). Patterns of volunteering may fluctuate related to availability. For example, if personal abilities change or an increase in family caregiving responsibilities occurs, volunteers need to adapt to realistic use of time and energy.

Along with responding to identified community needs, volunteers may have many personal motivations for volunteering. For some, it is a permanent or temporary transition to retirement. They seek a position related to former paid employment that serves to retain a sense of a worker role. If seeking a return to paid work, the volunteer experience serves as a bridge back to employment (Carr & Kail, 2013).

Choices of volunteer positions ideally reflect an individual's unique interests and skills. Motivators often include giving back to the community and altruistic values. However, careful determination needs to be made to match personality and skill sets to needed tasks. Investigating volunteers who worked in psychiatric settings, researchers learned that the most highly committed volunteers had former experience in volunteering, interest in mass media, a social professional background, recognized the existence of discrimination toward the mentally ill, and a positive attitude toward community psychiatry (Lauber, Nordt, Falcato, & Rossler, 2002).

A variety of feelings about volunteering were studied by Costa Guerra, Demain, and Marques de Sousa (2012). Some experienced feelings of inadequacy when leading activities for an intervention program for people with dementia and their families. They sensed an increased competence with experience but wished to learn more about possible intervention strategies and relate them to family members' needs. They expressed motives of developing friendship and a sense of community, desire to help others, and a wish to experience personal development. Their findings suggested a need for agencies to understand and adjust volunteer programs to maintain volunteers' satisfaction and commitment.

Volunteer Retention and Rewards

Merrell (2000) explains that volunteers also have some level of expectation of getting something out of volunteer experiences. Studying volunteers who assisted paid health care providers, they had an increased sense of empowerment as they gained skills through specialty training; through feedback and recognition, they had an increased sense of the positive value of contributing their time and effort. This was described as a balanced reciprocity. To sustain valued volunteers, attention needs to be given to avoidance of exploitation.

Korda (1995) states that when positive rewards are known for the body, mind, and spirit, it is helpful to retain current volunteers and recruit new people. Working in a hospice program, the positive rewards need to be promoted and supported to meet the needs of volunteer retention.

Recognizing individual and societal benefits of volunteering, an additional level of consideration is raised by Warburton, Paynter, and Petriwskyj (2007). They recommend that incentives be developed by government agencies and private organizations to promote volunteerism, such as increased training, flexible hours, diverse task operations, and possibilities for intergenerational contacts.

According to Hoad (2002), volunteers expressed a need for clarification of duties when working in the homes of frail and confused elders. There were unclear boundaries with paid workers, leading to a need for a defined division of labor. Considerations included the complexity of a case and the amount of professional health care provided. Hoad (2002) recommends attention to state and local legal and policy constraints on the "job description" of volunteers in specialized settings.

Some incentives include a small stipend to promote volunteer services in lower economic groups (Kleyman, 2003). This allows for a method of promoting and attracting individuals to a service area in need of additional human resources.

Baby Boomers and Volunteering

Shifting demographics and attitudes about volunteering have offered challenges to predicting the availability of volunteer help. Recent decades of volunteers have represented individuals who were community minded and had lifelong habits of participating in activities and social groups. Baby Boomers who are now retiring view volunteering differently (Harvard School of Public Health, 2003; Prisuta, 2003). They expect many years of healthy activity with goals of participating in self-fulfilling activities. Others look forward to post-retirement as a new chapter of finding creative ways to utilize former career skills. The volunteer workforce of older adults could double in upcoming years (Kleyman, 2003). In recent decades, children through high school years have been encouraged to participate in community service projects. Perhaps this early exposure will lead to lifelong habits of finding many rewards in volunteer roles.

Volunteering for Occupational Therapists

A survey conducted by Cole and Macdonald (2011) explored the actions, thoughts, and feelings of retired OTs who participated in volunteer activities. During volunteer exploration, issues of meaningfulness included life priorities, time use, application of professional skills, and knowledge that volunteering has health benefits. Feelings were identified as a wish to help others, an urge to give back to the community, excitement about new involvements, away to meet personal social needs, a desire to feel needed, a spiritual calling, and concern about learning new things and fitting into a new role.

Through the actual volunteer experience, the respondents identified a shift in thoughts and feelings. Thoughts included reflecting about fulfillment; determining how to apply skills to new roles; a variety of issues related to learning the culture of a work environment, a new expertise, new roles and policies, and new ways to solve problems; and considering how to propose change or respond to supervision. Feelings were reported as enjoyment, connection, need for avoiding emotional overload, wanting a support system to discuss experiences, limiting stress, receiving credit and recognition for efforts, and avoiding physical strain.

These findings supported evidence by others regarding the need to understand and provide for the special needs of volunteers. Johnson (2003) recommends development of systems to effectively attract and engage potential volunteers, especially when recently retired. The Harvard School of Public Health (2003) identified specific recommendations to increase the variety and management of volunteer positions. This included suggestions to offer time-limited projects, opportunities to work in groups, flexible scheduling, and matching tasks to skills and interests.

APPLICATIONS ACROSS THE CONTINUUM OF CARE

The Centennial Vision promotes the development of OT roles in the community in new avenues of involvement. OT entrepreneurs could design consultant roles addressing many aspects of volunteer exploration and participation. In medical model settings, OTs could work cooperatively with administrators and volunteer department heads to address the issues of volunteer training and the provision of ongoing support. Offering services as volunteers themselves, OTs could introduce agencies with many volunteers, such as senior centers, schools, and places of worship, to the possibilities of applying OT expertise to their volunteer programs.

Community and Home Care

Volunteering might be an ideal way for older clients to reintegrate into their communities following a health event. As a productive occupation, there is much more flexibility in scheduling and responsibility than there is with paid employment. There is ample evidence that volunteering serves a protective role against physical and mental decline with aging, and OTs could share this information with clients as an effective wellness and prevention strategy. Most volunteer positions also offer opportunities for social interaction, helping clients build their social networks, which is another protective layer against the harmful effects of aging.

When clients in the community are evaluated in a home care or a primary care setting, the OT should inquire about past and current volunteer activities. Many older adults build their social contacts and friendships through volunteering and find this a meaningful, productive occupation in many aspects. In constructing an occupational profile for the client, engagement in volunteering should not be overlooked. The approach OT might take can be similar to returning to paid work, with similar attention to adapting tasks, schedules, environments, and social and work expectations. OTs could reclaim this important occupation that has long been a part of their domain.

Learning Activity 71: Designing Educational Sessions for Senior Center Volunteers

Imagine being asked to provide an in-service to a group of volunteers at a senior center. They will be working as assistants in the crafts department. Use the content from other chapters in this book to help design group sessions for each of the following topics:

1. Their own body mechanics and safety considerations, as well as safety considerations for seniors attending the craft sessions (see Chapter 6: Self-Manager)

2. How to most effectively communicate with older adults who have varying health conditions (see Chapter 5: Occupational Therapist's Roles in Productive Aging)

3. How to teach craft skills to older adults (see Chapter 11: Lifelong Learner)

Hospitals and Rehabilitation Facilities

Hospitals rely on a large contingency of volunteers. An OT employee can meet with the Director of Volunteers to offer to provide in-service training to volunteers. In these sessions, real-life situations may be discussed or simulated, such as maneuvering a wheelchair in an elevator, or proper position of assisting in feeding a patient. Preventive measures could be taught, such as proper body mechanics for the volunteer to use if moving a heavy cart. Skills for clear and appropriate communication and support may be taught for volunteers to effectively serve as "friendly visitors," with goals to maintain or promote the patient's positive perspective.

Furthermore, in serving older clients as an OT in hospitals and rehabilitation settings, volunteering as a productive occupation needs to be considered along with other meaningful occupations. OTs need to ask the following questions: What volunteer positions have brought meaning to your life? What do you do for others informally that you would like to continue to do? Could returning to volunteer activities or exploring new opportunities be a long-term goal? How could you help the client prepare for volunteer participation?

Learning Activity 72: Creating Volunteer Roles in an Occupational Therapy Department

Suppose you are an OT at a busy inpatient facility. An older adult, a former public school teacher, is assigned to volunteer for you two afternoons each week as an aide in the clinic:

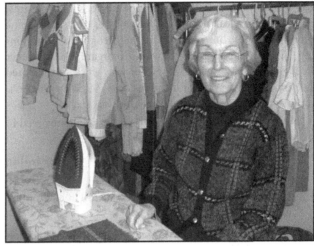

Figure 9-4. Maxine irons clothes to be sold at a thrift shop.

1. What responsibilities could you assign? Describe three and give your reasons.

2. What training would be required for your new volunteer?

3. How would you orient, communicate with, and supervise your volunteer?

4. What would be the benefits of this volunteer arrangement for you and your volunteer?

Assisted Living and Retirement Communities

In an assisted living setting, residents are typically mobile and able to drive. Many have moved to a new community. An OT could be a consultant to assist volunteer exploration. Prepared with listings of community agencies seeking volunteers, the OT could provide basic screening of interests and skills. A single afternoon workshop could be designed to identify potential jobs and analyze job requirements (requires prolonged standing or repetitive clerical tasks). Sample projects might be available to "try on for size." For example, a church thrift store may have placed a "Volunteers Needed" sign on the clubhouse bulletin board. A simulated task of sorting, labeling, and pricing garments could be arranged. The OT could be especially helpful in suggesting any modifications that might enhance performance in a proposed work site. These may include printed sequence of job steps for a new learner or careful selection of chair style and back rest for an individual with chronic back pain (Figure 9-4).

Learning Activity 73: Volunteers in an Assisted Living Facility

Imagine that you are a consultant at an over 55 assisted living facility and one of your roles is to advise the activity coordinator about designing skill-based activity programs, and how to grade activities for success. Residents have some mobility issues, but most retain high cognitive functioning. The activity coordinator wants to organize a Volunteer Recognition Day for 30 volunteers who work in the gated community. She wishes for the residents to create the invitations, decorations, party favors, and snacks.

1. What might be a good way to get residents involved in decision making and planning?

2. How could you encourage creative expression within the activities?

3. What would you recommend as a timeline, supplies, and approaches?

4. How could you apply your knowledge of group facilitation to support resident involvement and satisfaction with their experience?

Volunteering in Long-Term Care

In long-term care facilities, an OT may supervise volunteers who wish to be of assistance in a rehabilitative setting. Possible roles may include transporting residents to the clinic, assisting with management of equipment and supplies, or aiding in a group exercise program. Some volunteers prefer a single long-term commitment, while others want a variety of short-term projects.

The supervising clinician has many obligations to ensure the training, ability, and satisfaction of a volunteer. Sensitivity is required to determine the individual needs and motivation of volunteers. Some are seeking meaningful avenues for giving of special skills, while others have deep personal drives for feeling needed and acknowledged. Whatever the underlying motivation, the OT supervisor must be aware of the time and levels of interaction that foster a valued experience by the volunteer.

Because I enjoy inventing therapeutic activity equipment, I was asked over the years to interview two senior volunteers as prospective workers in the OT department. The first, Ernie, was a skilled woodworker. Whatever I would design, he would build at home. A favorite was a three-dimensional stacking puzzle of a deli sandwich. He was a quiet man who appeared angry, withdrawn, or depressed. A man of very few words, he would deliver his latest creation with, "Here it is," and before I could rave about it, he would ask, "What's next?" and then leave the second I gave him the next drawing of a design. After I marveled over many dozens of items, it occurred to me to send him a thank you note acknowledging his special skills, and how appreciative I was. He arrived the next week, very upset and wondering why I was "letting him go." I was shocked. I would never have interpreted my thank you as a "goodbye." I reassured him that I still had ideas, and urged him to continue coming. After over 100 inventions over several years, his health changed and he couldn't continue. I dared to send him a

"thinking of you" card on occasion, hoping that was acceptable to him.

Another volunteer, Sarah, had a daughter who was an OT and lived far away. She had always loved hearing about her daughter's training and experiences, and stated she would like to be a part of an OT department. Her special skill was sewing. She was a delightful, energetic person who especially liked encouraging residents as they participated in therapy. With her brightness and enthusiasm, I wondered if she could lead a small reminiscing group during a quiet time in the schedule of the special care unit for dementia. When coleading with me, she was perfection. If I asked her to lead while I only observed, she was perfect. When transitioned to independently leading, she was lost and very upset. I realized she needed to be in connection with me. Over time, I designed sewing projects, from decorative banners to pillows to a parachute for group exercises. She enjoyed doing the sewing projects at home. One week, she arrived and rather quickly broke into tears. She explained that she was a Holocaust survivor and just couldn't come back anymore to this Jewish facility. I had no idea of the inner strength and torment that she was struggling with just to arrive at this setting each week or her inner desire to honor her cultural heritage through volunteering. I offered support and thanks and expressed understanding and appreciation.

Therapeutic use of self has many dimensions, including sensitively recognizing a volunteer's personal needs and capabilities, and adjusting one's approaches to match even unexpected situations. Creativity for developing new possibilities for volunteer participation can lead to meaningful roles that continue to grow in possibilities and benefit others in unexpected ways.

JOURNAL ENTRY (K. M.)

As a volunteer for decades, I have enjoyed a variety of short- and long-term roles. Knowing the many benefits to self and society, I wondered why a person might intentionally choose not to be a volunteer, especially following retirement. Volunteering has so many opportunities for personal growth, learning skills, and meeting people. In qualitative research, to explore a construct in more depth, a suggestion is made to identify a "negative case." The negative case represents an example of someone who does not match the criteria or findings of the study. This brought to mind an acquaintance who had retired years ago. He was lively and active—a real "people person." As he approached retirement, I assumed he would segue into interesting volunteer opportunities. Time passed, and he never really connected to any form of productive work again. At some point, I inquired about whether he might someday be interested in some sort of volunteer work. He almost defensively blurted out sentiments about how he had spent almost

50 years of his life getting dressed, getting to work on time, following schedules and rules, and having a boss and that he would never want to do any of that again. I was rather startled at the time, realizing I had touched upon a sensitive subject. Now years later, I can analyze his perspective of volunteering and concur that it did in fact parallel his description of his paid work life. Would there ever be any way to engage someone like him in volunteering? Wouldn't he love it if he tried it? I realized my own personal values and biases were interfering with understanding and respecting his personal perspective.

EXPERT'S EXPERIENCE—
ELLEN RABINOWITZ, MPS, OTR

Ellen Rabinowitz is a retired OT who specialized in adult and geriatric practice in New York. She worked in long-term care facilities, adult day care, and home care settings. She is now a very active volunteer OT in a large metropolitan zoo. The perspective of her interview was analyzing the population of older volunteers at the zoo and the environment and services that promote their ongoing participation. The intent was to relate this to how an OT could apply similar principles to understand a large community organization, and aid in promoting appropriate volunteer services for older adults. One goal is for the reader to recognize how engagement in volunteer activities promotes many levels of health and ability. Another goal is to describe how OTs may utilize extensive task analysis skills when consulting with local agencies to evaluate program needs and recommend approaches for meeting participant needs.

In a telephone interview, Ms. Rabinowitz described how the demographics of volunteers have changed due to several factors. While the average age in this cosmopolitan area is 34, the "graying of America" means that many volunteers are in their 70s and 80s. There has also been an influx of new middle-aged volunteers who are unable to locate jobs and are therefore volunteering; many of them are attracted to working in an animal-related setting as an enjoyable occupation separate from paid work. Additionally, over 100 teenagers volunteer during the summer, so volunteer services are sensitive to multigenerational interests and abilities. The older adult volunteers have a variety of roles and may choose assignments within a specified category of services. Examples of these include public education of visitors, providing directions, office work (such as answering phones), outreach into the community, and preparation of specialized diets for the animals.

She explained that the older adults often initiate their involvement due to a desire to stay active. Many enjoy interacting with the public, especially with children. They enjoy the exercise, fresh air, and various forms of socialization. The location of the zoo is also convenient for access

by car, bus, bike, or on foot. She continued, "they have a determination. The dropout rate is high in young people but low in the older volunteers. Many proudly wear their 15- or 20-year badges. They enjoy giving back to the community, and demonstrate an ability to teach others. Part of the retention is also an ability to choose their own schedules. Each volunteer knows, if you sign up, you had better show up—people are depending on you."

She shared that "recruitment is formal, with a level 1 open house providing general information. If a person is interested, he or she signs up, and is interviewed by two experienced volunteers and one staff member. If accepted, he or she participates in a 3-day general overview training session. Level 2 is 3 additional days of advanced instruction related to the volunteer's specialized role. Level 3 encompasses an additional 8 months of training and supervision, with the goal of working independently. Each individual chooses his or her personal level of commitment and service. For each job, there is continuing education and mini-classes that are job specific. For most jobs, there is ongoing support, both formal and informal. New volunteers have the opportunity to shadow a veteran volunteer to see if a specific job is appealing. The staff really wants to ensure that volunteers feel comfortable. Once a volunteer is established, supervision is less formal, but the Director of Volunteers always keeps in touch."

"Each program area has a Volunteer Liaison. There is a team consisting of both staff and volunteers who stay on top of it all. This includes scheduling, ongoing training and support, and recognition to show appreciation for volunteers. In addition, special lectures and events are held throughout the year, open to all volunteers and staff members. There are holiday parties, and acknowledgment when a milestone number of hours has been completed." Serving as a volunteer also includes some other perks. During the city's Volunteer Week, other educational and cultural institutions offer free admission to zoo volunteers. Groups of volunteer colleagues/friends enjoy carpooling and visiting the other venues.

Ms. Rabinowitz gave an example of task analysis. "People think that answering the phones, for instance, sounds like a simple job. But not just anyone can answer phones. It isn't just answering phones. You have to understand the system, be able to answer or redirect questions, stay calm and organized…it is an important combination of cognitive, social, and motor skills…you have to be able to push the right buttons, be able to relate to people, understand and have a good attention span…take notes and make sure to follow up with messages." She stated that an OT could have a key role in any volunteer setting to assist with task analysis. It would be helpful if a breakdown was provided of the job requirements and necessary skills within written job descriptions. That would lead to better informed decisions for matching an individual's abilities with a specific set of volunteer opportunities.

An OT could play a number of roles in assisting with volunteer services. This could include evaluation of environment and consideration of adaptations to enable work performance. At the zoo, they offer a variety of accommodations for special needs. For example, a volunteer may be set up with a partner to job share. Responsibilities may be shifted to allow for indoor and/or seated tasks. They also adjust time expectations to maintain volunteer status: adults must provide a minimum of 50 hours per year of service, while for senior volunteers the requirement is 20 hours. Other roles for OT expertise could be consultation about training, with attention to how information is disseminated to an older population (e.g., understanding the learning needs and styles of older adults). Demonstration and hands-on practice may be more effective than lecture or assigned reading. The OT may also use his or her training in health promotion toward any adaptations needed for individuals with special needs, whether visitors or volunteers.

She continued that the "status" of being involved as part of a large group is important and offers many opportunities for socialization, as well as for meeting like-minded people who love animals. She said, "we jokingly refer to ourselves as a cult" and noted that many volunteer relationships extend beyond the zoo setting, sharing lunches together, visiting other zoos, or enjoying holiday celebrations.

When the time comes for a volunteer to consider retirement from service, if the need is not apparent to the individual, a liaison may talk to the Director of Volunteers. The Director may contact a family member or neighbor to continue to be part of a support system if a volunteer is exhibiting physical or mental decline. The Director of Volunteers is very involved in any critical situation, ensuring the safety of all volunteers while on the premises. There has also been some follow up to determine that former volunteers are doing well, especially individuals known to be living alone.

Ms. Rabinowitz expressed that OTs could have a valued role in consulting for community programs that offer volunteer services. She recommended that to explore this as a role, the OT should select a specialty in which she is passionate and an organization whose mission is clear and realistic. Then, she suggested volunteering within the organization, even on a small scale, and beginning to analyze the tasks, performance expectations, training, and environment and offer pro bono professional expertise and recommendations at that level. This would serve as a foundation for establishing the therapist's experience, which could then be applied to other facilities and organizations on a more formal paid consultant basis.

IMPLICATIONS FOR OCCUPATIONAL THERAPY PRACTICE

Opportunities for OT roles exist on many levels, working with clients both inside and outside the medical model. Therapy may include reconnecting with a volunteer role following illness or injury or a new involvement to initiate a volunteer role may be recommended following intervention for depression. If the client expresses a desire to volunteer, planning may occur to initiate volunteer exploration, with the OT offering information and support. This process could include steps to encourage personal contact with organizations, interviews, observing other volunteers, and online research (Cole & Macdonald, 2011).

Consulting With Organizations to Define Volunteer Roles

Another layer of OT involvement could be at the institutional or organizational level. An OT could be hired as a consultant to recruit and screen volunteers through a career fair. An OT could offer specialized skills for training new volunteers for effective and efficient job performance. Other roles could include environment assessment to determine potential safety risks or designing volunteer recognition programs. OTs could also have significant roles to match individuals with volunteer roles that include "relationships with a purpose" (Freedman, 1999). Because OTs are skilled in respecting the importance of social connections and an understanding of group dynamics, roles as consultants are possible. Recommendations could be made through activity analysis and the interpretation of group development or interpersonal issues (Cole, 2012; Donohue, 2013; Mosey, 1986).

Grading Volunteer Activities to Accommodate Advancing Age

OTs could be helpful in assessing skills for potential volunteer tasks and suggest adaptations or task modification techniques to maximize successful performance and evaluate for energy conservation and work simplification. Advice about transportation, scheduling, positioning, pacing, and planning could be helpful in enabling independent work skills. From the organization's perspective, adapting work tasks would enable older volunteers to remain productive, which concurrently helps the organization retain their trained volunteers and to get more of their important work done.

Some volunteers may need assistance in determining methods to grade activities as performance may decrease with age. Many senior volunteers retain those roles for many years, proud of their contributions and identity as a worker. On other occasions, life circumstances may change, making it difficult to retain a cherished role. For example, death of a spouse may change the volunteer's ability to continue in that role as new demands arise for unfamiliar home management responsibilities. The OT could consult with volunteers and their supervisors about appropriate timing for retiring from a volunteer position. Reasons could range from needing less commitment to changes in cognitive status.

Learning Activity 74: Enabling Client Volunteer Exploration

Some individuals have difficulty initiating a new or unfamiliar task. If you had a client who had a therapy goal of finding a volunteer position, how would you approach the topic of volunteer exploration?

1. Summarize the benefits of volunteering for health and wellness in layman's language. Be convincing.

2. How could you and the client begin to explore volunteer options? What steps would be involved?

3. How could you help to increase the client's comfort level in taking on a new occupational role?

Occupational Therapist's Support for the Productive Occupations of Volunteering

Because many volunteers are in the health care arena, OTs could have a helpful role in teaching basic communication skills, boundaries and precautions, self-protection from injury, and maintaining appropriate levels of emotional correctness. Because many volunteers expressed a desire for support, OTs could offer to lead a regularly scheduled discussion session where ideas and concerns could be raised (Cole & Macdonald, 2011).

The survey by Cole and Macdonald (2011) included a section of qualitative data. One of the questions asked was, "If you could make one change in the world of volunteering, what would it be?" The authors appreciated the retired OT's critical thinking. A recommendation was made for new retirees to take some time to finish old "to do" or bucket list projects, and then take a clear look at the "whole picture." This implied careful consideration of where to devote time and skills as a volunteer. They suggested identifying preferences to continue with variations of former professional responsibilities versus an entirely new endeavor. Many expressed a desire to continue with paid work for fewer hours, concurrently with volunteering. Their suggestions

paralleled with The Harvard School of Public Health's (2003) findings of suggesting better defined roles, increasing schedule flexibility, offering varied options for tasks, allowing for structured peer support, and providing means for recognition and appreciation.

Advocating for Occupational Therapist's Roles in Volunteering

Knowing the health benefits of volunteering, the OT as a private individual may advocate for increasing volunteer opportunities in his or her local community. Acting as a "go between" for different populations of older adults (senior center, places of worship, AARP meeting, and area agencies), an OT might raise public awareness of the need to establish or increase opportunities for volunteer services.

Because OTs are encouraged to expand upon and develop community-based services, volunteer issues create many opportunities. OTs could have strong single or ongoing roles in matching community needs to prospective volunteers. Whether creating openings for volunteer commitments, matching environment to volunteer performance, or advocating for volunteer training and recognition, OTs may have creative and flexible roles.

Case Example: Ben

Ben is a 70-year-old retired high school biology teacher in Washington state. He is a widower who lives alone and had been enjoying many post-retirement activities until he was in a motor vehicle accident 6 months ago. He sustained a concussion, which continues to pose challenges to his usual occupations. He received OT intervention for 2 months, and then was discharged with a recommendation to continue the principles learned in OT.

He has residual symptoms related to vestibular, sensory, and cognitive issues. He experiences dizziness with movements such as turning, leaning, or bending. Ben is sensitive to visual or auditory stimulation, especially when fatigued (bright lights, loud noises, and crowded spaces like in a concert hall lobby). He also has difficulty with mild confusion when in an unfamiliar or rushed situation. He knows that he must carefully plan and follow a "one thing at a time, one step at a time" lifestyle or his symptoms are exacerbated.

When discharged from OT, his therapist explained that he could return for services on a private pay basis. He arranged to meet with her in her private office for a single visit. When speaking on the phone, he described a need for assistance in planning a special upcoming trip. He knew he would need support and guidance for anticipating challenges and planning approaches to help manage his symptoms.

Ben was planning a trip with his 15-year-old grandson, Jason. Ben would be one of the chaperones for a youth group in their synagogue who would be participating in a service project during summer vacation from school. The group of 12 youth and adults would be flying to New York City to join other youth groups for a 5-day renovation project. The setting was a historic synagogue known for serving lunch to local homeless individuals. To refurbish the large cafeteria and kitchen, the volunteers would be responsible for scraping, washing, spackling, priming, and painting the walls and trim. The schedule was to work from 9 a.m. to 3 p.m. with a lunch break, and then have a 1-hour group "debriefing." Evenings were free time.

Anticipating that many aspects of this trip might be challenging, he contacted his physician, who approved his trip and sent a referral to the OT. Ben explained that the trip was planned 3 months ago and he had assumed he would "be fine" by now. He was eagerly looking forward to this opportunity to go to New York, a lifelong dream of his. He was excited to share time and work with Jason. Their rabbi was familiar with Ben's challenges and promised to offer assistance in any way necessary.

Learning Activity 75: Lessons From Ben

After reading Ben's scenario, brainstorm potential areas of difficulty for Ben. Create an outline with the following topics and expand on these headings:

1. Planning a trip (travel, packing, to-do lists and calendar, adaptations, such as a walking stick)

2. Airport experience (airport itself, travel)

3. Getting settled in New York

4. Role as chaperone/grandfather

5. Role as volunteer participant

6. Support as needed, self-disclosure issues

7. Leisure time in New York (balance of work, leisure, rest)

8. Prevention of symptoms (energy conservation, pacing, body mechanics/positioning to prevent disabling vestibular discomfort)

9. Preserving energy and ability for return trip.

10. Determine system for Ben to independently assess results of his adaptations and anticipate changes needed for future similar experiences

Group Discussion and Problem Solving: The OT will address strategies for the above considerations identified by Ben. Break into small groups, assigning one of the above 10 topics to each group. Brainstorm for areas of functional challenges. List and prepare to share with the full class. Brainstorm for possible OT recommendations, including considerations for promoting his successful compliance and follow up. For example, verbal instruction alone would not be appropriate for Ben. Compare notes for this extensive task analysis and treatment planning. Consider adaptations, alternatives, priorities, and what would be realistic

for Ben. Review the role of a private practice OT who offers intervention as needed for functional challenges. Reflect on identified strategies and determine if they are considered principles of client-centered practice.

SUMMARY

The role of volunteering has many meanings for older adults, from skill maintenance to new learning, and from social interaction to giving back to the community. Whatever the personal motivation and meaning, OTs may have a role and function in promoting volunteer activity participation. This may range from accessing appropriate volunteer opportunities, to grading tasks for successful performance, to consulting with agencies about how to maximize effectiveness of volunteer services. From volunteer exploration to volunteer participation, OTs may use their skills in task analysis, group dynamics, and program development to enhance volunteer service opportunities.

REFERENCES

American Occupational Therapy Association. (2014). *Occupational therapy practice framework: Domain & Process.* (3rd ed.). Bethesda, MD: Author.

Backes, G. M. (1993). Importance of social volunteering for elderly and aged women. *Zeitschrift für Gerontologie, 26,* 349-354.

Brown, J. W., Chen, S., Mefford, L., Brown, A., Callen, B., & McArthur, P. (2011). Becoming an older volunteer: A grounded theory study. *Nursing Research and Practice.* 2011;2011, 361250. doi: 10.1155/2011/361250.

Caro, F. G., & Morris, R. (2001). Maximizing the contributions of older people as volunteers. In S. E. Levekoff, Y. K. Chee, & S. Noguchi, (Eds.), *Successful and productive aging* (pp. 71-96). New York, NY: Springer.

Carr, D. C., & Kail, B. L. (2013). The influence of unpaid work on the transition out of full time paid work. *The Gerontologist, 53,* 92-101.

Cavanaugh, G. (2005). Civic engagement—ASA helps lead new approach to retirement. *Aging Today, 36*(2), 16.

Cole, M. B. (2007). Volunteering for older adults: Roles for occupational therapy. *American Occupational Therapist Association, Gerontology Special Interest Section Quarterly, 30,* 1-3.

Cole, M. B. (2012). *Group dynamics in occupational therapy* (4th ed.). Thorofare, NJ: SLACK Incorporated.

Cole, M. B., & Macdonald, K. C. (2011). Retired occupational therapists' experiences in volunteer occupations. *Occupational Therapy International, 18,* 18-31.

Cornwell, B., Laumann, E. O., & Schumm, L. P. (2008). The social connectedness of older adults: A natural profile. *American Sociology Review, 73,* 185-203.

Costa Guerra, S. R., Demain, S. H., & Marques de Sousa, L. X. (2012). Being a volunteer: Motivations, fears, and benefits of volunteering in an intervention program for people with dementia and their families. *Activities, Adaptation & Aging, 36,* 55-78.

Donohue, M. (2013). *Social profile: Assessment of social participation in children, adolescents, and adults.* Bethesda, MD: AOTA Press.

Freedman, M. (1999). *Prime time: How baby boomers will revolutionize retirement and transform America.* New York, NY: Public Affairs.

Fried, L. (2005). Volunteer: The right dose. In fifty ways to fix your life. *US News & World Report, 137*, 84.

Harvard School of Public Health. (2003). Reinventing aging: Baby Boomers and civic engagement. *Report highlights*. Retrieved from www.hsph.harvard.edu/chc/reinventingaging/report.

Hawkley, L., & Cacioppo, J. (2004). Stress and the aging immune system. *Brain Behavior Immunology, 18*,114-119.

Hawkley, L., Masi, C., Berry, J., & Cacioppo, J. (2006). Loneliness is a unique predictor of age-related differences in systolic blood pressure. *Psychological Aging, 21*, 152-164.

Hoad, P. (2002). Drawing the line: The boundaries of volunteering in the community: Care of older people. *Health Social Care Community, 10*, 239-246.

Johnson, C. (2003). Infrastructure of volunteer agencies: Capacity to absorb boomer volunteers. In Harvard School of Public Health, Report of Conference on baby boomers and retirement: Impact on civic engagement. Retrieved from www.hsph.harvard.edu/chc/reinventingaging/report.

Knight, J., Ball, V., Corr, S., Turner, A., Lowis, M., & Ekberg, M. (2007). An empirical study to identify older adults' engagement in productivity occupations. *Journal of Occupational Science, 14*, 145-153.

Kleyman, P. (2003). Study shows how older volunteer force in US could double. *Aging Today, 24*, 1. Retrieved from www.agingtoday.org/at-241/Study_Shows_How.cfm.

Korda, L. J. (1995). The benefits of beneficence: Rewards of hospice volunteering. *American Journal of Hospital Palliative Care, 12*, 17-18.

Lauber, C., Nordt, C., Falcato, L., & Rossler, W. (2002). Determinants of attitude to volunteering in psychiatry: Results of a public opinion survey in Switzerland. *International Journal of Social Psychiatry, 48*, 209-219.

Merrell, J. (2000). You don't do it for nothing: Women's experiences of volunteering in two community Well Women Clinics. *Health Society Care Community, 8*, 31-39.

Morrow-Howell, N., Hinterlong, J., Rozario, P., & Tang, F. (2003). Effects of volunteering on the well-being of older adults. *The Journals of Gerontology Series B: Psychological Sciences and Social Sciences. 58*, S137-45.

Mosey, A. C. (1986). *Psychosocial components of occupational therapy.* New York: Raven Press.

Musick, M. A., Herzog, A. R., & House, J. S. (1999). Volunteering and mortality among older adults: Findings from a national sample. *The Journals of Gerontology Series B: Psychological Sciences and Social Sciences, 54*, S173-180.

Mutchler, J. E., Burr, J. A., & Caro, F. G. (2003). From paid worker to volunteer: Leaving the paid workforce and volunteering in later life. *Social Forces, 81*, 1267-1293.

Okun, M., & Schultz, A. (2003). Age and motives for volunteering: Testing hypotheses derived from socioemotional selectivity theory. *Psychological Aging, 18*, 231-239.

O'Reilly, P., & Caro, F. (1994). Productive aging: An overview of the literature. *Journal of Aging & Social Policy, 6*(3), 39-71.

Prisuta, R. (2003). Enhancing volunteerism among aging boomers. In Harvard School of Public Health, Report of Conference on baby boomers and retirement: Impact on civic engagement. Retrieved from www.hsph.harvard.edu/chc/reinventingaging/report.

Rook, K. S., & Sorkin, D. H. (2003). Fostering social ties through volunteer role: Implications for older adults' psychological health. *International Journal of Aging and Human Development, 57*, 313-337.

Ruler, A. J. (1998). Integrating life themes of work in the care of older people. *Contemporary Nursing, 7*, 205-211.

Tanz, J., & Spencer, T. (2000). Candy striper my ass! *Fortune, 142*,156-160.

Tavares, J. L., Burr, J. A., & Mutchler, J. E. (2013). Race differences in the relationship between formal volunteering and hypertension. *Journals of Gerontology, Psychological Sciences and Social Sciences, 68*, 310-318.

Tomas Sancho, A., Kennedy, L., & Colomer Revuelta, C. (1998). Volunteerism and the reorientation of health services. *Atención Primaria, 31*, 450-456.

U.S. Bureau of Labor Statistics. (2004). Volunteering in the United States, 2004. Retrieved from www.bls.gov/news.release/volun.nro.htm.

Van Willigen, M. (2000). Differential benefits of volunteering across the life course. *Journal of Gerontol B Psychol Sci Soc Sci, 55*, S308-s318.

Warburton, J., Paynter, J., & Petriwskyj, K. (2007). Volunteering as a productive aging activity: Incentives and barriers to volunteering by Australian seniors. *Journal of Applied Gerontology, 26*, 333-354.

Wheeler, J. A., Gorey, K. M., & Greenblatt, B. (1998). The beneficial effects of volunteering for older volunteers and the people they serve: A meta-analysis. *International Journal of Aging & Human Development, 47*, 69-79.

10

Older Worker

Marilyn B. Cole, MS, OTR/L, FAOTA

"Keep doing what you love." (Participant, Johanna)

Although the official retirement age is 65 (soon increasing to 67.5) in the United States, statistics show that many older adults continue to work for pay well beyond that age. In Chapter 2, the demographics of retirement describe a wide range of patterns, including multiple exits and re-entries into the work force throughout older adulthood. As reviewed in Chapter 2, Baby Boomers, those born between 1946 and 1964, are due to retire in increasing numbers over the next several decades, yet their unique characteristics make them more likely to choose paid work over other productive occupations (hard working/workaholics) and less likely to be financially prepared (due to high credit card debt, large houses, nice cars) to retire. A Pew Research Center (2011) report confirms that two-thirds of Baby Boomers are not retired, and those ages 50 to 61 said they "may have to delay their retirement because of current economic conditions" (para 14). Of the latter group, 23% plan to work until at least age 70 and 12% say they never plan to retire (Pew Research Center, 2011, para. 13). Furthermore, the U.S. Bureau of Labor Statistics (2008) predicts that the number of workers age 55 to 64 are expected to increase 36% by 2016, while the number of workers over 75 will increase by 80%. Reasons given for continued paid employment may be largely financial, especially for the Baby Boomer generation, for whom Social Security and Medicare benefits are becoming more questionable. Because more Baby Boomers will become OT clients in the

upcoming decades, OT professionals need to be prepared to assist older workers to make the necessary adaptations to continue paid work when that is their chosen productive occupation. Traditionalists who have retired from career jobs may be more likely to return to employment for different reasons, such as socialization, feeling useful and needed, or giving structure to their day, rather than strictly financial reasons. Either way, evidence supports working as beneficial to health and well-being, and aging productively.

The AOTA's OTPF III defines work as "labor or exertion to make, construct, manufacture, form, fashion, or shape objects; to organize, plan, or evaluate services or processes of living or governing; committed occupations that are performed with or without financial reward (Christiansen & Townsend, 2010, p. 423)" (AOTA, 2014, p. S20). Working at a job generally means performing tasks for someone else and implies collecting a paycheck after the required tasks are completed. However, the term *work* encompasses a broad range of activities that are categorized in various ways. For example, a laborer may rely heavily on physical ability and may work for low pay or minimum wage. A *blue collar worker* typically refers to a tradesman, such as a carpenter, plumber, welder, or mason—jobs that require a specific set of skills often learned through apprenticeships in addition to schooling. Older tradesmen can make very good pay, an incentive to continue working well into older adulthood. White collar workers usually have a higher level

Cole MB, Macdonald KC.
Productive Aging: An Occupational Perspective (pp 171-182).
© 2015 Taylor & Francis Group.

of education and earn higher pay than laborers or trades-men, but this is not always true. Working in the professions used to mean doctors, lawyers, teachers, and clergymen, but that too has expanded to cover a broad range of work roles. Furthermore, Western cultures place a high value on any kind of work. Therefore, in the United States, a person's work position and the status it provides throughout his or her life often becomes an important part of individual and social identity.

Another way to categorize work is by the meaning it holds for the individual. One's vocation, or "calling," implies a spiritual connection, one's purpose for living that is seen by some as a message from God. From this viewpoint, it is work, or "occupation," that gives meaning to one's life. If older adults find spiritual meaning in their work, it is easy to see why they may choose to continue even after it is no longer financially necessary. Conversely, when an older worker is forced to retire or becomes physically unable to continue working, he or she may feel useless or marginalized, increasing the likelihood of depression.

The OTPF III (AOTA, 2014) lists the following three categories of work-related occupations:

1. *Employment interests and pursuits*: Identifying and selecting work opportunities based on assets, limita-tions, and likes and dislikes relative to work (adapted from Mosey, 1996, p. 342).

2. *Employment seeking and acquisition*: Advocating for oneself; completing, submitting, and reviewing appro-priate application materials; preparing for interviews, participating in interviews, and following up after-ward; discussing job benefits and finalizing negotia-tions.

3. *Job performance*: Performing the requirements of a job, including work skills and patterns; time management; relationships with coworkers, managers, and custom-ers; creation, production, and distribution of products and services; initiation, sustainment, and completion of work; and compliance with work norms and proce-dures (AOTA, 2014, p. S20).

While these categories seem more geared to younger and middle-aged adults, they can also apply to older workers who become unemployed involuntarily, choose to change jobs, or leave career jobs for bridge jobs and may have a need to adapt their work situations to accommodate changes in health, decreased stamina, or other changes that affect job performance. Most of our participants who continued paid employment described the adaptations they have made, including part-time hours, less stressful working condi-tions, flexibility of job requirements, and a greater focus on social relationships with clients, coworkers, or students.

Retirement preparation and adjustment is defined by the OTPF III as "determining aptitudes, developing inter-ests and skills, selecting appropriate avocational pursuits and adjusting lifestyle in the absence of the worker role"

(AOTA, 2014, p. S20). Because the evidence shows that so many older adults prefer continued paid work after retire-ment, OT professionals need to include this option in retirement planning discussions with clients.

Learning Activity 76: Analyzing a Prior Job

Write a description for a job you have held in the past. This is a good opportunity to use your OT activity analysis skills.

1. What are the physical requirements for this job?

2. What training was necessary?

3. What mental abilities are necessary for this job?

4. If you were the boss, and a healthy 65-year-old person applied for this job, what concerns would you have and why?

PARTICIPANT PERSPECTIVES

Of our 40 participants, 15 had worked for pay within the past year. Most of them continued working in a modi-fied way within their lifelong careers. Only one participant, Johanna (age 71), continued to work 40 or more hours per week, and she did so by choice because it gave her life meaning. She practices elder law, despite fighting ovarian cancer. Her advice: "Keep doing what you love. Mostly women call me with problems…legal situations. How can I say no? I want to keep helping them as long as I am able to. My daughter [a paralegal in her office] helps me by bring-ing home files so I can work from home. Sometimes, I am working all day. I wish I could find a way to cut down to 20 hours per week. This work keeps me going. It gives me a reason to get up every morning."

Four of our participants were university professors who continued teaching because they enjoyed it. Pearl, an English professor for over 30 years, still teaches 2 courses a semester—writing and English literature. "This is what I know how to do. I don't know how I would spend my time otherwise. I have made adaptations. I sit while lecturing, I cut back on assignments that need more extensive feedback. [But] it is important to stay in contact with younger genera-tions. Teaching keeps me connected." Ken, a biology pro-fessor for over 40 years, teaches a freshman seminar each fall and spring. "I attempt to balance work obligations with outside life. I try to make the work fun." Signian teaches 6 credits each semester as a part-timer. She combines her academic expertise with her lifelong interest in quilting through involving students with quilting as service learn-ing in two fieldwork settings. Mary continues her interest in research through thesis and dissertation advisory roles at two local universities.

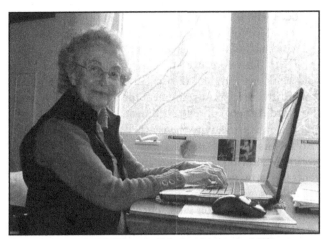

Figure 10-1. At age 86, Mildred still finds writing to be fulfilling.

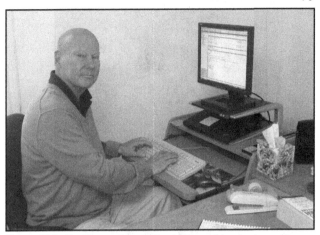

Figure 10-2. Charlie spends each day writing at his suburban office.

Mildred has continued her lifelong career through writing. She has published four books since her retirement, including a historical memoir (Figure 10-1). She continues her editorial role, as well as revising chapters in books. "I want to keep writing and revising my chapters on the Five Stages [a group technique she has developed] because I still believe in them. For the latest revision, I had to do something new. So I volunteered to run a group with young autism spectrum and mentally-challenged clients...something I had not done before. It was a challenge! They do not respond the same way as adults with mental illness or older adults with dementia. I learned a great deal from them that I could convey in my revisions. It would not occur to me not to do this." Mary also has continued her career through writing about something in which she believes. She has just published a manual about an assessment tool she developed earlier called the Social Profile. Charlie, a former TV comedy writer, still maintains his suburban office, where he arrives early each morning and writes crime novels until midafternoon. He has completed two novels that he self-published on Amazon: *Wall Street Killers* and *The Bennington Murders*, both set in New York City, his former place of employment. "It is important to be self-disciplined when you want to accomplish your goal." Charlie rewards himself by making sure he arrives back home by 5 p.m. for happy hour each day with his wife and friends (Figure 10-2).

Peggie, at age 78, still covers for vacationing nurses in her former place of employment. She participates in temporary paid projects, such as giving flu shots at local area corporations and health fairs. "I see the extra dollars as found money to invest." Mary V. also continues her nursing career: "I get up early and do part-time work offering private duty care. It is more than I planned on." Nettie still works part-time: "I had worked in geriatrics with so many agencies and organizations. Now I work in pediatrics, doing consulting."

Some participants have found employment in areas different from their former careers. Sue, a former banker, has worked 6 hours per day as a church administrator for 25 years. At age 65, she still needs the income, but she also continues because she loves helping people. "This work keeps me busy and involved with people outside home." Linval, a former maintenance worker, works "12 hours a week, and I also get hired by people to do small house or yard jobs" (Figure 10-3). Judi does "some babysitting. I make some pocket money so I don't have to go into my savings. I also house sit." Jim has found an interesting job as a product demonstrator. "I am working part-time up to 4 days a week, 6 hours a day. I am on my feet, I didn't know I could do that, but I can with a half hour break in the middle. I do product demonstration in a grocery store. I rotate around 13 stores, interacting with people and the store personnel, 99% terrific and also the shoppers...that's another story!" Dave continues working just because it keeps him busy and active. "Why do I stay at my job? It's a routine...get up in the morning, you have something to do. You have to fill that time. If I don't have something to do, I'm in trouble."

While some participants admit to needing the extra income, working into older adulthood was mostly by choice, with other benefits taking precedence over earning a living. Some continued their "life work" because it gave their life meaning and because it reinforced their social identity as a professional, a teacher, or a helper. For most, working made them feel needed and valued, allowing them to apply their lifelong skills in ways that benefited others. At the very least, working gave their day structure, a routine that kept them busy, physically active, and socially connected.

LITERATURE REVIEW

Persons over age 65 in the United States have an average life expectancy of an additional 18.8 years (20 years for females and 17.3 years for males) (U.S. Administration on Aging, 2011). Even if they choose to retire at age 65 while

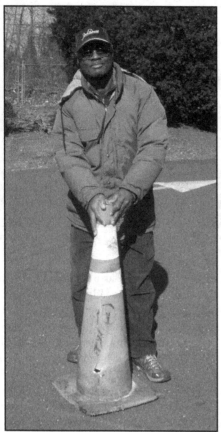

Figure 10-3. Linval does outdoor maintenance work on church grounds.

tive occupations in Laslett's Third Age is the goal of self-fulfillment. Most of our participants who worked for pay and did so because of the satisfaction and meaning it brought to their lives. Therefore, even though it sounds contradictory, paid work as a productive occupation in older adulthood can greatly enrich post-retirement life when it helps to meet the Third Age goal of self-fulfillment.

Erikson's generativity theory (Erikson & Erikson, 1997) also factors into the reasons many older adults continue working. Showing concern for and commitment to future generations by passing on knowledge, wisdom, and skills exemplifies generativity in the workplace as a defining factor in continued job satisfaction (Dendinger, Adams, & Jacobson, 2005; Mor Barak, 1995). A MetLife Foundation/Civic Ventures (2005) survey, identifies four post retirement trends for retiring Boomers seeking continued employment:

1. Want to do work that helps others, now and in retirement.

2. Want careers that are about people, purpose, and community.

3. Have divergent attitudes about post-retirement work based on gender and race.

4. Don't think it will be very easy to find second careers doing good work, and strongly support public policy changes to remove obstacles.

For recent retirees, including Baby Boomers with full-time career jobs, a one-time, permanent retirement was found to be the exception rather than the rule. Instead, about half transition to "bridge job" employment, including part-time consulting work, self-employment, or switching jobs in a related field. Of these, 80% experienced a cut in pay from 11% to 50% in bridge jobs (Cahill, Giandrea, & Quinn, 2012).

Risk Factors for Older Workers

Some research has focused on risk factors for work-related injury among older workers. In 2011, 16.7% of all older adults in the United States were employed (U.S. Bureau of Labor Statistics, 2012). Workers over age 65 are at increased risk for more severe work-related injury, requiring longer recovery times and more days lost from work than their younger peers. The median days lost from work over age 65 was 16 days. Furthermore, fatal work injuries for older workers is more than three times that of those younger than age 65 (U.S. Bureau of Labor Statistics, 2012). Risk of bone fracture was found to be higher for women age 55 and older, especially with comorbid obesity (Compston et al., 2011). Older workers had higher levels of hypotension, making them more likely to sustain a traumatic brain injury due to a fall, as well as hemothorax, pelvic fractures, cervical fractures, and upper and lower extremity fractures (Konstantinidis et al., 2011). In a study linking heart disease with job stress, older workers who had a coronary event

still in good health, most of their remaining years can potentially be spent in productive occupations. Furthermore, attitudes toward retirement are changing. "The idea of Americans at age 65 saying goodbye to the workplace and spending hours with a long-desired leisure occupation is no longer realistic or even necessarily desirable" (Womack, 2008, p. 76). Womack (2008) notes that earlier studies indicated that "the meaning and satisfaction derived from work tended to be a better predictor of work longevity and productivity than did age or any other factor" (p. 76). Other purposes served by continued work for older adults include social status, social interaction, structured use of time, and a sense of productivity (Sanders & McCready, 2010).

Theory and Older Workers

From a theoretical perspective, paid employment categorizes an older adult in Laslett's Second Age because it precedes retirement. Laslett (1989) defined the Third Age as beginning with retirement and lasting until the onset of disability or dependency in at least one ADL. However, the key feature of paid work in the Second Age is economic necessity. Most of our participants fit into Laslett's Third Age category because they engaged in paid work by choice not by financial necessity. Another key feature of produc-

were four times more likely to experience high job strain and more likely to report low job control (McCarthy, Perry, & Greiner, 2012). Employees with inflammatory bowel disease are more likely to take sick time, at a high cost to employers (Gunnarsson et al., 2012).

Cognitive health or impairment in older workers has been a growing concern. The Centers for Disease Control and Prevention (CDC) (2011) found that perceptions of "what defines a healthy brain" or "staying sharp" included living to an advanced age, having good physical health, having a positive outlook, being alert, having a good memory, and being socially involved. Their analysis of 55 cross-cultural focus groups concluded that maintaining a healthy lifestyle, healthy diet, social involvement, participation in enjoyable activities, a positive mental attitude, spiritual activities, and accepting and adapting to physical and cognitive changes are all needed to promote cognitive health in aging (CDC, 2011). While workers may take longer to solve complex problems, they are usually able to perform the cognitive demands of their jobs (CDC, 2011).

Learning Activity 77: Older Workers as Depicted in the Media

1. Find three recent stories of older workers in newspapers, magazines, or online and summarize them. Note sources.

2. Discuss the positive and negative implications portrayed in the stories you found.

3. What did you learn from these articles about older adults in the work force?

4. What is your opinion about older people continuing to work as they age?

Adaptations for Health Conditions at Work

Several studies addressed the process of adaptation for workers with health problems. Older workers age 46 to 63 with self-reported health conditions varied widely in their ability to remain productive at work, based on visibility of the health problem, work-related autonomy, relational support, and ability to ask for help (Leijten et al., 2013). From an employer's perspective, the most effective strategies for helping older employees return to work after injury or illness were offering a graded return to normal job activity and employee participation in cognitive behavioral therapy (Odeen et al., 2012). The same systematic review study found little evidence of decreased sick leave after workplace health education or physical fitness programs. However, workplace programs that reduce work-related stress, based on a review of longitudinal data across 11 European countries, were found helpful in "maintaining

workability in early old age" (Reinhardt, Wahrendorf, & Siegrist, 2012, p. 156).

Learning Activity 78: Disabled Older Worker Interview

Visit an older worker who is coping with a chronic health condition.

1. What type of work does this person do and how does he or she feel about the job?

2. What functional limitations exist? List and describe. How do these limit his or her ability to perform tasks at work?

3. What adaptations are necessary for this person to continue working? What problems or issues still exist? Give an example.

4. How might you, as an OT, advise this person to address problems or facilitate his or her occupational performance?

APPLICATIONS TO CONTINUUM OF CARE

Community dwelling older workers do not always get the help OTs could offer, because this role falls between the cracks of medical reimbursement systems. OTs could consult with employers in providing assessment and interventions for older workers, helping them make adaptations to their work situations and environments. For example, older workers with lower back pain may need to adapt their work stations using ergonomic principles for seating positions, computer and telephone use, and other technologies. Learning good body mechanics may help older workers who have more physically demanding jobs. Prevention is the key to workers' ability to continue employment as they age.

Community and Employer Consultation

Advocacy in the workplace helps older workers negotiate better working conditions that accommodate age-related changes, such as better lighting, flexible hours, and more frequent breaks. Other wellness and prevention strategies also may be incorporated into the typical work day. OT practitioners may consult with employers or with community agencies in providing educational sessions that support the needs of older workers.

Fran is a good example of a community-dwelling older adult who needed the income of paid work. In her younger years, she did not work long enough to qualify for Social

Security, but spent many years building her homemaking skills. At age 66, Fran was hired at a local senior center and now works 4 hours each day preparing and serving nutritional lunches to center members and guests. The income, along with free lunches and transportation, keeps Fran living independently and off of public assistance, a source of pride for her.

Helping Older Workers in Primary Care Settings

When an injury or illness causes absence from work, the primary care physician makes recommendations as to when the client might safely return to the job. Depending on the situation, a worker's medical expenses could be covered by employer-based insurance or workman's compensation. If the client is self-employed, a part-time worker without benefits, or paid by the hour, day, or upon task completion, then he or she loses income while recovering from an illness. In requesting referrals from a primary care physician's office, an OT might seize the opportunity to assist older clients with self-management of illness or injury, including advocating for flexibility in job requirements and adapting work tasks to allow for an earlier return to work. For example, Sue has functional mobility issues. In her position as church administrator, she enters the building and walks to her ground level office. Because she must use a cane for balance, she cannot carry heavy items or use both hands for carrying. Her chair has wheels so she can move around the office without standing up. Sue has learned to ask for help when needed—a deacon often carries items in from her car or assists her with storing larger items (copy paper, paper supplies for the coffee hour on Sundays). Older individuals with illnesses or disabilities can often complete work tasks by adapting their environments and adjusting their schedules to facilitate this important and meaningful productive occupation.

Rehabilitation Facilities

Older clients encountered in rehabilitation centers have usually experienced an unexpected injury or acute health condition that requires specialized medical intervention to restore function and/or prevent long-term disability. Both inpatients and outpatients in this situation have an expectation of recovery and returning to their former occupations. OTs need to know whether clients expect to return to paid work and to learn what functional abilities their jobs require. In some instances, older workers who have bone fractures or other physical injuries that do not affect their mental abilities will be able to return to work with adaptations to their seating, positioning, and workstation technology. Jobs requiring physical strength and skills may require longer medical leaves to allow for work hardening (building up strength, ROM, and endurance), and job requirements may need to be altered to accommodate a slower healing time.

Within the protocols for rehabilitation in ADL following the onset of more complex disabilities, OTs also need to determine whether an older adult has a long-term goal of returning to work or working in any capacity. When the work role is central to the older adult's social identity, giving up hope of recovery of that role, even when it seems impossible from a medical viewpoint, may have devastating effects for the motivation and well-being of the client. The OT practitioner, while respecting the client's occupational priorities, uses therapeutic use of self to motivate the client to work on the skills of self-management, including self-care and functional mobility, as the initial step in the recovery of other productive occupational roles. Incorporating some aspects of important work roles, such as enabling e-mail communication, using a familiar computer program for building perceptual skills, or using work-related objects or situations to develop problem-solving skills, may result in higher client engagement in OT interventions.

Assisted Living to Long-Term Care

Older adults may have part-time jobs for pay even within their institutions. For example, they might work in a gift shop or make craft items to sell to others there. As they are capable, they may leave an assisted living facility to work elsewhere in the community or do work in their rooms or apartments, such as editing the writing of others or communicating using a computer or Smartphone. Some long-term care facilities offer sheltered workshop types of employment. Piece work is provided by local factories or corporations, and residents are paid according to the quantity of work completed.

IMPLICATIONS FOR OCCUPATIONAL THERAPY PRACTICE— DR. MARTHA SANDERS, PHD, MSOSH, OTR/L, CPE

OT consultation for older workers should consider the system or organization in which the older worker is employed. OTs should promote a positive organizational culture for older workers, in which other employees respect and appreciate the special skills older workers bring to the workplace. OTs must specifically address the job tasks performed, and the individual worker within the context of his or her life roles.

Organizational Culture: Older Workers' Generational Strengths

Stereotypes exist relative to older workers being grouchy, slow, short-tempered, and averse to learning technology (Smola & Sutton, 2002). Such stereotypes have been debunked repeatedly, with studies demonstrating the value of older workers in customer service centers, reservation centers, and retail jobs. In fact, older workers outperformed younger workers in the volume of reservations at a Days Inn reservation center because they took time with customers and quickly established a relationship (McNaught & Barth, 1992). Older workers' abilities to understand customers' needs in the homebuilding industry has created positive experiences for older workers where they can mentor or teach younger workers, and establish a loyal customer base in the process (Sanders & McCready, 2010, 2011). These experiences contribute to generativity and successful aging (Erikson & Erikson, 1997). Thus, OTs can highlight older workers' generational strengths, which creates value for the organization as a whole.

Optimizing Job Design: Training, Work Teams, and Mentoring

OTs also can provide recommendations for the *optimal job design* for older adults. Sanders and McCready (2010) and Wahlstedt, Nygard, Kemmlert, Torgen, and Bjorksten (2000) found that older workers benefit from a team-oriented organizational structure that promotes social support, camaraderie, and autonomy in decision making. Although older workers tend to be less interested in climbing the career ladder, older workers can lead work groups, special project teams, and mentor younger workers to utilize their skills and interact with others (Desmette & Gaillard, 2008). This social support provides benefits beyond the workplace to contribute to overall self-efficacy and control over one's life (Sanders & McCready, 2010).

Specific to job tasks, OTs should emphasize the importance of designing jobs so that workers use a variety of skills and are retrained alongside younger workers. Although older workers do not always receive the same ongoing job training as younger workers (Brooke, 2003), Schooler, Mulatu, and Oates (1999) found that performing cognitively complex work increased the intellectual functioning of older workers even late in their careers. Continual training promotes not only cognitive health, cognitive engagement, and stimulation, but also a feeling of empowerment and control over their lives.

Job Tasks Modification

The primary focus of job modification for older workers is minimizing the risk of injury from physical demands,

promoting comfort and safety, and maximizing the environment to promote optimal productivity. Table 10-1 highlights key modifications recommended for older workers based on typical age-related changes.

Sensory Changes

Visual and hearing changes are most commonly acknowledged as impacting older workers' jobs. Many options exist for compensating for visual losses. Older workers can wear computer glasses or safety glasses (for physically demanding jobs) with magnification or progressive lenses. Such glasses, along with large font lettering on measuring devices and large font signage, are increasingly recognized as a benefit to all workers, not just older workers. One of the most effective ways to promote vision is to increase illumination levels. Older adults require approximately 30% more light than younger counterparts to effectively utilize visual abilities. Thus, higher illumination levels for overhead lighting, headlamps for fine work, and task lighting for desk activities can promote visual abilities along with natural lighting provided by work environments with windows.

Musculoskeletal Changes

Older workers generally experience gradually reduced strength capabilities after age 50, which may be hastened by working in physically demanding jobs over the course of their lifetime. While workers are typically able to meet job demands, the performance of tasks may take a higher percentage of their capabilities, creating fatigue or risk over a period of time. Ways to minimize older workers' energy expenditure and risk for injuries include using mechanical assists (overhead lifts, dollies, pallet jacks), reducing load carried, and developing a team lift policy to decrease the weight an older worker typically lifts. Older workers can be encouraged to use good body mechanics, powered ergonomic tools, and break down larger loads into small parcels (take more trips) to lessen the loads lifted. Aerobic endurance can be maximized by pacing oneself during the day, taking short "pause" breaks between tasks, and by having a seat option close by for those with primarily standing and walking tasks (Sanders & McCready, 2009).

An area of increasing concern is falls in the workplace. Risk factors for falls include myriad factors, such as low vision, low lighting, changes in balance reactions, trunk control, decreased lower extremity strength, medication side effects, and clutter in the employee's work environment, among others. OTs are well positioned to recommend environmental modifications that carry over from the home to the workplace, such as reducing clutter in the environment (good housekeeping!), improving lighting, promoting optimal conditioning of the employee, avoiding the use of step ladders or precarious walking on unstable surfaces if possible, and even installing hand rails where

TABLE 10-1		
CONSIDERATIONS FOR OLDER WORKERS		
SENSORY SYSTEMS	**IMPACT OF AGE-RELATED CHANGES ON WORK**	**ENVIRONMENTAL OR JOB ADAPTATIONS**
Visual	Difficulty reading small print Difficulty seeing in low light Sensitivity to glare Changes in depth perception Changes in ability to discern contrasts in backgrounds	Magnification, reading glasses Safety glasses with progressive lens low vision assists Larger signage in environment Increased illumination levels Task lighting Contrasting environment and stairs
Hearing	High frequency hearing loss and inability to hear speech or emergency alarms Sensitive to background noise	Low frequency warnings Minimal background noise Acoustic panels Personal workspace
Temperature	Less able to regulate temperature	Sweat-wicking or protective clothing Adequate winter protection for hands, face Periodic breaks from heat or cold Adequate hydration
MUSCULOSKELETAL SYSTEMS		
Strength	Decreased strength 25% to 30% by age 65	Use of mechanical assists Team lift policy Powered ergonomic tools Break down loads Lifts at waist height
Grip strength	Arthritis; decreased strength	Powered tools Ergonomic hand tools Joint protection
Balance	Instability; difficulty catching self	Increased lighting Remove clutter Minimize walking on unstable surfaces Avoid climbing or secure ladders Install rails Lower extremity conditioning
Reaction time	Slower reaction time	Keep items in close reach Provide more time between repetitive tasks Larger targets

(continued)

TABLE 10-1 (CONTINUED)		
CONSIDERATIONS FOR OLDER WORKERS		
	IMPACT OF AGE-RELATED CHANGES ON WORK	**ENVIRONMENTAL OR JOB ADAPTATIONS**
COGNITIVE FUNCTIONS		
Aerobic capacity	Decreased endurance	Pace self Alternate light and heavy work Take "pause breaks"
Cognition	Changes in working memory, complex problem solving, prioritizing	Simple directions Written or verbal cues Time to complete tasks Practice Ongoing training
Driving	Changes in motion perception Slower braking time Slower signal selection Changes in scanning at intersections	Ample space between cars Minimize left hand turns Clearly labeled controls Wide maneuvering area
Adapted from M. Sanders, personal communication, 2013.		

needed. Such principles will become increasingly important as more Baby Boomers remain at industrial jobs.

Work Task Training

Fisk, Rogers, Charness, Czaja, and Sharit (2009) suggests that training for older adults should be thorough, yet self-paced, with ample time to learn and practice tasks prior to performing them on the job. Training programs should build on previous experiences of older workers to enable them to make cognitive associations for new job tasks. Progressing an older worker from simple to complex tasks in a training program may facilitate the older worker's adaptation to new work environments. Good training should include time, practice, simple instructions, self-paced learning, and access to help.

Personal Work-Life Balance

As discussed in Chapter 8, older adults have increasingly complex home responsibilities that may impact their jobs. They may have dependent or elder care (grandchildren, adult children, or spouses) issues that affect their work schedules, and may benefit from flexible scheduling or part-time work due to caretaking. Just as work environments are increasingly offering pre-tax spending options for dependent childcare, human resource departments may

be encouraged to provide information on broader life planning needs for older workers related to assisted living, home care options, and retirement planning. Finally, workplaces can offer health promotion programs that include diet, nutrition, exercise, energy conservation, and stress management. Referral to Employee Assistance Programs may help coordinate the individual needs of older workers with community and corporate resources.

Learning Activity 79: Adapting Worker Roles

Choose a specific occupation, such as office workers, construction workers, or nurses.

1. Search online for articles about how workers age 60 and older in these fields can continue to perform the tasks required. Summarize your findings, with references.

2. How does increased age impact their ability to work in the area you have chosen? List three factors that might limit their ability.

3. How could these be adapted? What do the articles suggest, and what can you add?

Recommendations From Interdisciplinary Literature

The interdisciplinary literature also addresses workplace issues for older workers. For example, consultants to employers might suggest initiating programs and policies that encourage aging employees to remain on the job. Melillo (2013) compiled a list of factors to "enhance workplace climate for older workers" as follows:

1. Retirement planning

   - Provide organizational support (including retirement planning policies, volunteering opportunities).
   - Offer flexible retirement options.

2. Working conditions

   - Ensure nondiscriminatory practice (ageism).
   - Target training opportunities for enhancing skills/knowledge.
   - Recognize and acknowledge institutional history/value and expertise of older adults.
   - Provide information and referral assistance with management of grandchild care and elder care responsibilities through formal care networks/referrals.
   - Have older workers mentor younger workers.
   - Promote a culture of caring and teamwork.

3. Work adaptations

   - Provide flexible work schedules and varied work arrangements.
   - Educate on incorporating adult learning principles; build on making a connection with past learning and experience.
   - Provide supervision specifically geared toward older workers.
   - Encourage employee feedback on aging issues by surveying employees and listening to concerns or suggestions (Adapted from Melillo, 2013, citing the following sources: Bal & Visser, 2011; Loy, 2011; Koopman-Boyden & MacDonald, 2003; Work Safe Alberta, 2006).

Group Occupational Therapy Interventions for Older Workers

As an OT consultant to a company or corporation, you could arrange wellness days for groups of older workers to inform them about successful aging and the value of exercise, a healthy diet, lifestyle choices, and work-life balance. Groups might also benefit from instruction about the adaptation of workstations using ergonomic principles

and strategies to prevent overuse syndromes, such as carpel tunnel or lower back strain.

For older adults in the community who might wish to work for pay, job seeking groups might advise older adults about what to look for in a part-time job, and how to advocate for themselves as older workers. OTs might also partner with community organizations to promote productive aging in all of its forms by educating older adults about the benefits of remaining productive, whether in paid work, volunteering, caregiving, or lifelong learning.

Learning Activity 80: Group Design for Older Workers

Design a group for older office workers who have problems with hearing and vision loss. List and describe six topics you might address to help these older workers self-manage on the job. Write two discussion questions for each topic that encourage members to generalize learning and to apply strategies to their own employment situations.

1.
2.
3.
4.
5.
6.

JOURNAL ENTRY (M. C.)

At first I was confused about this role because we wanted to focus on productive roles after retirement, as in no longer working for pay. But this was not the reality we found. People retire from one job, but often find another. They like the added income, and they like how it makes them feel to be able to work. Many expressed pride in their ability to continue working, even with many adaptations to tasks, environments, hours, and working conditions. This is consistent with Laslett's Third Age; after they stop working to support themselves and their families, people continue to work for different reasons after retirement.

When I first interviewed Johanna, she was 71. With a full-time law practice, she didn't think she would qualify for our study: "I wish I knew how to cut back to 40 hours a week, never mind 20!" I wondered about this too, but I realized that what she had done in middle adulthood to support her family after her husband's heart attack and premature retirement, she now did because she loved it. It was mostly women she helped to get out of legal jams, messy divorces, probate, and unfair lawsuits. Johanna died a few weeks ago at age 73, finally losing her battle with ovarian cancer. Her daughter told me she was still reviewing files, signing papers, and making phone calls from her hospital bed as recently as 3 weeks before her death. At her funeral, the church overflowed with people she had helped, and many testified to this—that she often asked for little in return and sometimes she didn't get paid at all. It didn't matter to her, because she felt this was her life work, and she loved doing it. She remained a productive ager, living in the Third Age right up to the end. What a wonderful example she was for her children and grandchildren, and for all of us.

SUMMARY

Because of the tendency for older adults to work longer, and to reenter the work force after their initial retirement, OTs will likely encounter many older workers as clients in the future. Like workers at younger ages, older workers have issues with stress, physical strength and endurance, time management at work, and balancing work with other occupational roles. While they may have more chronic health conditions, older workers also may enjoy the benefits of longer experience, well-established social and work-related networks, and a stronger work ethic than younger workers. Some of our study participants continued working because they found more enjoyment and meaning in their work roles than in other occupations they might have chosen in retirement. OTs have much to offer older workers in helping them adapt tasks, schedules, and physical and social contexts. OTs can serve as advocates for older workers and can consult with places of employment to establish or enhance age-friendly working conditions.

REFERENCES

American Occupational Therapy Association. (2014). The occupational therapy practice framework 3rd Edition: Domain and process. *American Journal of Occupational Therapy, 68*, S1-S48.

Bal, P. M., & Visser, M. S. (2011). When are teachers motivated to work beyond retirement age? The importance of support, change of work role and money. *Educational Management Administration & Leadership, 39*, 590-602.

Brooke, L. (2003). Human resource costs and benefits of maintaining a mature-age workforce. *International Journal of Manpower, 24*, 260-283.

Cahill, K., Giandrea, M., & Quinn, J. (2012). Older workers and short-term jobs: Patterns and determinants. *Monthly Labor Review, 135*(5), 19-32.

Christiansen, C., & Townsend, E. (2010). *Introduction to occupation: The art and science of living* (2nd ed.). Cranbury, NJ: Pearson Education.

Compston, J. E., Watts, N. B., Chapurlat, R., Cooper, C., Boonen, S., Greenspan, S,... Siris, E. S. (2011). Obesity is not protective against fracture in postmenopausal women: GLOW. *American Journal of Medicine, 124*, 1043-1050.

Center for Disease Control and Prevention. (2011). *Healthy aging: What is a healthy brain? New research explores perceptions of cognitive health among diverse older adults*. Retrieved from http://www.cdc.gov/aging/pdf/Perceptions_of_Cog_Hlth_factsheet.pdf.

Dendinger, V. M., Adams, G. A., & Jacobson, J. D. (2005). Reasons for working and their relationship to retirement attitudes, job satisfaction, and occupational self-efficacy of bridge employees. *International Journal of Aging and Human Development, 61*, 21-35.

Desmette, D., & Gaillard, M. (2008). When a "worker" becomes an "older worker": The effects of age-related social identity on attitudes towards retirement and work. *Career Development International, 13*, 168-185.

Erikson, E. H., & Erikson, J. M. (1997). *The life cycle completed*. New York: Norton.

Fisk, A. D., Rogers, W. A, Charness, N., Czaja, S. J., & Sharit, J. (2004). *Designing for older adults*. Boca Raton, FL: CRC Press.

Gunnarsson, C., Chen, J., Rizzo, J. A., Ladapo, J. A., Naim, A., & Lofland, J. H. (2012). The employee absenteeism costs of IBD: Evidence from US National Survey Data. *Journal of Occupational and Environmental Medicine, 55*, 393-401.

Koopman-Boyden, P. G., & MacDonald, L. (2011). Ageing, work performance and managing ageing academics. *Journal of Higher Education Policy and Management, 25*, 29-40.

Konstantinidis, A., Talving, P., Kobayashi, L., Barmparas, G., Plurad, D., Lam, L., Demetriades, D. (2011). Work-related inquiries: Injury characteristics, survival, and age effect. *The American Surgeon, 77*, 702-707.

Laslett, P. (1989). *A fresh map of life: The emergence of the Third Age*. Cambridge, MA: Harvard University Press.

Leijten, F., Heuvel, S., Geuskens, G., Ybema, J., Wind, A., Burdorf, A., Robroek, S. (2013). How do older employees with health problems remain productive at work? A qualitative study. *Journal of Occupational Rehabilitation, 23*, 115.

Loy, B. (2011). *Accommodation and compliance series: Employees who are aging*. Retrieved from http://www.askjan.org/media/aging.html.

McCarthy, V. J., Perry, I. J., & Greiner, B. A. (2012). Age, job characteristics and coronary health. *Occupational Medicine, 62*, 613-619.

McNaught, W., & Barth, M. C. (1992). Are older workers "good buys"? A case study of Days Inns of America. *Sloan Management Review, 33*(3), 53-63.

Melillo, K. D. (2013). Cognitive health and older workers: Policy implications. *Journal of Gerontological Nursing, 39*, 6, 13-18.

MetLife Foundation/Civic Ventures. (2005). *The new face of work survey*. Retrieved from http://www.encore.org/find/resources/new-face-work-survey.

Mor Barak, M. E. (1995). The meaning of work for older adults seeking employment. *International Journal of Aging and Human Development, 41*, 325-344.

Mosey, A. C. (1996). *Applied scientific inquiry in the health professions: An epistemological orientation* (2nd ed.). Bethesda, MD: American Occupational Therapy Association.

Odeen, M., Magnussen, L. H., Maeland, S., Larun, L., Eriksen, H. R., & Tveito, T. H. (2012). Systematic review of active workplace interventions to reduce sickness absence. *Occupational Medicine, 63*(1), 7-16.

Pew Research Center. (2011). *The generation gap and the 2012 election. Section 5: Generations and the great recession*. Retrieved from http://www.people-press.org/2011/11/03/section5-generations-and-the-great-recession/.

Reinhardt, J. D., Wahrendorf, M., & Siegrist, J. (2012). Socioeconomic position, psychosocial work environment and disability in an aging workforce: A longitudinal analysis of SHARE data from 11 European countries. *Occupational and Environmental Medicine, 70*, 156-163.

Sanders, M., & McCready, J. (2009). A qualitative study of two older workers' adaptation to physically demanding work. *Work, 32*, 111-122.

Sanders, M., & McCready, J. W. (2010). Does work contribute to successful aging in older workers? *The International Journal of Aging and Human Development, 71*, 209-229.

Sanders, M., & McCready, J. W. (2011). Meeting the challenge of supervising older workers in the retail homebuilding industry. *Journal of Business and Retail Management Research, 5,* 17 - 30.

Schooler, C., Mulatu, M. S., & Oates, G. (1999). The continuing effects of substantively complex work on the intellectual functioning of older workers. *Psychology and Aging, 14,* 483-506.

Smola, K. W., & Sutton, C. D. (2002). Generational differences: Revisiting generational work values for the new millennium. *Journal of Organizational Behavior, 23,* 363-384.

U.S. Administration on Aging (2011). *Aging statistics: Profile of older Americans.* Retrieved from http://www.aoa.gov/AoARoot/Aging_Statistics/Profile/2013/2.aspx.

U.S. Bureau of Labor Statistics (2008). *Older workers.* Retrieved from http://www.bls.gov/spotlight/2008/older_workers/.

U.S. Bureau of Labor Statistics (2012). *Labor force statistics from the current population survey: Demographics: Age.* Retrieved from http://www.bls.gov/cpw/demographics.htm#age.

Wahlstedt, K., Nygard, G.I., Kemmlert, C.H., Torgen, K., & Bjorksten, M. G. (2000). The effects of a change in work organization upon the work environment and musculoskeletal symptoms among letter carriers. *International Journal of Occupational Safety and Ergonomics, 6,* 237-255.

Womack, J. L. (2008). Occupations of older adults. In S. Coppola, S. Elliott & P. Toto (Eds.), *Strategies to advance gerontology excellence: Promoting best practice in occupational therapy* (pp. 59-90). Bethesda, MD: AOTA Press.

Work Safe Alberta. (2006). *Safe and healthy: A guide to managing an aging work force.* Retrieved from http://alis.alberta.ca/pdf/cshop/safehealthy.pdf.

Lifelong Learner

Marilyn B. Cole, MS, OTR/L, FAOTA

"Have an insatiable desire to learn." (Participant, Peggie)

In older adulthood, motivation for learning serves a different purpose than it did during childhood and adolescence. Retirees often seek self-fulfillment through learning new skills; gaining knowledge about topics of interest; increasing their understanding of local, national, or world events; or discovering new forms of creative self-expression. Some older adults we interviewed had even completed training for an entirely different career in their retirement, one that helped them to better serve others, and to which they felt more emotionally connected. But taking formal classes represents only one of many forms learning can take. Other forms of adult learning include volunteer on-the-job training, focused reading or online searches, traveling to learn about other cultures, and participating in discussion groups such as book clubs, religious study groups, and groups that focus on specific interests such as cooking, gardening, local history, or health-related issues.

Learning in later life has been called *educational gerontology* (Withnall, 2002). An acknowledged need for learning in older adulthood has spawned thousands of Third Age Universities across the globe, so named because of their focus on the learning needs of retirees. They thrive because older adults retiring in their 60s now look forward to 20 to 30 years of continued health and productivity and are seeking inspiration for new forms of self-fulfillment through creative expression and service to society. Third Age Universities, more popular in other developed countries than in the United States, offer adult education in topics of interest to elders, as well as the latest information on wellness and prevention of the harmful effects of aging. Continued learning about how to stay healthy in older adulthood can be understood as an essential prerequisite for performance of other productive roles in aging. Older adults who have acquired skills in the use of technology find a greater access to knowledge and services through the Internet, which some research predicts will keep them connected socially as well.

The AOTA's (2014) OTPF III defines education as an occupation that includes "activities needed for learning and participating in the educational environment" (p. S20). Three categories of educational activity are defined as follows:

1. *Formal educational participation:* Participating in academic (e.g., math, reading, degree coursework), nonacademic (e.g., recess, lunchroom, hallway), extracurricular (e.g., sports, band, cheerleading, dances), and vocational (prevocational and vocational) educational activities.

2. *Informal personal educational needs or interests exploration (beyond formal education):* Identifying topics

Cole MB, Macdonald KC.
Productive Aging: An Occupational Perspective (pp 183-196).
© 2015 Taylor & Francis Group.

and methods for obtaining topic-related information or skills.

3. *Informal personal education participation:* Participating in informal classes, programs, and activities that provide instruction or training in identified areas of interest (AOTA, 2014, p. S20).

PARTICIPANT PERSPECTIVES

Most of our participants gave multiple examples of ongoing learning activities, ranging from formal classroom learning to online courses; learning while traveling, volunteering, or working; and informal learning through reading, television, or interacting with others.

For some participants, the motivation to learn became a driving force in their future planning. Peggie gave this as one of her secrets: "have an insatiable desire to learn and improve oneself." Bob C. likes to "keep moving and doing different things…seniors in New York City can take college classes free of charge. I'm now auditing an economics class." He recommends "following your curiosity by reading…following interests in the news…following politics is interesting because it has a big influence on economics and investments." Ann M. viewed retirement as an opportunity to expand her horizons by "being able to take trips I never had time for."

Taking Classes

Ken's retirement planning included preparation for a new, more satisfying career. As he cut down teaching hours, Ken had time to follow his lifelong love of animals, taking classes to become a veterinary assistant and completing his degree before he retired. Signian, who also continues teaching part-time, takes adult education classes in pencil sketching, art appreciation, and Asian cooking. Malcolm enjoys "being in a classroom and watching college level, primarily liberal arts, lectures from Teaching Company and Yale University [on the web]. I enjoy solving problems, especially writing and debugging computer programs [currently taking a class in JavaScript, a computer programming language]." Patricia, at age 91, attends lectures on astronomy and paleontology given at her retirement community. She also teaches poetry writing to others in her community and has just completed writing a memoir of her experiences living in India during and following World War II. Phyllis, following her bypass surgery, "enrolled in educational courses through the local university and senior center. They were most interesting and informative." June takes classes in oil pastels and rug hooking. She advises "Learning to do something new."

Learning at Work or Volunteering

On-the-job training and volunteer training were additional avenues to new learning. Sue has taken on new responsibilities at her job as church administrator. "I taught myself to use a computer using the latest technology, one of the perks of continuing to work." Sue's supervisor also paid for her to be trained as a bookkeeper as she took over more financial responsibility and record keeping. Betty continues to volunteer at Carnegie Hall and the Metropolitan Museum of Art, partly because she gets to go to concerts and lectures for free. She also participates in fundraising for political organizations, stating, "It's important to keep yourself informed about politics. I want to learn more about international events. I would love to learn to be a guide to the United Nations."

Informal Learning

More informal ways to learn include watching cable TV, participating in book discussions, focused reading, and learning by watching others. June points out that living within a budget forces you to "learn to fix things yourself." "Whenever I hire skilled workers, I watch them very carefully and ask a lot of questions." Malcolm studies French by reading lessons from textbooks and listening to audiotapes: "I have enjoyed many years of French language and culture, in spite of having a very limited ability to soak up French vocabulary and grammar. It is salutary to me to have to work so hard to accomplish so little in this area. I love it but I'm slower here than anything else I try." Mary reports holding many volunteer board positions in her former profession (Figure 11-1). "I'm always reading, attending conferences, and learning from online discussions."

Pearl recognized her need for continued intellectual stimulation after she retired and organized a book discussion group with her colleagues who had retired from university teaching in a variety of disciplines. "Meeting with the book club every 2 months provides good intellectual discussions with colleagues. It takes a lot of reading, and also sometimes we see the movie and compare impressions." Vi belongs to two book groups. "You are forced to read books you wouldn't read otherwise, then you are able to discuss them with others." Other participants who actively participate in book clubs are Valnere, Signian, Patricia, Peggie, Gloria, Johanna, and Jan. All take their turns hosting and choosing what books their group will read. Other community organizations offer interesting topics for discussion. Geno reports, "I do research on the computer for giving lectures at my organizations. I belong to several community groups [Grange, Toastmasters]. They are interesting, challenging, and stimulating." Peggie attends an investment club as well as Bible study and other church activities.

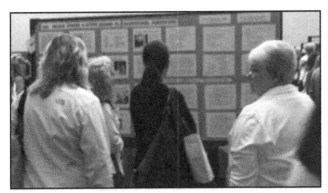

Figure 11-1. Conferences keep professionals informed about the latest developments in their fields, with the added bonus of social interaction (Johanna on right).

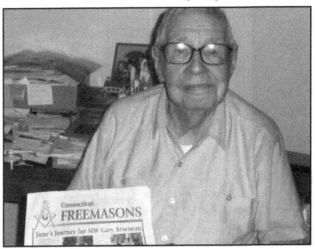

Figure 11-2. Ray keeps up with current events through reading the newspaper.

Charlie belongs to three social clubs. Gloria organizes and moderates political debates with local and state candidates through her role as Steering Committee Chair for the League of Women Voters. Betty loves to interact with the cultural, artistic, and political community in New York City. Margie leads a bilingual (Spanish-English) Bible study group in Atlanta. There were many other examples of group participation given that provided both intellectual stimulation and social connections.

Current Events

It almost seems impossible to avoid exposure to media and news coverage in modern American society. News is available in many forms, from traditional word of mouth to newspapers and radio (Figure 11-2). Now, news is also available 24/7 on television and online, and many forms of printed publications including books and magazines. Many family-style restaurants feature television sets that are playing news channels, even if on a mute setting. A number of the participants stated how it was very important for them to keep up with current events and to be informed with what is happening in the world. Many read a daily newspaper and most commented on some period of watching news on the television on a regular basis. Bob M. reflected on how he likes to "keep up with politics. I like to listen to politics, but not more than 1 hour a day. I follow national, international, and local events. I make sure to vote."

Learning Activity 81: Importance of Current Events

A finding of the PAS was the tendency for the participants to have a strong interest in the news.

1. How do you relate to current media avenues for local, national, and world news?

2. Considering its importance for the study participants, how does that compare with your generation or other generations? Explain your reasoning.

Traveling as Learning

Traveling was another important way participants sought to learn new things. Malcolm has traveled widely both in the United States and abroad: "Elderhostel offers reasonably priced programs blending the travel experience with classroom time. They offer the opportunity to discuss both the material of the lectures and travel experiences with other mature seekers of wisdom." Mary V. traveled to Ireland in search of her roots: "I traveled to my ancestor's home...we had worked on genealogy. We were able to go to the ship area where she traveled at age 19 to come to America and build a new life. I hope I am from some of that stock." Maxine and her gentleman friend travel considerably, "visiting friends and for pleasure...just got back from Hawaii for an Army reunion, now planning an upcoming trip to Switzerland." Nettie just enjoys the process of traveling: "I can't believe it, but I fly in an airplane, a small one. My friend knows a pilot and he takes us up!...I enjoy any kind of traveling." Margie comes from a large Puerto Rican family. She stays in contact by going on "sister trips" with her three sisters. This year they are going to tour the Greek Islands. Jack and Peggie spend 3 or 4 months each year traveling (Figure 11-3). They have time shares in Maui and Palm Desert, California, but love to trade for more exotic destinations (Costa Rica, Thailand) and enjoy cruising with family and friends.

Self-Help and Self-Directed Learning

Following one's own interests is one of the privileges of being retired, according to some of our participants. They may work just as hard and find themselves just as busy as when they were working, but their daily pursuits tend to be much more self-directed. Our participants seem to apply the same work ethic to learning and planning meaningful experiences with others that they once did at

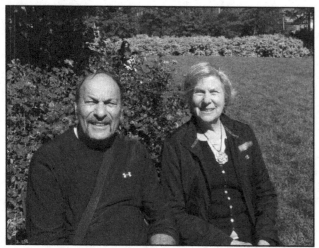

Figure 11-3. Peggie and Jack explore Rose Kennedy's garden in Boston.

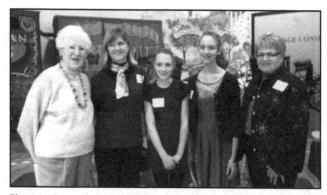

Figure 11-4. Johanna and Gloria attend a lecture for American Association of University Women, February 2013. (Left to right: Gloria Francesconi, Johanna's daughter Robin Dougherty, two grandchildren Kathryn and Meghan, and Johanna Malinowski at a lecture given at the P.T. Barnum Museum.)

their full-time jobs. For example, Valnere practices Tai Chi daily, takes several classes through adult education, and attends weekend retreats. She has also hired a computer coach who comes to her home to help her to keep abreast of new technology. Malcolm disciplines himself to learn and practice new French vocabulary nearly every day. Signian continues to plan and lead annual student educational trips to Guatemala through the Albert Schweitzer Institute at her former university. This experience helps her to make connections with another culture through humanitarian roles such as providing educational lectures and materials to students and health care educators in that country, which is personally satisfying on many levels. Margie seeks spiritual growth through her leadership roles within her church. In preparing Bible study lessons in Spanish, she also extends her own knowledge and exchanges personal stories with other group members.

Many participants combined learning and socialization through attending educational programs together with their families or friends. The American Association of University Women, with branches in almost every town across the country, has the specific mission of educating women. This and many other community organizations provide educational programs for the public (Figure 11-4).

LITERATURE REVIEW

The field of educational gerontology has expanded to incorporate many diverse disciplines, including sociology, psychology, business administration, economics, and the health professions. Some areas of research related to productive aging include the following sections: adult education theory, Third Age University Movement, Adult Development and Learning (post-conventional thought), cognition and aging in Older Adulthood, and the impact of learning on health and well-being.

Adult Education Theory

Adult learning takes many forms, as our participants have told us. The formal educational model used for kindergarten through high school and beyond has become known as *pedagogy*, defined by Merriam and Caffarella (1999) as "the art and science of helping children learn (p. 292)." In pedagogy, the teacher (who is the expert) instructs the students (who are the learners) according to a predetermined curriculum. This is necessary when children must learn basic skills, such as reading, writing, and arithmetic—the tools they will need to get along in a civilized world. In contrast, Knowles (1990) defines *andragogy* as "the art and science of helping adults learn" (p. 43). Andragogy is based on the following six principles of adult learning:

1. Motivation for learning is internal and self-directed

2. Adults draw upon their experiences to aid learning

3. Adults plan their own learning experiences and evaluate their instruction

4. Readiness to learn often accompanies the assumption of new social roles

5. Adult learning is closely related to application for solving immediate problems

6. Adult learners like to be respected for their life experience (Adapted from Knowles, 1990)

These principles contrast sharply with childhood learning experiences in that they integrate adult learning with life roles and experience, such as working, caregiving, maintaining a home, being a good citizen, and participating in one's community.

Transformational learning has emerged from Knowles' earlier work, adding the additional factor that learning should encourage further development of the adult learner through experience and critical reflection and analysis (Merriam & Caffarella, 1999). In other words, adult learners need to go beyond memorizing facts and think about the relevance of new knowledge and its potential to increase their understanding of their own experiences in the world around them. Learning has a different purpose for adults in that they are mainly interested in learning things that will make them more effective participants in life. Organizational learning follows these principles by providing learning experiences for workers that are intended to make them more effective at their jobs. The concept of transformation implies that learning results in significant change for the learner.

Most current proponents of adult or lifelong learning contend that adults learn best through experience. Renowned learning theorist Jarvis (1987) suggests that "all learning begins with experience" (p. 16). Experiential learning has the advantage of taking a new concept beyond cognitive understanding and adding affective and behavioral elements through its immediate application in a learning activity. Often, experiential learning is accomplished in small groups in which the adult learners participate together in a real life situation. In this type of learning, immediate or concrete experience becomes the basis for observation and reflection. A good example of this is Yalom's self-reflective loop (Yalom & Leszcz, 2005) in the process of group dynamics. Yalom, as group facilitator/therapist, points out specific group interactions among members and asks them to examine their feelings about it and reflect on its meaning for them. For example, if one member of a group insults another, that interaction becomes the basis of new learning about how to more effectively communicate with other people in each member's own relationships outside the group.

For older adults, experience takes on another dimension in learning—that of contributing their own expertise and wisdom to others, while also learning from the experiences of others in an educational group environment. For this type of learning to occur, "classes" need to rely heavily on directed group discussions, within which "students" can openly discuss, analyze, and reflect upon the topics, concepts, and ideas being taught. In such educational experiences, the "teacher" must become more of an equal member of the group of learners; his or her role goes beyond imparting knowledge into facilitating discussions about the meaning of new ideas, knowledge, or skills and exploring potential applications in the lives of each learner. In the British model of Third Age universities described in the next section, great importance is given to respecting the life experience of older adult learners and allowing them the freedom to participate in planning the direction and methods used to achieve educational goals.

Universities of the Third Age

Universities of the Third Age (UTAs) actually began in the 1960s and 1970s, well before Laslett's (1989) developmental theory. The first one emerged at the University of Toulouse, France, in 1973, in accordance with a government mandate requiring universities to provide lifelong learning opportunities to retirees. The French model, begun by Professor Pierre Vellas, proposed 4 objectives: (1) raise the level of physical, mental, and social health of older people; (2) provide a permanent educational program for older adults; (3) coordinate gerontological research programs; and (4) provide all students with current knowledge about gerontology (Formosa, 2010). UTAs following this model soon spread all over Europe, with over 100 campuses, most affiliated with existing universities. Courses included topics of interest to retirees, such as wine tasting, music appreciation, watercolor painting, and organic gardening, in addition to more traditional liberal arts topics. UTAs have since expanded internationally; for example, China had established 19,300 UTA centers by 2002 (Thompson, 2002).

The first British UTA began in 1981 at Cambridge with an entirely different model that rejected prepackaged courses and incorporated a more democratic approach that recognized the extensive knowledge elder students could offer from their life experience. This model promoted the organization of small groups of peers with similar learning needs and interests in which members equally shared in both learning and teaching or otherwise participated in organizing self-directed learning experiences. These self-help groups often developed around specific goals of desired personal or social change, such as overcoming grief over loss of a spouse or instituting safety measures aimed at reducing the incidence of crime in their neighborhoods. The British model, now utilizing the acronym "U3A" has produced upward of 731 such units in the United Kingdom, 211 in Australia, and 60 in New Zealand (The Third Age Trust, 2009; U3A Online, 2009). The United States is one of the few countries without established U3As, perhaps because it had previously established Lifelong Learning Institutes with a similar purpose stemming from the 1960s and mostly based at existing universities (Formosa, 2010).

According to surveys of UTA and U3A membership, nearly half are between ages 60 to 69, over half were married, and the majority were educated (70%) and female (85%) (AIUTA, 2006). Members' motivation for participating in U3A activities often included not only learning, but also associated social outcomes, such as making new friends or finding needed support for challenging life problems. Many reported essential learning about managing their own health conditions and measures to help them prevent disease and disability. Ideally, UTAs and U3As can help to meet the developmental goals for Third Agers, who are seeking both self-fulfillment through creative and satisfying occupations and meaningful roles that serve the needs of society.

As technology has advanced, Third Age universities now offer online courses through several websites, including Virtual University of the Third Age (vU3A) (http://vu3a.org). This website, run entirely by volunteers, offers learning experiences, support, and interaction strategies to anyone who logs on, although there is a small fee to participate.

In a critique of the current status of UTAs, Formosa (2010) notes the following concerns.

- *Cultural bias*: Current UTAs often focus only on the educational needs of a specific segment of the population, which is mostly middle class and predominantly female. They need to consider the interests and learning needs of working class elders and older men.

- *Top-down model*: Many UTAs still operate under a formal educational model, which assumes the teacher as expert and the students as subordinates. UTAs need to recognize the unique characteristics of older learners, and take advantage of their life experience using a democratic approach more akin to the British model.

- *Exclusion of Fourth Agers*: Many UTAs do not consider the ongoing learning needs of elders who are housebound or physically dependent. This is not in society's best interests because current research shows that engagement in intellectually and socially stimulating activities actually reduces dependency and its related costs.

- *Unaware of contemporary social change*: Need to keep up with the widening diversity of post-retirement lifestyles and preferences. UTAs are too focused on liberal arts, rather than directly addressing the practical problems of older learners. Furthermore, there must be avenues of intergenerational engagement, highlighting the unique knowledge that young and old have to offer one another.

In summary, "Nowadays retirees are embracing the philosophies of active and productive aging by engaging in consumer lifestyles, and some, even seeking to re-enter the labor market. Hence, UTAs must expand their learning focus to include consumer education, financial literacy, and skill development training" (Formosa, 2010, p. 8).

Adult Development and Learning

Virtually all theories of adult development view learning as a lifelong process. While Jung and Erikson focused on emotional and social maturation throughout one's life, Piaget (1972) and Kohlberg (1990) focused on the growing complexity of intellectual and moral reasoning as adults interacted with others and with the world around them. From an educational standpoint, Daloz (1999) emphasized the importance of mentoring for adults seeking further growth and development. He grouped these theories into the following collective stages:

1. *Preconventional stage* focuses on survival.

2. *Conventional stage* focuses on reflection and analysis.

3. *Postconventional stage* focuses on evaluating events critically.

Daloz (1986) further states:

> Significant learning entails development. Development means successfully asking broader and deeper questions of the relationship between oneself and the world...education should promote development. A good education ought to help people become both more receptive and more discriminating about the world: seeing, feeling, and understanding more, yet sorting the pertinent from the irrelevant with [an] even finer touch, increasingly able to integrate what they see and to make meaning of it in ways that enhance their ability to go on growing... We develop by progressively taking apart and putting together structures that give our lives meaning (p. 27).

This suggests that teaching adults also incorporates a mentoring role, influencing and encouraging rather than merely imparting information. It suggests that teachers ask questions rather than giving answers, respecting the adults' need to direct their own learning and to incorporate that learning into their own life experience.

Learning Activity 82: What Is Adult Learning?

1. What is the difference between teaching and mentoring?

2. As an OT, how might you use the principles of adult learning to educate a client about one of these topics: physical fitness, fall prevention, home safety, preventing social isolation?

3. Write three questions you might ask to encourage a client to think more deeply about the importance of the information you want him or her to learn.

    a.

    b.

    c.

Cognition and Wisdom in Older Adulthood

In recent years, much research effort has focused on the effects of aging on cognitive decline. Researchers at the National Institutes of Health reviewed hundreds of large-scale studies to identify both risk factors and factors that could possibly prevent cognitive decline in later life (Plassman, Williams, & Burke, 2010). They found that current tobacco use, genetic markers, and certain medical conditions, such as diabetes and depression, increased the risk of cognitive decline, while only cognitive training (processing speed and reasoning) and physical exercise were effective in helping to maintain cognition.

The most compelling research related to lifelong learning links engagement in brain-stimulating activities with the prevention of Alzheimer's disease later in life (Yang, 2012). In an extensive study of healthy older adults at age 60, Landau et al. (2012), researchers at University of California, Berkeley, found that brain positron emission tomography (PET) scans of older adults who reported a lifelong habit of engaging in cognitively challenging pursuits, such as reading to acquire new information, playing games and puzzles, or coping with complex problems both inside and outside their workplace, had fewer deposits of beta-amyloid, a destructive protein that is the hallmark of Alzheimer's disease. About one third of people over age 60 have some beta-amyloid deposits in their brain, a process that is influenced by genes and aging. However, those with a habit of lifelong learning showed brain scans with significantly less of the destructive protein believed to cause Alzheimer's disease in later life (Landau et al., 2012). Alzheimer's disease, which causes a predictable stepwise decline in memory and cognition in older adulthood, is predicted to affect up to 50% of older adults. Between 2000 and 2008, deaths from Alzheimer's increased 66%, making it the sixth leading killer in the country (Yang, 2012, p. 2). While no known medical treatment yet exists for Alzheimer's disease, a recent study has found an effective prevention strategy. University of California, Berkeley, researchers (Landau et al., 2012) studied PET scans of the brains of cognitively normal persons 60 years and older. When they controlled for gender, self-rated memory function, physical activity, and level of education, they found that brain scans revealed that only those who engaged in cognitively stimulating activities throughout their lives were independently linked to fewer deposits of beta-amyloid (Yang, 2012). This finding gives greater importance to including in one's lifestyle the productive role of lifelong learning as a way to preserve cognition and prevent this debilitating disease in older adulthood.

Learning Activity 83: Maintaining Mental Fitness

Concerns about cognitive decline in aging have inspired many new mental fitness programs on the internet. Find three "brain training" websites and try them out. Describe each briefly below.

1.

2.

3.

Which specific mental abilities were challenged for each? Which exercises or games would you recommend for older adult clients and why?

Wisdom and Learning

The adage "older and wiser" may have added credibility as adult learning and developmental theories are tested and revised. Recent studies in adult cognitive development have expanded Piaget's theory beyond the formal operations stage. Piaget (1972) identified formal thought as the highest cognitive level, which he perceived to be applied throughout adulthood to adapt to changing life circumstances through the processes of assimilation (fitting new information into existing concepts) and accommodation (changing existing knowledge structures to account for new information) to balance internal needs with demands of the environment. However, several new theories have been proposed, called post-formal stages (Birney & Sternberg, 2006; Sinnott, 1993). Adults apply the newly identified stages in problem-solving and decision-making strategies within social, interpersonal, moral, political, and scientific domains in ways that cannot be explained by Piaget's construct of formal operations. Adult developmental theorists have proposed that post-formal reasoning is more complex and involves multiple ways of knowing. Using mathematical axioms, Commons and Richards (2003) identified 4 post-formal stages as follows:

1. *Systematic order*: Define relationships between various parts of a system, including multivariate causes, and building matrixes or models to describe complex interrelationships. They estimate about 20% of the adult population are capable of thinking on this level.

2. *Metasystematic order*: Conceptualize entire systems interacting with each other and identify metasystematic actions that can compare, contrast, transform, and synthesize systems into metasystems. Professors at top research universities might function at the metasystematic level.

3. *Paradigmatic order*: Create new fields from multiple metasystems by comparing, combining, reorganizing, or coordinating very large and seemingly unrelated fields of knowledge. When facing problems unexplainable through existing paradigms, these thinkers create new paradigms that account for previously unexplained phenomenon. The authors give the examples of Einstein (physics) and Euclid (mathematics) from scientific disciplines.

4. *Cross-paradigmatic order*: Paradigms applied in fields for which they were not created can profoundly transform large areas of knowledge. The authors state that interdisciplinary studies do not qualify for this level of thought and are mostly at the paradigmatic order level. Few people have achieved this level of intellect. The example given is Charles Darwin, who intertwined the fields of biology, paleontology, geology, and ecology to form his theory of evolution, an entirely new relationship among paradigms.

Clearly, these complex levels of thinking demonstrate that learning and cognitive ability continue to grow throughout one's life and may indeed result in older adults seeking and achieving a higher level of knowledge and understanding of themselves and the world. For example, OTs now recognize complexity theory, chaos theory, and complex (dynamic) systems theory, which have recently been applied across academic and health sciences, including OT. The new discipline of occupational science, or the concept of OT in "high definition," might be represented by one of these higher levels of thought.

In considering post-formal theories, OTs need to remember that clients have multiple ways of thinking, learning, and communicating, and that we as OTs need to consider this when trying to understand their problem-solving strategies, judgments, and life decisions. Older adults who have continued to learn over their lives have been better able to adapt to age-related changes as they grow older. Some theories of aging have linked this fact with the need to encourage lifelong learning through adult education or Third Age universities (Baltes & Smith, 2001).

Learning Activity 84: What Is Wisdom?

1. Define wisdom in your own words.

2. How do you think older people achieve wisdom?

3. Describe an older adult you know who is wise. Why do you think so? To what extent has this person reached a post-formal level of thinking?

4. How are wisdom and lifelong learning related? How are they different?

APPLICATIONS TO CONTINUUM OF CARE

We have already discussed the multiple ways that community dwelling older adults continue to learn after they retire: formal classes, volunteer on-the-job training, focused reading or Internet searches, traveling to learn about other cultures, and participating in discussion groups such as book clubs, religious study groups, and groups that focus on specific interests such as cooking, gardening, local history, or health-related issues. It is important for the well elderly to be aware, and to take advantage of the many opportunities for learning that become available to them in their communities.

Community Programs and Primary Care

Most communities have senior centers that offer multiple services and opportunities to learn. For example, Baldwin Senior Center in Stratford, Connecticut offers daily exercise at various fitness levels, from step aerobics to seated exercise, as well as groups in memoir writing, quilting, woodworking, card and board games, and bocce ball. The center provides assistance with Medicare, Medicaid, or other public assistance applications; income tax preparation; various health screenings; and outside guest speakers on a variety of topics, and they sponsor monthly bus trips to places of interest. OTs in home care often educate clients with various health conditions in ways to overcome obstacles to their educational goals. It may be necessary to assist clients in accessing community resources, such as mentoring them in using the Internet to find local educational opportunities or suggesting ways to arrange transportation.

Staff at the Baldwin Senior Center welcome any guest speakers or programs addressing wellness and prevention, citing these as their best attended events. This might be a good opportunity for an OT to establish a role with productive aging outside of the medical model. People coming to senior centers such as the Baldwin Senior Center are often asked to pay a moderate fee for specialized learning sessions and many do so willingly.

Currently, there may be opportunities within primary care for OTs to design interventions for prevention, wellness, and self-management programs and educational groups for older adults related to aging in place. Title III of the Affordable Care Act, Improving Quality and Efficiency of Healthcare "creates program initiatives to link payment to quality programs that, among other things, help contain health care costs and reduce hospital admissions" (DeRosa, 2013, p. CE1). This provides an incentive for OTs to partner with primary care physicians to provide educational and self-management programs for their older patients, either individually or in groups, with the goal of enabling them to make needed lifestyle changes and overcome barriers caused by health conditions, so that they might continue to participate in the occupations that help them to age productively.

Learning Activity 85: Reliable Sources on the Internet

Find three reliable sources of health information on the Internet for older clients with *one* of these health conditions: arthritis, chronic obstructive pulmonary disease, diabetes, spinal cord injury, head trauma, depression, or post-traumatic stress disorder. Your client will use the recommended websites to gather the latest information on relevant health conditions and their treatment.

1. Briefly describe each website chosen.

2. Select five topics that are relevant to the client's occupational performance from the websites. How might you use this information to design an individual or group intervention in primary care?

    a.

    b.

    c.

    d.

    e.

Assisted Living and Retirement Communities

Assisted living and retirement communities are also known for offering a large and varied program of educational and learning opportunities, some even sponsoring in-house concerts and plays, along with multiple shopping and sightseeing trips. Residents in these centers may have isolated areas of dependency, such as being unable to drive or having poor hearing or vision—obstacles they may need help to overcome to fully benefit from their educational opportunities.

Tsao (2004) studied two university-linked retirement communities in the United States—University Commons at University of Michigan and Holy Cross Village at Notre Dame. Through interviews the participants demonstrated four behavioral patterns post-retirement: learning while aging, working while aging, leisure while aging, and intergenerational interactions. A "high overall satisfaction of these residents is attributed to the congruence between their motivations and the environmental resources that colleges and universities provide…giving them new opportunities to pursue personal growth and self-actualization" (Tsao, 2004, p. 3511).

Long-Term Care

Nursing home residents have a wide range of disabilities and an equally wide variety of educational interests and abilities. Some residents are motivated to seek out learning opportunities within the facility or to organize their own groups, while others may need encouragement and assistance to participate in any learning or recreational activities. Both professionals and volunteers can develop and offer educational programs to meet the needs of nursing home residents, but these must be adapted to varying levels of cognitive ability so all have an opportunity to participate as they wish. For example, residents with mild to moderate dementia can benefit from reminiscence activities that rely on long-term memory and offer a means of socialization in ways that de-emphasize their short-term memory issues (Haslam, Jetten, Haslam, & Knight, 2012).

IMPLICATIONS FOR OCCUPATIONAL THERAPY PRACTICE

Consider for a moment how much cognitive or mental ability is needed for working, caregiving, self-management, volunteering, and managing a home, as well as being a successful student. In fact, all of our productive occupations depend on our ability to continually learn and integrate new information. For this reason, maintaining cognitive mental abilities has high priority among occupational goals for older adults. For example, what happens when a client becomes unable to predict the consequences of his or her actions? As Claudia Allen (Allen & Earhart, 1992) once taught us, anticipating consequences and being able to plan ahead are high-level cognitive skills. People functioning at Allen Cognitive Level (ACL) 6 are capable of active and effective self-management, but even ACL 5, one level down, gets them into trouble when they begin to make poor financial decisions, neglect their own health needs, act or speak without thinking, or take unnecessary risks.

Facilitating the Occupation of Learning

OT practitioners take on a variety of roles in the productive occupation of lifelong learning. In working with individual clients, OTs identify facilitators and barriers to achieving learning goals, addressing the client's mental functioning, and adapting learning environments. OTs have also designed educational programming for both individuals and community groups around specific occupational interests, such as computer training, fall prevention, and home safety.

Given the close association between lifelong learning as a productive occupation and the mental functions (affective, cognitive, and perceptual) that interface with it, we include here a review of the OTPF III definitions of higher level cognition as one of the client factors necessary for occupational participation. *Specific mental functions* appears in the OTPF under client factors (AOTA, 2014, p. S22) with the following subcategories:

- "Higher-level cognitive: Judgment, concept formation, metacognition, praxis, cognitive flexibility, insight.

- Attention: Sustained, shifting and divided attention, concentration, distractibility.

- Memory: Short-term, long-term, and working memory.

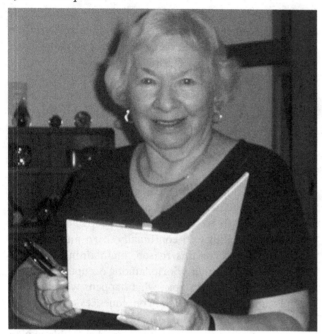

Figure 11-5. Phyllis finds it convenient to use her tablet to search the Internet.

- Perception: Discrimination of sensations (e.g., auditory, tactile, visual, olfactory, gustatory, vestibular-proprioception).

- Thought: Control and content of thought, awareness of reality vs. delusions, logical and coherent thought.

- Mental functions of sequencing complex movement: Mental functions that regulate the speed, response, quality, and time of motor production, such as restlessness, toe tapping, or hand wringing, in response to inner tension.

- Emotional: Regulation and range of emotions; appropriateness of emotions, including anger, love, tension, and anxiety, lability of emotions.

- Experience of self and time: Awareness of one's identity, body, and position in the reality of one's environment and of time."

One could argue that all of these mental functions, as well as some others, are required within the occupation of lifelong learning. Therefore, older adults who demonstrate deficits in any of these areas would likely have limitations to their ability to benefit from educational experiences. When clients set specific learning goals as priorities, OT practitioners need to identify and evaluate the limitations in mental functioning that may create barriers to desired learning and to explore ways to remediate, adapt, or compensate for them.

Developing Computer Skills

Suppose an older adult client wishes to learn how to use a computer to keep in touch with family and friends or to access needed health information via the Internet. The OT practitioner needs to determine what skills and abilities are necessary to operate a computer for these purposes, such as eye-hand coordination, good visual perception and discrimination, short-term memory, ability to sequence actions, and the like. A client with visual issues may need to practice finding relevant words and symbols on the computer screen and to recognize which aspects to avoid. When a client reports difficulty in using the computer, the technology must also be analyzed to help the client to simplify the process (setting up files or shortcuts on the desktop) or to make computer functions more accessible (enlarging font size, installing a mouse to replace a touchpad). Operating a computer may not be a traditional task addressed in OT, but its use is becoming increasingly important for older adults to perform essential tasks such as banking, paying bills, shopping, communicating, making appointments, getting things fixed, and solving many problems when their mobility becomes more limited with age (Figure 11-5).

Although computer technology has become integral to communication, social interaction, information retrieval, and daily living tasks, currently only 60% of older Americans use computers (AARP, 2009). The computer tasks in the AARP survey include the following: e-mail friends (56%), find information (57%), purchase products (44%), and make travel arrangements (38%). A review of computer training formats revealed that a variety of training formats revealed improved computer skills, as well as higher scores in measures of self-efficacy, confidence, and attitudes toward computers (Czaja et al., 2006). However, an overall critique of computer "courses" was the standard format and hierarchical skill-based curriculum without regard for existing skill levels or personal goals (Kim, 2008; Mayhorn, Stronge, McLaughlin, & Rogers, 2004). In one recent study, OT students and educators partnered with community senior centers in providing a 4-week computer training program for older adults who had not previously learned to use a computer. In this program, 92 clients ages 62 and older rated their own computer skill level, volunteered for the training, and set their own goals for computer use. Students provided four 1-hour sessions of individualized instruction to each participant, using his or her own goals as a focus for the sessions. Some examples of goals were e-mailing grandchildren; learning the basics of computer navigation; gaining confidence in common tasks, such as saving recipes, lists, or notes; creating projects using MS Word, Excel, or PowerPoint; searching for information; purchasing items; and uploading photographs and attaching them to e-mails for family and friends. The outcome of this OT intervention was 100% client goal achievement, with significant increases in comfort and confidence level with computers and an overall belief that they could learn to control computers and use them to perform productive tasks (Sanders, O'Sullivan, DeBurra, & Fedner, 2013).

Occupational Therapy Educational Programs for Community-Dwelling Older Adults

Another way OTs can contribute to older adult wellness is through consulting, educator, and advocacy roles. Painter and Elliott (2003) describe three educational group programs designed and led by OT students in partnership with a local community senior center in North Carolina. The first, called "Fall Prevention and Home Safety," addressed the following topics: factors that increase fall risk; personal factors such as increasing age, history of falls, decreased mobility, poor muscle strength, and decreased visual acuity. Extrinsic risk factors included uneven door thresholds, unstable furniture, bumps in carpets or floors, and cluttered floors and stairs. Participants learned and discussed strategies for preventing falls, modifications for their own homes, and resources for further help and information. The second group, entitled "Maximizing Your Memory," defined the various types of memory, gave an overview of the memory process, and included factors affecting memory such as medications, sensory and neurological changes, sleep, emotions, physical and mental activities, diet, and overall health. Participants learned memory strategies such as organizing and categorizing information, keeping a memory notebook, and being aware of why remembering may be difficult (e.g., feeling stressed and not paying attention). Presenters help group members to problem solve their own situations, and identify memory strategies that will work for them.

The third group, entitled "Memory and Safety Suggestions," was designed specifically for caregivers of individuals with Alzheimer's disease. Important components of this program included creating a consistent daily schedule, communication strategies, and organizing tasks such as bathing, dressing, and mealtimes to help maintain existing skills. Appropriate adaptations and responses to predictable levels of cognitive decline and their impact on ADL are discussed, along with safeguarding the home and outside environment to prevent unintentional dangers, such as installing fences or gates, restricting use of appliances and machinery, and handling telephone calls and mail (Painter & Elliott, 2003).

Case Example: Malcolm

"My first college, SUNY Maritime Fort Schuyler, was a military school in the same sense that West Point and Kings Point are. In my freshman year, I was frequently punished for very minor infractions associated with my not being sufficiently deferential. Then I would be restricted to the campus for the weekend while most of my classmates frolicked at their homes. This proved to be a great boon to me. I spent many weekend hours studying. I also got to read some

books that totally reshaped and broadened my outlook. The first such book was *Using Your Mind Effectively* by James L. Mursell. It provided me with a strategy for approaching study in any field. I still use its techniques. It worked. At the end of the academic year, I had the second highest GPA of the 96 engineers who started with me. More importantly, I laid a solid foundation for my future studies. Much technical knowledge is cumulative. It's very difficult to learn new material if you haven't mastered the prerequisite material. The second book that had a profound influence on me was *The Conduct of Life*, by Lewis Mumford. Mumford was an idealist philosopher and architecture critic. He attempted to show how modern governments erect impediments to our enjoyment of life, and what we can do to overcome these problems. It was a mind-expanding experience for me. Finally, I'll mention Robert Maynard Hutchins. He wrote a book about all the changes he, as chancellor, made to shake up the University of Chicago and why he made them. He was, of course, the foremost proponent in his time of Great Books and Socratic dialogs. He also favored in-depth study of epochs, such as the American and French Revolutions, and comprehensive exams covering great swaths of learning. I learned from him that there was a world of liberal arts that I would love to learn about that was far beyond my reach in my 4 years in an engineering school. I would have to do it on my own.

"My devotion to learning has played a very big part in my life. I seized every chance I could to further my studies both in technology and in liberal arts. When I was employed, I probably spent 90% of my time in technical pursuits and 10% in nontechnical. These days those numbers are probably reversed, but my ardor hasn't changed. I worked in the extremely competitive field of real-time computer software. Many of the people I worked with got laid off, usually at the end of projects. I did not want to join them. I wanted to be so knowledgeable and productive that I would be the last one laid off—I would turn out the lights. I spent a lot of time in technical institute classrooms, mostly in the evening, with my companies picking up the tab. This provided me with exposure to brilliant professors and bright students. I acquired five master's degrees, three of which were straight A. After that I audited another 14 tech classes. I was nearly 60 when I took my last class. While working, I was frequently my company's representative at 4- and 5-day Users' Conferences all over the country where we were briefed on what was new in software and hardware from our suppliers. I was also sponsored for short courses of 2 weeks at MIT, Stanford, and Michigan, 1 week at Penn State, and 4 days at Pheasant Run, and the Doral. I never had any difficulty convincing my bosses to accept my offer to trade the highest pay possible for the chance to further my knowledge and work with the best brains in the several job-related fields of interest to me. However, I made it a point to never spend a day in my 37 years in computers where I wasn't on some company's payroll. My wife's 20 years teaching helped greatly. Probably the best thing I got out of my MBA was learning why and how one should invest. I really socked away every dollar I could. That has allowed me a financially worry-free retirement. On the non-tech side, I enjoyed 4 years of Great Book discussions. I loved riding my exercise bike in the morning while watching a variety of liberal arts courses for many years on 'Sunrise Semester' from New York University and others. I attended about 20 Elderhostel courses from Virginia to New York.

"One of my goals in retirement is to do everything I can to maintain high levels of physical and mental health, to allow me to continue to enjoy every day of my life. I believe that if I continue to pay my dues I will boost the odds of living a long, healthy, and happy life. Although my wife died more than 20 years ago, for last 13 years I have been blessed with a warm and profound relationship with another wonderfully gifted woman. She and I share many values and interests, although we each have our own fields of interest. She is a first-rate cook and prepares healthy meals. We also go out often to the many fine restaurants in our area. We enjoy sailing with friends. We enjoy watching and listening to low priced but high quality performances by professional and student musicians and actors at the two state colleges near us. We enjoy watching several critically acclaimed movies from Netflix each week. We then discuss them. I then get three reviews (usually Ebert, Berardinelli, and a New York Times staffer). After we read the reviews, we discuss them. We usually make a 2-week or so tour (large ship, large sailboat, river boat, or land) to Europe annually. We've also visited many interesting areas of the United States with both my former shipmates and college buddies and their significant others.

"While in retirement, a key factor in my continuing good physical and mental health and zest for life is watching and listening to college-level lectures while doing early morning exercises with my Nordic Track and with very light weights. The Nordic Track is so noisy that I had to buy noise-canceling headphones to hear lectures coming out of my computer without blasting the rest of the house. I work out for at least an hour at least 5 days a week. I have two main sources for the lectures I watch. The Teaching Company does a terrific job of selecting and recording professors chosen both for their erudition and their lecturing abilities. Many of them have won awards in that category. Excellent graphics accompany some of the courses, although some of them are strictly talking heads. I have purchased more than 60 courses. Each course has a comprehensive manual summarizing the lectures and providing definitions, biographies, bibliographies, and significant dates. All lectures are 30 minutes so I usually watch three at a time. Courses may have 12, 24, 36, 48, 60, 72, or 84 lectures. I've watched courses in history, art, music, literature (of course Shakespeare), philosophy, religion, and science. I've done some of the readings but I've been much less intense than I would be if I were taking these courses for credit. My other primary source is college lectures from the web. These are free, live lectures from many of our best schools taped with much less fidelity than Teaching Company manages. My favorite is Yale. I have watched 14 courses of 24 or 26 lectures of 50 minutes to 115 minutes from Yale. Lectures are supplemented by many aids to learning: transcripts, reading lists (essential and optional), and supplemental notes. Whichever the source, when I have finished my morning physical and mental exercises I feel wonderful—ready for whatever the day brings."

Malcolm exemplifies the habit of lifelong learning by tracing it from adolescence and early adulthood, through his retirement years. The lesson we learn that could help clients is the variety of topics and the intentionality in knowledge seeking that has propelled Malcolm to succeed in many of his life goals, from promotions at work and financial security to the preservation of mental and physical fitness in older adulthood. He also demonstrates how learning environments have led him to meaningful social relationships with other "mature seekers of wisdom," including Mary, his significant life partner for over a decade.

Learning Activity 86: Learning From Malcolm

Considering Malcolm's case, answer the following:

1. How did Malcolm apply the principles of adult learning described earlier? Discuss three ways and give an example for each.

2. In what ways did Malcolm's learning activities change after he retired?

3. To what extent does lifelong learning contribute to Malcolm's continued health and well-being as he ages?

4. What lessons from this case might help you, as an OT, to design interventions for other older adults who are interested in learning but did not continue their education before retirement?

JOURNAL ENTRY (M. C.)

The PAS participants, almost without exception, placed a high value on staying informed about what is going on around them on some level, whether locally, globally, or nationally. However, there is a level of learning that is right for each of our clients, and we must be careful not to judge them for not having higher learning goals.

Some older adults resist new concepts, like using a computer. Two of our participants refused to own a computer or any electronic device beyond the simplest cell phone. Several others had a computer, thrust upon them by a well-meaning son or daughter, which they seldom if ever used. They preferred talking on the telephone to e-mail, reading the actual book to the electronic version, writing and mailing checks instead of using credit cards and online banking. Maybe it is just a habit of thinking or maybe it is a lack of trust in technology. I wonder, are they just unwilling to change or do they really know something the rest of us don't? Will they become marginalized as the rest of society progresses toward even greater dependence on technology? Or are we (younger folks) the ones being naïve, trusting when we shouldn't and minimizing the extent of our vulnerability? Maybe these older folks will eventually save us all by protecting their own identity and right to privacy and, by default or intention, ours too.

SUMMARY

Lifelong learning is the occupation that adults perform within the social role of student. Unlike when they were children, adults intentionally seek knowledge with a specific purpose in mind, based on the direction of their own lives. Although some older adults do register for formal education classes, much of their learning comes from in-service or on-the-job training, volunteer training, and self-improvement or self-paced programs through written manuals, DVDs, or over the Internet. Our participants defined learning broadly, encompassing traveling to learn about new countries and cultures, book discussion groups, informative TV programs like "60 Minutes," or informal conversations with others.

When clients identify learning goals, OTs help them to overcome barriers to achieving them. However, learning also takes on added importance as an essential skill for remaining productive. Clients need to understand how to access the latest health information in order to keep themselves well. For example, Johanna, Gloria, and June watch Dr. Oz on television to learn health-related information, while Malcolm and Mary D. search the Internet. Keeping one's brain sharp as one ages sometimes means challenging oneself by intentionally seeking out new learning experiences. Most importantly, OTs need to make sure their older clients are able to learn and apply the skills of self-management to continue living their lives to the fullest as they grow older.

REFERENCES

AARP. (2009). *Internet use among midlife and older adults: An AARP bulletin poll*. Washington, DC: AARP Knowledge Management.

AIUTA. (2006). *U3A balance after 30 years*. Retrieved from http://www.aiuta.org/documents/aiutappt.pdf.

Allen, C. K., & Earhart, C. (1992). *Occupational therapy treatment goals for the physically and cognitively disabled*. Bethesda, MD: American Occupational Therapy Association.

American Occupational Therapy Association. (2014). Occupational therapy practice framework: Domain and process, 3rd ed. *American Journal of Occupational Therapy, 68*, S1-48.

Baltes, P., & Smith, J. (2001). *New frontiers in the future of aging: From successful aging of the young old to the dilemmas of the Fourth Age*. Retrieved from www.valenciaforum.com/Keynotes/pb.html.

Birney, D., & Sternberg, R. (2006). Intelligence and cognitive abilities as competencies in development. In E. Bialystok & F. Craik (Eds.), *Lifespan cognition* (pp. 315-330). New York: Oxford University Press.

Commons, M. L., & Richards, F. A. (2003). Four postformal stages. In J. Demick & C. Andreoletti (eds.). *Handbook of adult development* (pp. 199-220). New York, NY: Plenum Series by Springer.

Czaja, S., Charness, N., Fisk, A., Hertzog, C., Nair, S., Rogers, W., Sharit, J. (2006). University of Miami factors predicting the use of technology: Findings from the Center for Research and Education on Aging and Technology Enhancement (CREATE). *Psychology of Aging, 21*, 333-352.

Daloz, L. (1986). *Effective teaching and mentoring*. San Francisco: Jossey-Bass, Inc.

Daloz, L. (1999). *Mentor: Guiding the journey of adult learners*. San Francisco: Jossey-Bass, Inc.

DeRosa, J. (2013). Providing self-management support to people living with chronic conditions. *OT Practice*, CE1-CE8.

Formosa, M. (2010). Lifelong learning in later life: The universities of the Third Age. *Lifelong Learning Institute Review, 5*, 1-12.

Haslam, C., Jetten, J., Haslam, A., & Knight, C. (2012). The importance of remembering and deciding together: Enhancing the health and well-being of older adults in care. In J. Jetten, C. Haslam, & A. Haslam (Eds.) *The social cure* (pp. 297-315). New York: Psychology Press.

Jarvis, P. (1987). *Adult learning in the social context*. London: Croom Helm.

Kim, Y. S. (2008). Reviewing and critiquing computer learning and usage among older adults. *Educational Gerontology, 34*, 709-735.

Knowles, M. (1990). *The adult learner: A neglected species* (4th ed.). Houston, TX: Gulf Publishing.

Kohlberg, L. (1990). Which postformal levels are stages? In M. L. Commons, C. Armon, L. Kohlberg, F. A. Richards, T. A. Grotzer, & J. D. Sinnott (Eds.), *Adult development: Vol 2. Models and methods in the study of adolescent and adult thought* (pp. 263-268). New York: Praeger.

Landau, S., Mintun, M., Joshi, A., Koeppe, R., Peterson, R., Aisen, P., ... Jagust, W. (2012). Amyloid deposition, hypometabolism, and longitudinal cognitive decline. *Annals of Neurology, 72*, 578-586.

Laslett, P. (1989). *A fresh map of life: The emergence of the Third Age*. Cambridge, MA: Harvard University Press.

Mayhorn, C. B., Stronge, A. J., McLaughlin, A. C., & Rogers, W. A. (2004). Older adults, computer training, and the systems approach: A formula for success. *Educational Gerontology, 30*, 185-203.

Merriam, S. B., & Caffarella, R. S. (1999). *Learning in adulthood* (2nd ed.). San Francisco, CA: Jossey-Bass.

Painter, J., & Elliott, S. (2003). Educational programs for community-dwelling seniors. *OT Practice*, Feb. 24, 25-26.

Piaget, J. (1972). Intellectual evolution from adolescence to adulthood. *Human Development, 15*, 1-12.

Plassman, B., Williams, J., & Burke, J. (2010). Systematic review: Factors associated with risk for and possible prevention of cognitive decline in later life. *Annals of Internal Medicine, 153*, 182-196.

Sanders, M., O'Sullivan, B., DeBurra, K., & Fedner, A. (2013). Computer training for seniors: An academic-community partnership. *Educational Gerontology, 39*, 179-193.

Sinnott, J. D. (1993). Yes, it's worth the trouble! Unique contributions from everyday cognition studies. In J. M. Puckett & H Reese (Eds.) *Mechanisms of everyday cognition* (pp. 73-95). Mahwah, NJ: Lawrence Erlbaum Associates.

The Third Age Trust. (2009). *The Third Age Trust*. Retrieved from http://www.3.griffith.edu.au/03/u3a.

Thompson, J. (2002). *The amazing universities of the Third Age in China today*. Retrieved from http://www.worldu3a.org/worldpapers/u3a-china.htm.

Tsao, T. (2004). New models for future retirement: A study of college/university-linked retirement communities. Dissertation Abstracts International Section A: Humanities & Social Sciences, 64(10A), 3511.

U3A Online. (2009). *Links – U3A related*. Retrieved from http://www3.griffith.edu.au/03/u3a.

Withnall, A. (2000). Three decades of educational gerontology: Achievements and challenges. *Education and Aging, 17*, 87-102.

Yalom, I., & Leszcz, M. (2005). *The theory and practice of group psychotherapy* (5th ed.). New York: Basic Books.

Yang, S. (2012). *Lifelong brain-stimulating habits linked to lower Alzheimer's protein levels*. Retrieved from http://newscenter.berkeley.edu/2012/01/23/engaged-brain-amyloid-alzheimers/.

Social Connections
Participation and Strategies

Marilyn B. Cole, MS, OTR/L, FAOTA

"Just as brains can do things that no single neuron can do, so can social networks do things that no single person can do."
(Christakis, 2009, p. xvi)

Social connections is the second main theme in our PAS. Connections are the ties people have to family, friends, coworkers, neighbors, and other people with whom they are familiar and often interact. Patterns of such interactions define social networks (Christakis & Fowler, 2009). As a theme, its thread runs through all of the productive occupations described earlier, but also occupies a central role in each person's life. Humans are social beings, living their lives within the context of social groups from birth (family), through childhood and adolescence (classrooms, sports teams, friendships, neighborhoods), and throughout adulthood (work groups, community groups, extended family groups, learning groups, leisure interest groups) until death. The need to maintain social connections does not end in retirement, but rather continues and, in some cases, increases with aging. The important difference described by our participants is intentionality. After retirement, older adults need to make a focused effort to keep in contact with former coworkers and friends and to reach out to make new friends in their neighborhoods and communities. Our participants all made the effort to stay connected.

Social participation is defined by the AOTA's OTPF III as "the interweaving of occupations to support desired engagement in community and family activities as well as those involving peers and friends (Gillen & Boyt Schell, 2014, p. 607); involvement in a subset of activities that involve social situations with others (Bedell, 2012); and that support social interdependence (Magasi & Hammel, 2004)." Social participation can occur in person or through remote technologies such as telephone calls, computer interaction, and video conferencing (AOTA, 2014, p. S21). Three types of social participation are included in this section:

- Community: Engaging in activities that result in successful interaction at the community level (e.g., neighborhood, organizations, workplace, school, religious or spiritual group).

- Family: Engaging in activities that result in "successful interaction in specific required and/or desired familial roles" (Mosey, 1996, p. 340).

- Peer, friend: Engaging in activities at different levels of interaction and intimacy, including engaging in desired sexual activity.

These definitions imply that people take on multiple social roles throughout their lives, within which they interact with others in customary or traditional ways. For example, a mother within the family, a mayor in the community, a supervisor in the workplace, or a priest or pastor at church each have specific roles and tasks to perform. The social expectations of each change within different cultures, but each plays some type of leadership role—directing, managing, or inspiring others within their organizations. What

Cole MB, Macdonald KC.
Productive Aging: An Occupational Perspective (pp 197-213).
© 2015 Taylor & Francis Group.

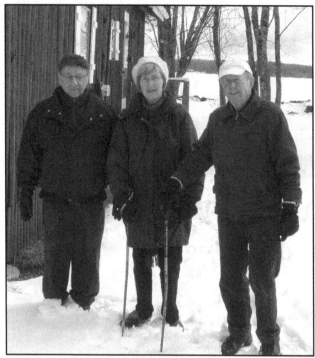

Figure 12-1. Taking a walk together makes staying fit a social activity.

are the social roles specified for older adults? For example, what might be the role of a grandparent? What are the social expectations for someone who is retired?

Four other elements within the OTPF III also impact social connections: communication management and community mobility, both from the category of IADLs; social context, one of six contexts or environments within which occupations are performed; and roles represent one of the performance patterns. These are defined as follows:

- *"Communication management:* Sending, receiving, and interpreting information using a variety of systems and equipment, including writing tools, telephones (cell phones and smartphones), keyboards, audiovisual recorders, computers, communication boards, call lights, emergency systems, Braille writers, telecommunication devices for deaf people, augmentative communication systems, and personal digital assistants" (AOTA, 2014, p. S19).

- *"Driving and community mobility:* Planning and moving around in the community and using public or private transportation, such as driving, walking, bicycling, or accessing and riding in buses, taxi cabs, or other transportation systems" (AOTA, 2014, p. S19).

- *"Social environments:* Presence of, relationships with, and expectations of persons, groups, or organizations with whom clients have contact. The social environment includes availability and expectations of significant individuals, such as spouse, friends, and caregivers; relationships with individuals, groups, or populations; and relationships with systems (e.g.,

political, legal, economic, institutional) that influence norms, role expectations, and social routines" (AOTA, 2014, p. S28).

- *"Roles:* Sets of behaviors expected by society and shaped by culture and context that may be further conceptualized and defined by the client. Roles are attributable to both persons and groups or populations" (AOTA, 2014, p. S27).

Interconnection of Social Roles and Productive Occupations

The inclusion of these IADLs clearly points to the overlap that exists between social connections and the various areas of occupation. It would be difficult to make a date with a friend or accept a party invitation without being able to communicate via telephone, e-mail, or in writing. Attending social events requires a level of functional mobility, by either driving oneself to the event location or arranging for a ride. Furthermore, when older persons reach a point where they can no longer drive safely, this creates a barrier to community mobility, which has a major impact on their ability to participate in social activities. They need to depend more than ever on communicating through other means to maintain their social connections in older adulthood. Occupations are also hard to separate from their social context because whether they are performed by a group (singing in a choir), they must nearly always meet the expectations set by social tradition (cleaning one's home) or by others outside the group (meeting job requirements). Roles also require interactions with others, and our participants gave examples such as a spouse, grandparent, caregiver, home maintainer, teacher, hairdresser, and friend, all of which contributed to the way they defined themselves (self-identity) and the way they perceived that others viewed them or how they wished to be viewed (social identity) (Figure 12-1).

Learning Activity 87: Explore Your Own Social Identities

1. In a group of people you have just met at a non-work related social gathering, what three things would you say to identify yourself after you say your name?

   a.

   b.

   c.

2. In each of the above items, discuss what social identity you are trying to convey.

   a.

   b.

   c.

3. What larger societal groups do you categorize yourself as belonging to (Christian/African American/college graduate/Midwesterner)?

4. How do work or social group memberships and self-categorizations contribute to your social identity?

5. How are social identities positive or negative? What is the impact of each on your occupational options and choices?

PARTICIPANT PERSPECTIVES

Social connections took prominence at many levels in the lives of all our participants. The top priorities were marriages or partners, friendships, and family roles, followed by group and organization memberships, including work, volunteer, or religious groups. Participants demonstrated the strength of their social identities through their multiple social roles.

Spouses or Partners

Many of our participants mentioned their relationships with one significant other, whether a spouse, partner, or friend. "I spend about half my time away from my house living with my significant other...I found a lady about 11 years ago to share my life. She is a perfect complement to me. Of course we don't agree about everything, but most of our interests dovetail extremely closely. That's half the battle" (Malcolm). "I live with a gentleman. We take care of each other and are very active and travel. We go with each other to many social functions and family gatherings" (Maxine). "I go out to lunch almost every day with my partner and friends" (Greg). "My wife loves to plan social activities for both of us" (Jack). "Each evening I go to Susan's [girlfriend of 25 years] for cocktails and dinner, we watch TV, and I sleep over. Most of our friends are her friends. I'm a loner. Susan keeps me involved with others socially. She plans outings with others, theater, concerts, or traveling" (Bob C.). "My main social identity is as a partner—we love to hang out together, share concerts, eat in or out, socialize, go sailing, travel together" (Mary D.). "I do a lot of things with my wife, we go out for dinner, have picnics, and go to concerts and plays" (Geno). Spouses and partners often enjoyed activities as a couple or socialized with others together and felt this to be a positive influence for the most part.

A few spouses or partners felt some conflict in their relationships. "As I age, the days get shorter with not enough time to get done what I want to do. Now I have a [newly] retired spouse who thrives on activity and reorganization" (Margie). This is a minor stress for her because her husband also helps her with caring for their grandchildren and accompanies her in traveling and family outings. Sue feels burdened by caregiving for a disabled husband. After his stroke, he "used to be violent, but now he's fairly docile." Alice (widowed) and Betty (divorced) also reported feeling burdened when caring for their disabled husbands. There is a strong connection and potential conflict between the social and caregiving roles for spouses, a phenomenon discussed more fully in Chapter 2.

Many currently married or partnered couples mention the sharing of household management. Vi states, "Ask a married person. Companionship raises your level of functioning and your quality of life."

Family

The next major connection, mentioned by almost all participants, was family. "Being in close contact via phone, e-mail, and meetings with friends and family is essential for me" (Mary D.). "I go to brunch with my family every week after church. I talk to my brother on the phone" (Mary V.). "We have a cabin to go to that my family shares. I do many projects there for decorating and keeping it up, and then we all enjoy entertaining and gathering there" (Nancy B.). "I try to attend grandkids' athletic games, and participate in their lives" (Vi). "I'm very active with my family, and now I am helping my brother at his work. He is doing the job I did before I retired" (Linval). "I enjoy visiting friends and family. Our whole family works together to organize tasks that need to be done" (Nancy B.). "I see my children and grandchildren when I can, 4 to 6 times a year (long distance)" (Maxine). Valnere spends much of each year traveling "visiting friends and family scattered all over—brother in Australia, sister in Germany, another sister in North Carolina...I must travel to New Hampshire at least one week each month to visit Mother, do finances, take her shopping or to medical appointments." "Currently, I spend most time with my family" (Ken). "We host weekly family dinners [4 sons, 1 daughter, 11 grandchildren, 1 great grandchild]...we make an effort to attend grandchildren's activities" (Peggie). "I am a grandmother who enjoys her family" (Johanna). Johanna, who is widowed, also travels with her sister, who is divorced. Mildred recently moved to a retirement community near her daughter's family, but no longer drives long distance to see her other daughter or her son.

Gloria and her sister Edna, both never married, live together and share home management tasks. They also travel together to visit with their large Italian family: "Family members often visit and stay over with us on their way somewhere. We call this the 'half-way house.' Charlie lives with his wife, and his daughter, son-in-law, and 3 grandchildren are nearby. He often vacations with his family. "I've got my woman and my craft. Every man needs both" (Charlie). "My main family role is as sister to my brothers and sisters—we call or check in every weekend. I'm also Aunt Mary to my 17 nieces and nephews. One family with 6 nieces and nephews has lived near me for

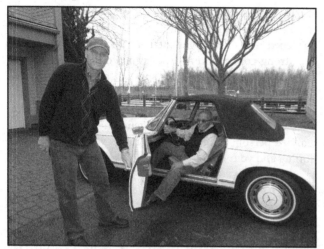

Figure 12-2. Greg's advice to other retirees: "Have lots of friends." He (driving) and partner Gary create a life structure around their social activities. Today they are off to lunch in style.

40-plus years, so we are very close. We celebrate holidays, birthdays, and now weddings together. Also, we volunteer together for a local food pantry" (Mary D.). Ellen speaks with her parents once weekly (phone) and they visit whenever possible (long distance). "I speak with my brother and niece periodically via phone or webcam" (Ellen).

June has a slightly different family perspective, advocating for a disabled adult son: "I experienced prejudice growing up, one of six Jews in my school. Now I intervene; you have to fight to protect your loved ones. Never let one of your children cope with discrimination as you did." Betty has a guarded relationship with one of her married sons. "Their two adopted boys are not well behaved…you must be savvy, choose your battles."

Friendships

Friendships were also highly valued among our participants. Ann M. reports, "I have enjoyed keeping friendships alive with people I used to work with. When I was widowed, I was alone…I had to take charge of my social life. I would follow up with people I hadn't seen." Her advice: "Join a social group. Don't be lonely and feel sorry for yourself and be depressed. Do something about it—visit [a friend] for coffee, go to a senior center. Just do something [with other people]." Likewise, Nancy states, "I am still involved with my work friends. We enjoy social activities, but we always go back and talk about work. We are still 'that group' even though we are retired…it's a clique." Maxine tells us, "I like to be with people in my own age bracket at the senior center or social gatherings." Ellen says "I socialize with neighbors and friends whenever possible—I enjoy entertaining in my own home or going out to theaters and restaurants." Vi reports, "I ask people to do things with me." Malcolm says, "I enjoy getting together with friends, and at events such as school and ship reunions, or club meetings." Jan recom-

mends, "Building strong and diverse communities. Keep up social contacts…Strengthen existing [networks] and build new ones." June no longer enjoys going to parties, "I prefer one-to-one relationships." Greg likes to plan each day around social activities. Betty (age 90) observes "friends are getting older and losing health, moving to assisted living." It makes her question "Why am I still here?" Gloria suggests retirees "Develop a network of family and friends that keep you involved. As you get older, it's harder to move to a new community." Alice recommends "Stay involved with friends and make new friends. Join a gym group—there are senior activities now. As you get into it, you gain strength. You'll be better off than sitting around doing nothing. And that's not going to happen to me!" Phyllis recommends, "Keep in touch with people." Maxine advises, "It is about associating with as many people as you can, good friends, and get out and meet people. The message from our participants is clear: older adults need to make an intentional effort to keep in touch with former colleagues and friends, and to reach out to others and develop new friendships (Figure 12-2).

Community Groups and Organizations

Participation in community groups and organizations helped many of our participants to stay connected to others. Gloria and Peggie both identify themselves as "joiners" and take on leadership roles in many community organizations. Charlie belongs to three social clubs and enjoys traveling with friends. Geno also belongs to several community groups and finds them "interesting, challenging, and stimulating." Mary reports, "In my church, I am involved in volunteering in the thrift store, but I have decreased my previous involvement. A new group came in, not the old established one. I still enjoy [volunteering] but now I let the younger group do what it needs to do." Bob M. (newly remarried) reports, "I used to belong to organizations, church, and groups related to Boy Scouts and Indian Guides. Now I go with my wife to some of her events." Dave H. also attends organizations, but "at this stage of the game, I don't want to be the head. I'm very willing to help [as a member]." Sue S. was active for years in the Grange: "I had so many creative ideas for programs and contests. It was a lot of hard work, helping clean up [after meetings]. I think I should have received a medal for all I did for so long." Sue S. is also a member of Widows and Widowers and does things with her church. Margie doesn't mind being the leader of multiple community groups (church, Girl Scouts); however, she does "get overcommitted and then overwhelmed." Clearly, there are overlaps between joining groups and organizations because of common interests, taking on leadership or volunteer roles within them, and forming social connections and friendships through participation.

Some participants mentioned support groups in particular. Nettie tells us, "I have a tremendous support group. I've been surrounded with a lot of love all my life." Bob M. attended "Widows and Widowers [support group]…it was very helpful in hearing other people's explanations and comments about the same situation, then we would go out socially for lunch, which was fun—1 guy with 10 girls! The ladies were faithful and often attended for too long. The men would come and go." Phyllis gives some insight to what might happen without social support, "people who make no effort to reach out or keep in touch—they wait for others to call them. Those people always talk about themselves, and never ask, 'How are *you* doing?' In closing yourself off to others, you become a shell unto yourself. These are my feelings of what one should *not* do!"

Social Identity

Social identity refers to the sense of self that people derive from their membership in social groups (e.g., family, work, community) (Jetten, Haslam, & Haslam, 2012; Tajfel, 1978). For our participants, that translated into two areas: the roles they play within various groups, and the larger social groups in which they consider themselves a member. Nearly all identified prominent *family roles* for themselves, such as daughter or son, spouse or partner, parent, grandparent, brother, sister, aunt, or uncle. Many also strongly identified with a particular *ethnic* group: Gerry, Mary D., and Jim talked about their strong Irish heritage, and Geno, Greg, Sue S., and Gloria come from large Italian families. Margie is one of eight siblings in an extensive Puerto Rican family. Linval, a Jamaican, states "I never knew prejudice [before I came here]. Where I came from, all the people there were all mixed. My grandmother, who passed away 41 years ago, said 'wherever you go, respect other people and they'll respect you.' When upset, don't just say anything out of mouth—cope, go home, calm down, and then go back and say 'what you did was wrong,' then they apologize… otherwise you might say the wrong thing and it becomes a conflict." Sue, although married to an American, still considers herself an Englishwoman. Valnere speaks with an accent like her Australian mother but considers herself very much an American. Vi identifies with her Japanese heritage, often speaking publicly about the plight of Japanese Americans during and after World War II.

Religion also figures largely in the social identities of many participants. Betty identifies herself as a "collapsed Jew," by which she means not observing except for high holy days. June and Mildred both speak about the discrimination they experienced as a result of being Jewish. Since Mildred moved into a retirement community, she has discovered that she is the only Jewish woman there, and she feels that others hesitate to include her in their social activities partly because of this. For many Catholics and Protestants, church activities play a central role in their social lives. Jan coordinates a large altar guild for her Episcopal church and takes charge of a church bazaar each year, which involves many subgroups for sewing, baking, and crafts, as well as used item sales, a silent auction, and other committees. Gloria plays similar roles at her Catholic church. Peggie (Catholic) sings in her church choir, while Margie (Episcopal) leads Bible study groups in Spanish and English, serves on a Diocesan Hispanic Ministry committee and as lay coordinator for St. David's Hispanic Ministry, teaches First Communion and Baptism classes, and translates for monthly Rector-Spanish Priest meetings. She is proudly bicultural and bilingual. Mary D. was once a Catholic nun and learned Italian while teaching at a Catholic school in Italy. Although she left that calling many years ago, her religion remains a strong part of her social identity. Ann M. (Catholic) states, "I practice my faith in many ways. I say grace before a meal. I am involved with prayer groups and lists near and far. Now I know that people are praying for me, and I think, this feels nice. I wonder if all that goodness is coming toward me and healing me." Dave H. (Protestant) has this to say: "I mostly do church activities, like the Council of Churches. It's a feeling—very grateful to be able to do it—give something to an organization. With my background (engineer, executive), I feel it's my duty…give something back…help people if you are able to."

Some participants also identified *political* ideologies: Bob T., a Midwesterner, is an outspoken conservative Republican, while Betty works on political campaigns for Democratic candidates. Gloria considers herself an Independent, prides herself on being a mediator among different ideologies, and moderates political debates between local candidates for the League of Women Voters in her community.

Lastly, important social identities very often came from the *work and professional* roles of our participants during middle adulthood. Signian, Ken, Mary, and Pearl are retired university professors; Dave, Malcolm, and Geno are retired engineers; and Gloria, Ann M., and Marylyn are retired public school teachers. Johanna still practices law. Retired health professionals include Nettie, Ellen, Nan, Vi, Peggie, Mary D., Jan, Valnere, and Mildred, while retired business professionals include Jack, Bob C., Bob M., Jim M., and Ray P. All of these participants have continued their associations with organizations related to their former employment or professional roles. Greg and Nancy were hairdressers. Bob T. was an international airline pilot and an ex-Navy B2 Bomber pilot. Malcolm, an ex-Naval engineer, also identifies strongly with that early work role and keeps in touch with his former military buddies through frequent reunions. Charlie was a comedy writer for CBS in New York City and a freelance TV writer. As Pearl states: "College teaching has been so much a part of my identity. It has centered me. It has been a way of defining myself." In social contexts, many of our participants still identify

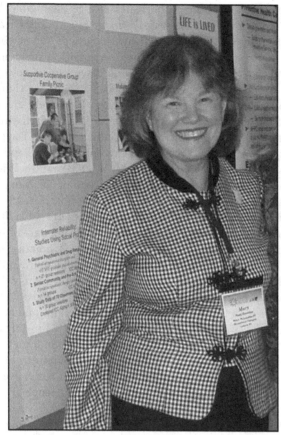

Figure 12-3. Mary demonstrates her social identity as a professional, here presenting a poster about her latest research study at a Centers for Disease Control conference in Washington, DC.

themselves with their former work title or position because it has become so much a part of who they are (Figure 12-3). Office workers and laborers were less likely to keep a strong work-related social identity after retirement but sometimes reported specific parts of their work experience as good preparation for volunteer positions.

Interestingly, some female participants who did not have careers of their own took great pride in the supportive roles they played in their homes. Marylyn reports, "I was a super mom…my husband worked. I took the kids to school, I took care of everything in the house, even if the water heater broke." June, after attending college only briefly, proudly received her "MRS." June's husband had a high-profile job, requiring her to constantly entertain his clients and colleagues, throwing dinner parties in addition to bring up their three boys: "Good thing I am a Hungarian Jew who knows how to cook!" Patricia also found her identity through her husband's work. Born in Australia and educated abroad, she became fluent in several languages. When she married an American oil company executive working in India, her role often involved entertaining foreign executives who did not speak English and acting as interpreter. In addition to caring for their four children, Patricia regularly played golf, bridge, or mahjong and entertained out of town

guests. In retirement, she has written and published a book of poetry and, more recently, a memoir of her life experiences living abroad, which is about to be published.

In summary, when we asked our participants what final recommendations they would make to others, *all* of them mentioned social connections as essential to their successful aging. Even more than participating in community groups, family relationships and friendships stood out as the most cherished. "Don't separate yourself from friends and family" (Gloria). "Have a lot of friends" (Greg). "Nurture social relationships. Stay involved with others" (Bob C.). "Keep in touch with friends and support the younger generation where possible to balance losses of people your age" (Mary D.). "Family is very important" (Patricia). "Reduce stress [by connecting with] friends and family, outside activities, volunteering. Rid yourself of emotional baggage and old hurts by making amends or cultivating new friends" (Peggie). "Interact with people of all ages" (Sue).

LITERATURE REVIEW

Social Connections and Health

Considering current research linking social connection with increased health and well-being, the PAS participants' recommendations seem to be on the right track. A meta-analytic review of 148 studies concluded that individuals with strong social relationships have a 50% lower risk of mortality, a finding that remained consistent across age, sex, initial health status, cause of death, and follow-up period (Holt-Lunstad, Smith, & Bradley Leyton, 2010). Additionally, this analysis determined that "the influence of social relationships on the risk of death are comparable with well-established risk factors for mortality such as smoking and alcohol consumption, and exceed the influence of other risk factors such as physical inactivity and obesity" (Holt-Lunstad, 2010, p. 3). Three aspects of social relationships have been shown to be associated with morbidity (illness) and mortality (death): (1) the degree of integration in social networks; (2) social interactions that are intended to be supportive; and (3) beliefs and perceptions of social support availability held by the individual. These researchers found that the association with morbidity and mortality was strongest for the first factor based on complex measures of social integration (Hold-Lunstad et al., 2010).

The identification of social isolation as a significant risk factor for illness, disability, and earlier death for older adults comes at a time when people across Western societies are becoming more isolated. More people are living alone rather than within extended families, and the global economy has sent younger workers farther away from their roots and origins (Holmes & Joseph, 2011). From a World Health Organization (WHO, 2001) perspective, four chronic conditions are responsible for premature mortality: cardiovascular disease, diabetes, cancer, and chronic respiratory disease. The WHO (2001) identifies four lifestyle risk factors that influence these chronic conditions: smoking, harmful alcohol use, lack of physical exercise, and high-salt, high-fat diets. However, social isolation, which has been shown to be a risk factor equal to these, has been largely neglected by the WHO, health policy makers in the United States and abroad, and the health community generally (Holmes & Joseph, 2011). These authors foresee the potential social roles for older adults: "They play important social, cultural, and economic roles in their families and communities. They look after grandchildren, enabling both parents to work outside the home, they undertake domestic and horticultural work; they buffer the effect of modern influences on young people, and pass on traditional rituals, skills and knowledge. They can provide emotional support, and a sense of continuity and belonging. But their contribution is often limited by chronic disability" (Holmes & Joseph, 2011, p. 2). This implies that the health care community should devote much greater attention, energy, and resources toward efforts that encourage greater social integration for older adults. Social connections should be regarded as an essential factor in healthy aging.

Social Support Theories

Social support "stems from social interactions and networks of relationships that are intended to strengthen the well-being of their members" (White, Philogene, Fine, & Sinha, 2009, p. 1873). Using the National Health and Nutrition Examination Survey, researchers studied the relationship between poor self-perceived health and the quality and quantity of social support available to them. This study found that adults age 60 and older across the United States who reported that they needed more social support were twice as likely to have poor health as those who were satisfied with their social support level (White et al., 2009). Social support serves different functions with regard to health and well-being: (1) emotional support, which is feeling understood by a confidant or close to another person; (2) instrumental support, such as providing financial or physical assistance; and (3) informational support, such as providing guidance, feedback, and additional resources (Berkman, 2000; Glass, Mendes de Leon, & Seeman, 1997). Of these, further evidence points to emotional support as the strongest predictor of health and well-being (Melchior, Berkman, Niedhammer, Chea, & Goldberg, 2003).

Social support theories have various titles, including social convoys (Rowe & Kahn, 1998), social exchange theory (Keyes, 2002), role theory (Kielhofner, 2008), social support banks (Antonucci & Jackson, 2002), and social capital (Stone, 2003; Veninga, 2006). Evidence shows that social relationships provide individuals with identity, social roles, and social support. The positive effects of social connections, including increased health, happiness, and longevity,

are well documented (Stone, 2003). *Role theory* has influenced the way occupations are selected and organized (Spencer, 2003). In OT, the Occupational Performance Model (PEOPM) (Baum & Christiansen, 2005) and the Model of Human Occupation (MOHO) (Kielhofner, 2008) are two occupation-based models that view roles as central ideas. Roles define the tasks or occupations that people do with or for one another, and the expectations and criteria for the performance of occupations may be socially and culturally determined.

Because the absence of social support has been associated with significantly higher mortality for older adults (Lyyra & Heikkinen, 2006), the formal and informal social networks of elderly people have been studied extensively. *Social support* for older adults may provide emotional comfort, guidance, companionship, information, and physical assistance. Exchange theories emphasize the reciprocity of social and emotional support given. Keyes (2002) reports that the discrepancy between hours given and received becomes more balanced with age, but for the oldest adults in the study, unequal exchanges produced worse emotional well-being. The *support bank theory* (Antonucci & Jackson, 2002) uses a similar exchange concept. The caregiving hours accrued in younger years can be "cashed in" in later life, making the receiving of care more acceptable. Such social exchange bank deposits and withdrawals may be used to explain intergenerational caring. Theoretically, parents who cared well for their children don't have to worry about becoming a "burden" in their time of dependency.

Social Networks Research

Another focus of research involves social networks of older adults. A national study based on data from the National Social Life, Health, and Aging Project, focused on older Americans ages 57 to 85 living in the community, found that age is negatively related to network size, closeness to network members, and number of non-primary group ties; conversely, age is positively related to frequency of socializing with neighbors, religious participation, and volunteering (Cornwell, Laumann, & Schumm, 2008). These results contradict the notion that "old age has a universal negative influence on social connectedness. Some later life transitions, like retirement and bereavement, may prompt greater connectedness" (Cornwell et al., 2008, p. 185). Another study of older adults in Montreal identified some types and predictors of social participation at the neighborhood level (Richard, Gauvin, Gosselin, & Laforest, 2008). The four variables they found to predict higher levels of engagement were (1) frequent walking outside the home, (2) high vitality, (3) good general health, and (4) perceived access to key resources for older adults. However, older age predicted lower levels of social engagement with neighbors.

More recently, research has focused on identifying different types of social networks in relation to subjective well-being for older Americans. Litwin and Shiovitz-Ezra (2010) identify five social network types: (1) diverse, (2) friend, (3) congregant, (4) family, and (5) restricted, each associated with different amounts of social capital. *Social capital* may be broadly defined as the resources available to individuals and groups through social connections and social relations with others (Cannuscio, Block, & Kawachi, 2003). Just as financial capital can be quantified for shareholders of a corporation, social capital quantifies the potential benefit in terms of social support for the members of a social network. The Litwin and Shiovitz-Ezra (2010) study based its investigation of social networks on seven social capital variables previously defined by Gray (2009): current marital status, number of children, number of close relatives, number of friends, frequency of getting together with neighbors, frequency of attendance at religious services, and frequency of attendance at organized group meetings. These seven compromise the main components of the social networks of older adults reported in the social network literature. Of the five network types identified in this study, diverse and friend networks produced the highest social capital and congregate (religious congregations), family (with few outside supports), and restricted types had the least social capital, in descending order. Those social networks with greater social capital tended to promote higher levels of well-being in terms of less loneliness, less anxiety, and greater happiness.

Social science researchers have recently used computer programs based on complex systems theory to study social networks (Christakis & Fowler, 2009). Generally, social networks operate according to the following five rules:

1. *We shape our social network*: We tend to connect with people like ourselves "homophily," choose how involved we want to be with each of our connections, and decide how centrally located we will be within the network (leader, follower, extravert, introvert).

2. *Our network shapes us*: The people we interact with in families, work places, and communities affect us in many surprising ways, from how smart we are (first-borns have a higher IQ), to our fashion sense, how much money we make, and for whom we vote.

3. *Our friends affect us*: All kinds of things flow through networks, from germs and viruses to obesity (diners who sit next to heavy eaters eat more food). Denser networks have more "transivity," which means that many of our friends are also friends with each other. In networks with low transivity, more central members tend to transmit flow between separate clusters.

4. *Our friends' friend's friends affect us*: Influence beyond our direct social ties are known as "hyperdyadic spread." If one neighbor keeps a manicured lawn, soon the whole neighborhood does the same, even if some of these people have never met. Christakis and Fowler (2009) have identified the three degrees of influence

rule: our own behavior, say the decision to vote, influences our friends, their friends, and their friends' friends to also vote. But after three hops, our influence peters out. Hypothetically, a person with 20 social contacts influences 400 people at 2 degrees of separation and 8,000 at 3 degrees.

5. Networks have a life of their own: For example, "la ola" (the human wave) that spreads through sports stadiums cannot be initiated by just one fan. Networks take on "emergent properties" (p. 26) apart from any single person. National and global trends can be understood this way, for better or worse (happiness, smoking habits, economic confidence, and ageism). Hence, the whole becomes more than the sum of its parts.

In summary, Christakis and Fowler (2009) write, "If we want to understand how society works, we need to fill in the missing links between individuals. We need to understand how interconnections and interactions between people give rise to wholly new aspects of human experience that are not present in the individuals themselves. If we do not understand social networks, we cannot hope to fully understand either ourselves or the world we inhabit" (p. 32).

Developmental Perspectives

Theories of adult development also have much to say about social connections. Erikson's (1963) socioemotional developmental stages extend well into older adulthood, representing a "widening social radius" across the life span, ending with the wider community and future generations. Many researchers have confirmed various stages (McAdams, Hart, & Maruna, 1998; Vaillant, 1993), adding the variation in timing of adult life stages. In the late midlife stage, generativity involves the social roles of teaching, mentoring, and coaching as ways of sharing wisdom learned from life experience. Erikson (1963) defined generativity as "primarily the concern in establishing and guiding the next generation" (p. 267). A classic longitudinal study supports Erikson's model, showing that generativity is significantly associated with successful marriage, work achievements, close friendships, altruistic behaviors, and overall mental health (Westermeyer, 2004). This study also found that favorable peer group relationships at midlife predicted the achievement of this advanced developmental stage in older adulthood. The latter part of Erikson's (1963) final stage, integrity vs. despair, while not specifically social in nature, has a potentially negative impact on social relationships. As some of our participants mentioned, people who are self-absorbed, "talk only about themselves" (Phyllis), or "complain all the time" (Gerry), are to be avoided and do not make desirable friends.

Adams (2004) has taken a closer look at Laslett's Third and Fourth Ages with regard to differences in their interest in and attitude toward social activities for young-old (60 to 80) vs. old-old (80 and older). She found that the younger group retains a high level of interest in the following social activities and issues: "entertaining others in my home, social events with new people, taking care of people and things, concern with others' opinions of me, feeling I should share opinions and advice" (p. 99). Those over age 85 had less interest in these things and more interest in the following: "hearing from family and friends, visits with family, religious services, worrying about friends or family problems, being a good neighbor, visiting with old friends and neighbors, and spending time alone." In a later study, Adams revised her Change in Activity Index (CAII-R) by clustering social and leisure activities into the following categories: active social, active instrumental, passive social spiritual, and transcendent attitudes (Adams, Roberts, & Cole, 2011). This study reported that Fourth Agers (age 80 and older) have a reduced interest in active instrumental and active social activities, and an increased interest in passive social spiritual domains when compared with Third Agers (ages 62 to 79). Furthermore, a reduced interest in active social activities had the strongest association with depression and mediated the relationship between poor health or functioning and depression. The part of this research that does not match our study is the ages in which changes in social interest take place. Most of our participants still fall into the category of Laslett's Third Age partly because they continue to lead productive lives despite their advanced chronological age.

A better fit with our results is socioemotional selectivity theory (SST), which predicts the voluntary narrowing of social circles at older ages as an adaptive mechanism, allowing elders to conserve limited energy for activities that are truly meaningful (Carstensen, Isaacowitz, & Charles, 1999). Older participants in our study did make conscious choices to limit their social contacts, such as no longer attending parties (June) or preferring the companionship of one special person over many. See Chapter 1 for a more extensive review of this theory.

Social Identity Theory and Research

Social identity theory (Jetten et al., 2012) holds perhaps the most relevance for our participants, as well as giving us some important guidelines for interventions for those less successful agers who might become OT clients. Historically, social identity theory stems from social psychology research beginning in the 1930s. George Herbert Mead argued that society shapes self-identity because self-conception is constantly modified through interpersonal interactions (Tajfel, 1978). Based on Mead's notion, Tajfel (1978) defined *social identity* as that part of an individual's self-perception that arises from the individual's knowledge that he belongs to certain groups that hold some emotional significance to himself. Current evidence, summarized by Jetten et al. (2012), supports the idea that both the physical

and mental health and the well-being of individuals directly relates to the strength of their social identity.

Most people belong to many groups and categorize themselves in many different ways at both a local and a societal level. At a local level, people seek out membership in groups that cast them in a positive light, attributing to them desirable qualities such as nurturing, compassionate, thorough, a good leader, a good problem solver, or a good friend. Interacting with such groups then reinforces these attributes as a part of that member's social identity. For example, large families might identify one older member as "matriarch" or "patriarch," meaning that person is looked to for guidance and wisdom, as well as being the keeper of family history and traditions—the "glue that holds the family together." The societal level group membership, however, has a different set of rules. For example, people might identify themselves as Irish (Gerry), Italian Catholic (Gloria), Polish American (Johanna), or Jewish (June, Mildred, Betty)—ethnic and/or religious identities that people do not choose because they come from family background. Some people categorize themselves within stigmatized societal groups that may not be positive, such as lower classes (factory worker), racial minorities (Black), or disability-related groups (autistic, alcoholic, mentally ill). Interestingly, people who resist associating with others in these groups because of their negative labels might actually be missing out on an important benefit. St. Claire and Clucas (2012) found that membership in a marginalized group actually offers a buffer against threats and accusations from outsiders, and that associating with others in disability group networks increases members' willingness to engage in health promoting behaviors.

Sexuality and Health in Older Adulthood

Sexual relationships and intimacy can enhance life satisfaction and well-being throughout adulthood. Many older married couples and sexual partners continue their intimate sexual relationships with sustained desire and enthusiasm. However, negative social attitudes about sex among elders and the onset of chronic health conditions discourages sexual encounters as one ages (Laumann, Nicolosi, & Glasser, 2005). A large-scale study of over 3,000 older Americans (Lindau et al., 2007) found that the majority of older adults are engaged in spousal or other intimate relationships and regard sexuality as an important part of life. Although the prevalence of sexual activity declined with age, a substantial number of men and women engage in vaginal intercourse, oral sex, and masturbation even in the eighth and ninth decades of life. Further findings of this study were the following:

- Women were significantly less likely than men to report sexual activity

- Of those sexually active, half reported at least one bothersome sexual problem

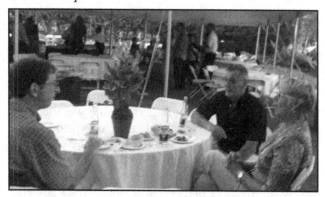

Figure 12-4. Ken and Signian networking at a social event at the university where they both teach part time.

- ○ Women's issues: Low desire, difficulty with vaginal lubrication, inability to climax

  - ○ Men's issues: Erectile difficulties, anxiety about performance

- Those with poor health reported less sexual activity

- Men masturbate (55%) more often than women (23%) without sexual partners

- Only 38% of men and 22% of women had discussed sexual issues with a physician after age 50

The reluctance to discuss sexual issues among older adults is problematic, because it can result in undiagnosed and untreated conditions or social withdrawal. Sexual problems can be a warning sign or a consequence of serious underlying illness, such as diabetes, infection, urogenital tract conditions, cancer, or depression (Lindau et al., 2007).

Through establishing a trusting therapeutic relationship with older clients, OT practitioners may become aware of such issues before other health professionals, and their input can assist clients in getting the medical attention they need. When open discussion is facilitated, other issues can also be addressed. For example, older adults with more than one sexual partner still need to use condoms as protection against unknown sexually transmitted diseases. Because chronic illness might also cause pain or other physical issues that interfere with sexual intimacy, the OT might engage the client (and spouse or partner) in problem solving, including discussions of positioning during sex to minimize pain or discomfort or other adaptations to overcome barriers to enjoyment of this important aspect of social participation.

Learning Activity 88: Discussing Sexuality With Older Adults

During a recent interview with a couple in their 90s on the television show "60 Minutes," the man told Leslie Stahl: "You should be asking us, 'How's your sex life?'" They both were eager to tell her it was active, thriving, and meaning-

ful. Think about how you might approach the topic of sexuality with an older adult client.

1. How might you discuss sexuality with a widow or widower who wishes to re-enter the dating scene?

2. What three questions might you ask an older client with a chronic disability who has a new live-in partner regarding their sexual relationship?

3. How does a client's sexuality relate to OT goals? List and describe three ways.

4. Discuss your own level of comfort in discussing this topic.

5. How do you think an older person might feel about discussing sex with an OT practitioner who is younger?

APPLICATIONS TO CONTINUUM OF CARE

Intentional Efforts in Staying Connected

Community dwelling seniors may continue to socialize as they always have, but when they transition from one phase of life to another, their social networks need to adapt. For example, when clients retire, they need to find ways to continue social relationships with coworkers and colleagues outside the workplace. Our participants have told us that retirees must make an intentional effort to preserve and nurture the connections they formed at work (Figure 12-4). There are many reasons why this is a priority. Work roles over young and middle adulthood often become an important part of a person's social identity. In later life, this social identity is best reinforced by people who remember retired workers at the height of their productivity and can confirm their best occupational performances in the workplace. Coworkers often share many common memories and keep their favorite work stories alive for younger generations to hear about, learn from, and enjoy.

Another common transition occurs when older adults lose a family member or close friend. For example, when an older woman's husband dies, she often finds herself alone, especially after the funeral and immediate formalities end. It is then that she must turn to her children and grandchildren, extended family members, and lifelong friends to support her through the grieving period and help her to build a new life structure. Some people have large networks of friends and family with whom they have nurtured relationships over the years. Others have lost touch and find themselves with no one to confide in after a life tragedy. Social isolation, as the evidence tells us, presents just as high a health risk as smoking and supersedes obesity and physical inactivity as determinants of physical and cognitive decline

(Holt-Lunstad et al., 2010). However, health care professionals and policies have not fully appreciated the importance of social connections as a protector of health and well-being as people age.

Driving and Social Connections

One occupation that facilitates social connections is the ability to drive. Researchers have recently studied the impact of driving cessation in older adulthood on social identity (Jetten & Pachana, 2012). They determined that driving cessation caused changes in both routines of social participation and social identity. Applying a social identity model of change, the best adaptation to any life-changing transition occurs when (1) membership in social groups is maintained, and (2) people take on new social identities to sufficiently replace the ones they leave behind. In this study, current older drivers projected devastating effects of driving cessation, such as "my independence would be horribly compromised," "I would be housebound. No bridge, no Toastmasters," and "marking the transition to the last phase of my life…it would make me feel handicapped and much older." Interestingly, those participants responding with the strongest negative emotions to the prospect of giving up driving were those who belonged to fewer social groups. Those with connections and social groups closer to their homes had fewer fears about making the transition to ex-driver. When comparing current older drivers with ex-drivers, these researchers found that anticipation was usually much worse that reality. Those who had accepted the transition to ex-driver had often rebuilt their lives, keeping their social networks intact, thus minimizing the social identity change and making the loss of driving far less stressful (Jetten & Pachana, 2012).

As part of AOTA's evidence-based practice initiative, Hunt and Arbesman (2008) did a systematic review of 19 studies supporting interventions to improve older driver performance and safety. Motor vehicle injuries are the leading cause of injury-related deaths among 65- to 74-year-olds and the second leading killer (after falls) for those 75 to 84 years (Gorina, Hoyert, Lentzner, & Goulding, 2006). Sources cited the skills required for driving are attention, visuospatial abilities, motor programming and function, judgment, memory, sequencing, and information processing. Of these, OT practitioners can design and use effective interventions focusing on cognition, visual function, motor function, self-regulation and awareness, and the role of passengers. Authors recommend that OTs collaborate with clients to raise their awareness of their own driving abilities and difficulties and to use a multisensory approach, rather than classroom or worksheet instruction (Hunt & Arbesman, 2008). When using computer programs for visual attention, field training, or cognitive training, clients need to understand the relationship between these skills and their ability to drive safely. On-the-road training or behind-the-wheel simulators work best because they require the client to attend to multiple perceptual cues and respond to unpredictable situations. Discussion about driving in challenging conditions, such as dawn or dusk, in heavy traffic, on unlit roads at night, or during rain or snowstorms, encourages older drivers' self-management in planning their road trips carefully. Passengers (two or more) can be distracting, but some studies identify the protective role of passengers, who may help to follow directions, read signs, watch for dangers, and provide guidance, especially at night (Hing, Stamatiadis, & Aultman-Hall, 2003).

The AOTA has identified driving and community mobility as an emerging OT specialty area, complete with an advanced certification course and credential (www.aota.org/olderdriver). For older drivers, OT practitioners can identify strengths, as well as physical, sensory, perceptual, and cognitive challenges, "and evaluate an individual's overall ability to operate a vehicle safely" (AOTA, 2008). OTs can also assess driver-vehicle fit and recommend assistive devices or behavioral changes to increase driving performance and to limit risks.

Learning Activity 89: Exploring Driving Cessation and Social Participation

1. Interview an older adult who can no longer drive. Describe the reasons given for this occurrence and its meaning for this individual.

2. How does driving cessation affect this older adult's socialization?

3. How might OT assist an older adult to continue valued social connections after he or she becomes unable to drive?

Adult Day Care: Expert's Experience— Diane Puterski, Director of Baldwin Senior Center, and Erin McLeod, Director of CARES Program

Older adults with mild disability, living with family caregivers who work, may find themselves alone most of the day. If the disability prevents them from driving, they are more or less housebound without much social interaction. Adult day care can meet the needs of these Fourth Agers need for social connections and activities by offering group programs such as The Community at Risk Elderly Service (CARES) program in Stratford, Connecticut. This subsidized community program accepts 27 to 30 participants at a cost of $15/day. Most participants come because family caregivers work or are seeking respite a few days each week. Many participants have mild to moderate dementia or have balance or mobility issues, making it unwise to leave them alone at home. Because this is a socially based program, participants must still have some level of physical independence. The program provides multiple opportunities for socialization in small groups for coffee hour, lunch, and craft projects, or larger groups for seated exercise, parachute games, or group games like bingo, wheel of fortune, the price is right, word games, or visits from a good citizen dog. The staff try to offer mentally stimulating activities, such as trivial pursuit with old movie themes or reminiscence (tapping into shared long-term memories of historic events). Sing-alongs are a favorite activity using a variety of sensory prompts, and a volunteer playing a donated piano. This program exemplifies a cost-effective method for communities to meet the social needs of both caregivers and those who require care. In addition to respite and support, caregivers benefit from the satisfaction their loved ones express when telling them about their activities at adult day care. Those they care for enjoy the benefit of both mental stimulation and social connection, two important protective mechanisms for health and well-being of older adults.

Assisted Living and Retirement Communities

Social programs offering an often vast array of activities are one of the main selling points of these 50 years and older communities and facilities. For some people, they provide more convenient socialization opportunities, with pools, clubhouses, and golf courses just a few steps outside their doors. For older adults who experience acute or chronic health conditions, OTs may need to provide assistance in self-management, home modification, or remedial interventions to "restore function, compensate for lost skills, adapt the environment or activity to facilitate independence and promote health" (AOTA, 2007). Because these residents still live independently, home health services are available to them just as if they were living in their own homes. The AOTA also suggests that OTs act as consultants to assisted living facilities to provide training to the staff, or to help managers to structure programs and environments that maximize residents' independence and participation. OT services are especially needed when serving older adults with dementia, allowing them to safely remain within such communities (Gitlin & Corcoran, 2005).

Rehabilitation Settings

Patients and clients encountered in rehabilitation facilities usually expect to recover functioning that was impaired because of an acute health condition. Their goals will include resuming some or all of their social and occupational roles, and they often continue to receive social support from family and friends throughout their rehabilitation. Even though some rehabilitation settings still have a narrow medical focus, many are now offering services to help clients transition back to their homes and communities. OT practitioners in these settings often work with family caregivers, perform home evaluations, and assist clients in locating needed services or social support groups in their communities. More could be done with this OT role to enable clients to make needed adaptations within home and community settings so that they could return to their former valued roles and productive occupations.

Because there are often clients in rehabilitation who share common disabilities and occupational issues, OTs could design helpful group interventions, although current reimbursement systems limit their ability to do so. Cotreating with several clients is currently reimbursable by Medicare, but cotreatment is not the same as a group intervention. Groups don't just happen, but rather are skillfully facilitated with the goal of modeling and encouraging supportive interaction and shared learning. OT practitioners have excellent training in group facilitation and would be very effective in this role. Some limited examples have been tried, such as a breakfast group for stroke survivors who are struggling to regain fine motor control in their dominant upper extremities. Groups help them to overcome embarrassment for their less than perfect performance, and the socialization serves as motivation for them to improve (Capasso, Gorman, & Blick, 2010).

Long-Term Care

In skilled nursing facilities, people may need help in connecting with others who are important to them. When Patricia suffered a stroke a few years ago, she moved from an independent apartment setting in her community to a single room in a building with a higher level of care. While her daughters still visited, the friends she had made near her apartment were no longer within walking distance, and because of the stroke she could no longer see well enough to drive. However, when she had recovered sufficiently, she made the effort each week to take the senior van to an exercise class near her old apartment, where she would visit with friends who could still engage in mentally stimulating conversation, as she could. Back in the long-term care setting, she felt more isolated. Surrounded as she was by people with multiple disabilities, Patricia often found herself in a helping role with residents sometimes younger than herself but less capable. While she didn't mind doing that part of the time, she missed the company of others more like herself. Professional staff should give priority to facilitate adaptations and arrangements that may be necessary, so that residents can continue the social connections most valuable and meaningful to them.

Social interaction and retaining social identities can also be facilitated for nursing home residents with dementia. In a recent experimental study, researchers wanted to use reminiscence to develop a "reconstructed identity" from remaining long-term memories in individuals with moderate to severe dementia in a residential care facility (Haslam, Jetten, Haslam, & Knight, 2012). They divided residents into 3 groups meeting over 6 weeks. The first facilitated reminiscence in a small group setting, the second received the same reminiscence one on one with a facilitator, and the third, the control group, played a social game of skittles having nothing to do with memory. Some of their findings were truly serendipity. First, they found that reminiscence improved memory and cognitive functioning *only* in the group format. In fact, for the one-on-one participants, both cognitive functioning and well-being actually declined over the 6 weeks. Next, when comparing both memory enhancement and well-being in the group reminiscence versus the group game of skittles, they found both had improved about equally. To summarize, they concluded that social interaction and the collective sharing of past memories were the critical factors for therapeutic benefit. Group activities involving interaction strengthened participants' social identity and sustained their sense of connection with others, regardless of the severity of their cognitive decline (Haslam et al., 2012).

In another study with nursing home residents, researchers wished to test how the empowerment of residents to make group decisions about their home's interior design might benefit their health and well-being (Knight et al., 2010). They worked with 2 floors, a total of 27 residents without dementia or any other serious diagnosis, who were about to move into a newly renovated building. Residents of the first floor made up an "identity empowered" group, which met formally and informally to make group decisions about colors (selected from a design palette), pictures, and plants to decorate their common areas (corridors, lounge, and dining room). For the control group of second floor residents, these communal spaces were designed for them by professionals, using a similar high standard of quality and an equal amount of money. Data were collected on the strength of their identification with other residents, their life satisfaction, and their physical health before, during, and 4 months after the intervention. They found that: all of these measures were consistently and significantly superior in the empowered condition—both residents and staff reported greater life satisfaction and better physical health over time. Additionally, they found a significant difference between the two groups' use of their redecorated communal spaces. The empowered group used their communal spaces 57% more often than before the intervention, while the control group used their communal spaces 60% less often. After 4 months, the empowered group continued to use their spaces twice as much as the control group. This study provides further evidence that social empowerment, interaction, engagement, and companionship can protect the health and well-being of residents in long-term care (Knight et al., 2012).

OTs have much to contribute regarding how groups are used to encourage social connection within long-term care. Just as OTs have a long history of group interactions within inpatient mental health settings, OT practitioners have also traditionally provided group interventions that help long-term care residents to maintain a feeling of connectedness and to reduce the sense of isolation that often comes with the onset of disability and dependence. One traditional model for long-term care is Ross's (2004) Five Stage Group, which applies sensory integration principles as a basis for group interaction for individuals with diminished cognitive functioning.

JOURNAL ENTRY (M. C.)

Our participants and our literature review have confirmed something I have always felt intuitively—that people have social reasons for almost everything they do. Even when getting dressed in the morning all by ourselves, we are thinking about our internalized social reference groups, our family, our friends, our coworkers—how will they respond to the way we look? Maybe we learn this as adolescents, when we did things that earned us approval or status in our chosen social groups. It seems we never outgrow our deep-seated need to belong. The cable TV show *What Not to Wear* often teaches "contributors" who are nominated for wardrobe makeovers that what they wear and how they feel about their appearance sends a plethora of social messages to others, often unintentional. For one lucky woman each week, this TV show demonstrates the process of gaining self-awareness and, ultimately, control over the messages her appearance sends out into the world. OTs can do the same thing with occupations—give clients "occupational makeovers" that will make them more likely to gain group acceptance and support and enable them to develop and enact meaningful roles in society.

In researching the topic of social connections, I was blown away by the strength of the evidence—that social connections can actually prevent illness, disability, and early death for older adults. As OTs, how can we continue to ignore this truth? Yes, our occupational focus makes us unique, but why do we keep trying to single it out? Occupations cannot realistically be separated from their social contexts because the relationship between them is transactional, engaging in occupation always affects social relationships while these relationships simultaneously change occupational performance. Say your client, Sam, goes bowling with a social club and they divide up into groups of four competing with each other. Even for inexperienced bowlers, what happens when their team is winning? People cheer! Team members offer advice and support. When Sam gets a strike, they might buy him food and drinks. Sam's self-confidence grows, and he feels the pressure to perform even better. Even when he gutters, he bounces back and tries harder to hit that sweet spot, pick up that spare. Whether winning or losing, team members watch and learn from each other. They carefully observe their opponents on other teams, too. And their occupational performance gets better, in part because of the social support they give one another. How can you begin to compare this group experience with someone bowling alone?

There are, of course, occupations that must be done alone. Painting a picture, reading a book, learning to play the piano. As our participant Charlie told me, his craft, writing crime novels, must be done alone. How, then, are these occupations socially embedded? Supposing someone met Charlie at a party, and asked him what he does? Just like when I first met him, he answered, "I'm a writer." He doesn't just say the words, he says them proudly because he's had some success as a writer, publishing his books on Amazon. People have read his books, paid for them, talked about them, reviewed them, and rated them. Being a writer has become an important part of his social identity, an identity that gets reinforced every time he has a conversation with someone about one of his books. As OTs, it is imperative that we find out what occupations make up our clients' social identities, even when they cannot be so easily named.

OTs already have a tried and true method for combining OT interventions within a social context: *groups!* Remember the bowling team? We can do the same for many other occupations, making our therapeutic activities so much more effective. Because a good OT group leader models and teaches the members to listen, empathize, encourage, and support one another in doing whatever is hard or challenging, group members solve together whatever problems they encounter with their occupational goals. As OTs, we should make every effort to offer OT group interventions whenever we can. OT groups can use activities to help members reconnect with others and to strengthen their social identities. Ask them to do activities that remind them of what they used to be good at, used to do well. When the occupation itself isn't possible, ask questions that get them to talk about it, draw it, tell stories about it, and bring photographs. Even people with cognitive disabilities in long-term care can retrieve some images of their former occupations from long-term memory, helping them to recreate at least a part of the social identity they had lost. No matter how low their level of mental functioning, they still crave and respond to social support, and they still need to feel a sense of belonging. OT groups can do this, given the opportunity. I hope all of the OT students and practitioners reading this will realize the critical importance of groups for the older adults we serve.

IMPLICATIONS FOR OCCUPATIONAL THERAPY PRACTICE

The importance of social connections has a central role in productive aging and for this reason needs to be promoted within the context of OT group design and facilitation, as has been suggested throughout this text. Group leadership has been defined as an extension of therapeutic use of self with groups of clients, and OT group facilitation has been structured around client-centered principles to maximize member participation (Cole, 2012). Groups, like all OT interventions, work differently within different frames of reference, and the design of the group depends on client functional status and occupational goals. However the common thread among all OT group interventions is the facilitation of client interaction.

Occupational Therapy Groups to Promote Social Skills and Participation

All of the productive occupations and roles, and the abilities and tasks implied within them, can become the focus of a group intervention. OTs are referred to Cole's (2012) *Group Dynamics in Occupational Therapy* for a deeper description of, and education and training in, the skills of OT group leadership, as well as the facilitation of positive client interactions to support and assist one another. Mosey (1986), and later Cole and Donohue (2011), defined 5 levels of group interaction: (1) parallel, (2) associative, (3) basic cooperative, (4) supportive cooperative, and (5) mature. These levels shift greater responsibility for member self-leadership as they move up the scale from parallel to mature, with mature groups able to operate on their own, cooperate with one another, and meet group goals within the limits of the sponsoring organization; examples would be a group of scientists and engineers working on research and development of new medications for a pharmaceutical corporation, or a group of engineers and programmers developing new computer software. Even these so-called mature groups have issues that interfere with their success when individual members exhibit less mature behaviors, such as trying to control others, dominate the group's work, or violate the groups' trust through outside influences. At a therapeutic level, OTs can openly discuss the group interaction skills that lead to successful outcomes, and the behaviors that can compromise group goals and those of individual members. Unlike work groups, OT groups generally have the goal of building the social interaction skills that enable members to support one another, empathize with one another, and offer assistance to one another, sharing their own successes and failures as lessons and working together on solving problems and overcoming barriers. A well-educated OT practitioner can design a group using any focus that relates to productive aging, use a variety of OT theories, models, and frames of reference along with supporting evidence, and build a group experience that enhances client learning by enabling the addition of social and emotional support for each other that comes from the other clients who are group members.

OT group interventions, designed in this way to support the occupations of productive aging, can also offer the added value of encouraging and modeling the skills that clients need to build and maintain the social relationships, networks, and connections that will sustain them through the natural or unexpected transitions of growing older. In this way, OT group participation can help older adults to continue to age productively.

Advocating Occupational Therapy Groups for Productive Aging in Communities

With the preponderance of evidence supporting social connections as a central factor in the prevention of illness and disability, it is surprising that more OT practitioners have not promoted their considerable educational background in group facilitation. Most communities do their best to reach out to older adults, but they need a professional such as an OT with the combination of medical knowledge and group facilitation skills to establish appropriate programming for older adults aging in place.

The OTPF III (AOTA, 2014) defines OT group interventions as: "Use of distinct knowledge and leadership techniques to facilitate learning and skill acquisition across the lifespan through the dynamics of group and social interaction. Groups may also be used as a method of service delivery" (p. S31). The OT group interventions listed are: "functional groups, activity groups, task groups, social groups, and other groups used on inpatient units, within the community, or in schools that allow clients to explore and develop skills for participation, including basic social interaction skills, tools for self-regulation, goal setting, and positive choice making" (AOTA, 2014, p. S31).

Learning Activity 90: Finding Occupational Therapy Group Examples

Search *OT Practice, Advance for OT,* or other publications for examples of OT group interventions with older adults. List and describe three here with references.

1.

2.

3.

Many of the published community programs for older adults have involved OT students from a local university; they often combine wellness and prevention programming for community members with research and fieldwork experiences for the students.

Other examples of groups offered by OTs are those used within the Well Elderly Studies (Clark et al., 1997, 2011; Mountain & Craig, 2011). See Chapter 1 for examples of OT group modules from these studies.

Learning Activity 91: Exploring Leisure Groups

1. Choose three leisure activities that older adults might enjoy, and search the Internet for groups that focus on this activity. Describe one such group for each leisure activity.

2. Explain how performing leisure occupations with the group helps older adults to expand their social connections.

SUMMARY

Our participants spoke extensively about the importance of social connections—a key factor for aging successfully. The evidence for staying connected with others in protecting against illness and disability as one ages is overwhelming, yet OTs and others in the health professions have not adequately addressed the social needs of older clients. Clearly, this needs to change. One way that OT can incorporate socialization into treatment is by designing group interventions. OTs can now advocate for payment for groups, armed with the strong evidence that now exists for its greater effectiveness within both OT (Well Elderly Studies) and interdisciplinary literature.

REFERENCES

Adams, K. B. (2004). Changing investment in activities and interests in elders' lives: Theory and measurement. *International Journal of Aging and Human Development, 58,* 87-108.

Adams, K. B., Roberts, A., & Cole, M. (2011). Changes in activity and interest in the Third and Fourth Age: Associations with health, functioning, and depressive symptoms. *Occupational Therapy International, 18,* 4-17.

American Occupational Therapy Association. (2007). *Occupational therapy's role in driving and community mobility across the lifespan: Driving and transportation alternatives for older adults. AOTA Fact Sheets.* Bethesda, MD: Author.

American Occupational Therapy Association. (2008). *Occupational therapy's role in assisted living facilities. AOTA Fact Sheets.* Bethesda, MD: Author.

American Occupational Therapy Association. (2014). *Occupational therapy practice framework: Domain & Process* (3rd ed.) *American Journal of Occupational Therapy, 68,* S1-S48.

Antonucci, T. C., & Jackson, J. S. (2002). Environmental factors, life events and coping abilities. In J. Copeland, M. Abou-Saleh, & D. Blazer (Eds.), *Principles and practice of geriatric psychiatry* (2nd ed., pp. 379-380). New York: Wiley.

Baum, C., & Christiansen, C. (2005). Person-environment-occupation-performance: An occupation based framework for practice. In C. Christiansen & C. Baum (Eds.), *Occupational therapy: Performance, participation, and well-being* (pp. 242-267). Thorofare, NJ: SLACK Incorporated.

Berkman, L. F. (2000). Social support, social networks, social cohesion and health. *Social Work Health Care, 31,* 3-14.

Cannuscio, C., Block, J., & Kawachi, I. (2003). Social capital and successful aging: The role of senior housing. *Annals of Internal Medicine, 139,* 395-399.

Capasso, N., Gorman, A., & Blick, C. (2010). Breakfast groups in an acute care setting: A restorative program for incorporating clients' hemiparetic upper extremities for function. *OT Practice,* May 10, 14-18.

Carstensen, L. L., Isaacowitz, D. M., & Charles, S. T. (1999). Taking time seriously: A theory of socioemotional selectivity. *American Psychologist, 54,* 165-181.

Christakis, N. (2009). Preface. In N. Christakis & J. Fowler (Eds.), *Connected: How your friends' friends' friends affect everything you feel, think, and do* (pp. xiii-xvii). New York, NY: Little, Brown & Co.

Christakis, N., & Fowler, J. (2009). *Connected: How your friends' friends' friends affect everything you feel, think, and do.* New York: Little, Brown & Co.

Clark, F., Azen, S., Carlson, M., Mandel, D., Zemke, R., Hay, J., … Lipson, L. (1997). Occupational therapy for independent living older adults: A randomized controlled trial. *Journal of the American Medical Association, 278,* 1321-1326.

Clark, F., Jackson, J., Carlson, M., Chou, C., Cherry, B., Jordan-Marsh, M., & Azen, S. (2011). Effectiveness of a lifestyle intervention in promoting the well-being of independently living older people: Results of the Well Elderly 2 Randomized Controlled Trial. *Journal of Epidemiology and Community Health.* Retrieved from http://jech.bmj.com/content/early/2011/06/01/jech.2009.099754.abstract.

Cole, M. (2012). *Group dynamics in occupational therapy* (4th ed.). Thorofare, NJ: SLACK Incorporated.

Cole, M., & Donohue, M. (2011). *Social participation in occupational contexts: In schools, clinics, and communities.* Thorofare, NJ: SLACK Incorporated.

Cornwell, B., Laumann, E., & Schumm, P. (2008). The social connectedness of older adults: A national profile. *American Sociology Review, 73,* 185-203.

Donohue, M. (2011). Social capital: A systems perspective. In *Social Participation in Occupational Therapy* (pp. 67-80). Thorofare, NJ: SLACK Incorporated.

Erikson, E. (1963). *Childhood and society.* New York: Norton.

Gitlin, L. N., & Corcoran, M. A. (2005). *Occupational therapy and dementia care: The home environmental skill-building program for individuals and families.* Bethesda, MD: American Occupational Therapy Association Press.

Glass, T. A., Mendes de Leon, C. F., Seeman, T. E., & Berkman, L. F. (1997). Beyond single indicators of social networks: A LISREL analysis of social ties among the elderly. *Social Science Medicine, 26,* 737-749.

Gorina, Y., Hoyert, D., Lentaner, H., & Goulding, M. (2006). *Trends in causes of death among older persons in the United States (Aging Trends #6).* Hyattville, MD: National Center for Health Statistics.

Gray, A. (2009). The social capital of older people. *Aging and Society, 29,* 5-31.

Haslam, C., Jetten, J., Haslam, S. A., & Knight, C. (2012). The importance of remembering and deciding together: Enhancing the health and well-being of older adults in care. In J. Jetten, A. Haslam, & C. Haslam (Eds.), *The social cure* (pp. 297-316). New York: Psychology Press.

Hing, J., Stamatiadis, N., & Aultman-Hall, L. (2003). Evaluating the impact of passengers on the safety of older drivers. *Journal of Safety Research, 34,* 343-351.

Holmes, W., & Joseph, J. (2011). Social participation and healthy aging: A neglected, significant protective factor for chronic non communicable conditions. *Globalization and Health.* Retrieved from http://www.globalizationandhealth.com/content/7/1/43.

Holt-Lunstad, J., Smith, T. B., & Bradley Layton, J. (2010). Social relationships and mortality risk: A meta-analytic review. *PLoS Med. 7*(7), e1000316. Doi:10.1371/journal.pmed.1000316. Retrieved from www.plosmedicine.org.

Hunt, L., & Arbesman, M. (2008). Evidence-based and occupational perspective of effective interventions for older clients that remediate or support improved driving performance. *American Journal of Occupational Therapy, 62,* 136-148.

Jetten, J., Haslam, A., & Haslam, C. (2012). *The social cure.* New York: Psychological Press.

Jetten, J., & Pachana, N. (2012). Not wanting to grow old: A social identity model of identity change (SIMIC) analysis of driving cessation among older adults. In J. Jetten, A. Haslam, & C. Haslam (Eds.), *The social cure* (pp. 97-114). New York: Psychological Press.

Keyes, C. L. (2002). The exchange of emotional support with age and its relationship with emotional well-being by age. *Journal of Gerontology Series B: Psychological and Social Sciences, 57,* P518-P525.

Kielhofner, G. (2008). *Model of human occupation* (4th ed.). Baltimore, MD: Lippincott, Williams & Wilkins.

Knight, C., Haslam, C., & Haslam, A. (2010). In home or at home: Evidence that collective decision making enhances older adults' social identification, well-being, and use of communal space when moving into a new care facility. *Aging and Society, 30,* 1393-1418.

Laumann, E., Nicolosi, A., Glasser, D.; and the GSSAB Investigators' Group. (2005). Sexual problems among women and men aged 40-80 years: Prevalence and correlates identified in the Global Study of Sexual Attitudes and Behaviors. *International Journal of Impotence Research, 17,* 39-57.

Lindau, S., Schumm, L. P., Laumann, E., Levinson, W., O'Muircheartaigh, C., & Waite, L. (2007). A study of sexuality and health among older adults in the United States. *New England Journal of Medicine, 357,* 762-774.

Litwin, H., & Shiovitz-Ezra, S. (2010). Social network type and subjective well-being in a national sample of older Americans. *The Gerontologist, 51,* 379-388.

Lyyra, T. M., & Heikkinen, R. I. (2006). Perceived social support and mortality in older people. *Journals of Gerontology: Series B, Psychological Sciences and Social Sciences, 61B,* S147-S152.

McAdams, D. P., Hart, H. M., & Maruna, A. S. (1998). The anatomy of generativity. In D. McAdams & E. de St. Aubin (Eds.), *Generativity and adult development* (pp. 7-43). Washington, DC: American Psychological Association.

Melchior, M., Berkman, L. F., Niedhammer, I., Chea, M., & Goldberg, M. (2003). Social relations and self-reported health: A prospective analysis of the French Gazel cohort. *Social Sciences Medicine, 56,* 1817-1830.

Mosey, A. C. (1986). *Psychosocial components of occupational therapy.* New York: Raven Press.

Mosey, A. (1996). *Applied scientific inquiry in the health professions: An epistemological orientation* (2nd ed.). Bethesda, MD: American Occupational Therapy Association.

Mountain, G., & Craig, C. (2011). The lived experience of redesigning lifestyle post-retirement in the UK. *Occupational Therapy International, 18,* 48-58.

Richard, L., Gauvin, L., Gosselin, C., & Laforest, S. (2008). Staying connected: Neighborhood correlates of social participation among older adults living in an urban environment in Montreal, Quebec. *Health Promotion International, 24,* 46-57.

Ross, M. (2004). A five-stage model for adults with developmental disabilities. In M. Ross & S. Bachner (Eds.), *Adults with developmental disabilities: Current approaches in occupational therapy* (pp. 250-267). Bethesda, MD: AOTA Press.

Rowe, J., & Kahn, R. (1998). *Successful aging.* New York: Pantheon.

Spencer, J. (2003). Evaluation of performance contexts. In E. Crepeau, E. Cohn, & B. Schell (Eds.), *Willard & Spackman's occupational therapy* (10th ed., pp. 427-449). Philadelphia, PA: Lippincott, Williams & Wilkins.

St. Claire, L., & Clucas, C. (2012). In sickness and in health: Influences of social categorizations on health-related outcomes. In. J. Jetten, A. Haslam, & C. Haslam (Eds.), *The social cure* (pp. 75-96). New York, NY: Psychological Press.

Stone, W. (2003). *Ageing, social capital and social support.* Australia Institute of Family Studies submission to the House of Representatives Committee on Ageing Inquiry. Retrieved from www.aifs.gov.au/institute/pubs/research.

Tajfel, H. (1978). *Social identity and intergroup relations.* Cambridge, MA: Cambridge University Press.

Vaillant, G. (1993). *Wisdom of the ego.* Cambridge, MA: Harvard University Press.

Veninga, J. (2006). *Social capital and health: Maximizing the benefits.* Health Canada Reports & Publications. Retrieved from www.hc-sc.gc.ca/sr-sr/hpr-rpms/bull/2006capital-social.

Westermeyer, J. (2004). Predictors and characteristics of Erikson's life cycle model among men: A 32 year longitudinal study. *International Journal of Aging and Human Development, 58,* 29-48.

White, A., Philogene, S., Fine, L., & Sinha, S. (2009). Social support and self-reported health status of older adults in the United States. *American Journal of Public Health, 99,* 1872-1878. Retrieved from www.medscape.com/viewarticle/714356_print.

World Health Organization. (2001). *International classification of functioning, disability and health.* Geneva: Author.

13

Self-Fulfilling Activities

Karen C. Macdonald, PhD, OTR/L

Self-fulfilling activities, the third main theme of the PAS, is an umbrella term selected to incorporate leisure, recreation, hobbies, sports, "play," and religious observance. The unique feature of self-fulfilling activities comes from their personal meaning, performed for the simple joy of doing them. Each activity is quite different in nature, but all contributed to a participant's sense of enjoyment, personal growth, satisfaction, and quality of life. Self-fulfillment comes from developmental theory, as an important life task of Laslett's Third Age (1989, 1997), incorporating that large segment of the older population who are retired but still healthy and engaged. This resonates with the participants in the PAS, who actively sought out self-fulfillment through their activity choices and described them as contributing to their own personal growth and satisfaction.

Self-fulfilling activities may also be called *avocational*, meaning they are performed for pleasure or diversion, outside of the context of one's work or vocation. Avocational is a broader term, encompassing hobbies, crafts, games, and sports, as well as other outside interests, such as collecting antiques, stamps, or coins. The term avocational implies an amateur status, something done for fun, often without prior training, experience or skill, and for which one does not get paid.

The AOTA's (2014) OTPF III identifies play and leisure as occupations within the OT domain. *Play* is defined as "any spontaneous or organized activity that provides enjoyment, entertainment, amusement, or diversion (Parham & Fazio, 1997, p. 150)" (AOTA, 2014, p. S21). *Leisure* is distinguished as "a nonobligatory activity that is intrinsically motivated and engaged in during discretionary time, that is time not committed to obligatory occupations such as work, self-care, or sleep" (Parham & Fazio, 1997, p. 250; AOTA, 2014). Both play and leisure imply self-directed participation in tasks that may or may not be connected to other areas of occupation (ADL, IADL, sleep, education, work, and social participation). Leisure includes two phases: exploration and participation. *Exploration* relates to identifying and planning for potential self-fulfilling occupations that meet individual client interests, including attention to matching skills to appropriate activity choices. *Participation* is described as actual engagement in the play or leisure activity, including attention to rules, use and care of tools or supplies, and need to balance with other life tasks.

JOURNAL ENTRY (K. M.)

As another layer of trustworthiness, I designed a homework assignment for my Task Analysis 2013 class at Housatonic Community College. The OTA students were asked to interview an older adult about leisure activity performance. The 11 individuals interviewed by the students confirmed many of the findings of the PAS:

- Leisure activities have consistently held importance.

- A variety of occupations are enjoyed by each person.

- Awareness of promoting health and ability through activities.

Cole MB, Macdonald KC.
Productive Aging: An Occupational Perspective (pp 215-230).
© 2015 Taylor & Francis Group.

- Found ways to modify or adapt to allow for continued engagement as needed with increasing age and/or emerging health conditions.
- "I will never give up what I love to do."
- Both solitary and social activities were selected.

They reinforced findings that leisure activities had deep meaning and were important pursuits for well-being and life satisfaction.

When I think of the broad spectrum of leisure activities that have had meaning to me over my lifetime, I feel very fortunate. Both my parents were always working on something, creating or building a project, learning a new art or craft. I always wanted to be watching and copying. As member of Girl Scouts from Brownie to high school graduation, which badge could I earn that related to making or creating something? Sunday School at church, and later Youth Group, often consisted of interesting craft or group projects. For holidays, my mother would give me a kit or supplies to challenge myself—candle-making, linoleum block printing, loom weaving, Icelandic knitting. All those 13 years of studying French left me with one special memory—the verb "faire," meaning "to make" or "to do." We don't have an English equivalent, but life has completely revolved around what I could make or do. I was destined to become an OT, where I could share this passion as a tool for therapy. I could create, design, and adapt activities to enhance a patient's personal patterns of doing. So often that assisted the patient in much more motivated participation in therapy and contributed to a sense of *feeling like myself* once again.

PARTICIPANT PERSPECTIVES

Self-fulfilling activities gave significant meaning to the participants' lives. Their choices reflected a spectrum from lifelong interests (reading) to recently acquired tasks (Sudoku). Leisure activities ranged from passive observation (television) to very active engagement (caning chairs). Some were seen as hobbies or interests, others as personal pursuits with ongoing skill development (quilting). Motivations included physical, social, and intellectual stimulation vs. relaxation. All were seen as personal pursuits with personal meaning. The occupations did not appear as a means to "fill time." Instead, they held an important place in the individuals' daily and weekly schedules.

Enjoying the Finer Things in Life

Cultural events were defined as entertainment or personal interests outside of the home, such as theater, concerts, opera, educational speakers, or museums and galleries, all reflecting some variety of visual or performance arts. Participants described how this could be a solitary and personal experience or shared with others as a social event. Although museums and galleries involved standing and walking to participate, they gave the sense of personally interacting with the objects on view.

Greg was representative of those who listed many areas of personal interest, with a diverse personal interpretation of the meaning of self-fulfilling activity. He identified that he "appreciate[s] beautiful things, loves traveling, music, art and theater…Fine dining, investing in collector's items and fine art. I believe in gay marriage but I am not an activist and am non-religious, politically conservative. I like to enjoy the finer things in life now that I am retired." He formerly cut hair for well-known actresses and enjoys telling stories from those experiences.

Peggie also identified a mixed bag of interests, stating that she continues with some professional activities as a nurse practitioner. She showed how she enjoys a balance of many interests, including big band music, singing in a choir, traveling to new places, and always learning. She spoke of participating in an investment club and following up on that. She stated that faith in God was important to her and believed in the benefit of prayer and helping the less fortunate.

Bob C. stated that he enjoys being a New Yorker, frequents the New York Library, and enjoys taking free college classes. Gloria appreciates having season tickets to the opera and ballet and enjoys New York City theater. Whether living in the theater capital of the world or a suburban community, participants found ways to enjoy the performing arts. Phyllis described how, "our local university has a 'Live at the Met' opera series to which I've subscribed. I also attend local live theater stage performances. There is also a local company that offers 1-day getaway trips by bus to area attractions. I love to go to museums and art galleries—my latest trip to Massachusetts included a visit to see the new wing of the Fine Arts Museum in Boston, and the Peabody/Essex museum in Salem for a special exhibit of Ansel Adams' photography; and in Maine, the Ogunquit Museum where a special collection of Charles H. Woodbury seascapes were on display."

Movies, Theater, and Television

Movies and theater were more sedentary and passive participation, yet contributed strongly to a sense of a meaningful and enjoyable planned activity, viewed either at home or in theaters. Some watched older movies and enjoyed reminiscing about classics they liked in the past or caught up on movies they had never seen over the years. Others appreciated more modern films and being able to relate to media coverage that often focuses on celebrities. They wished to keep up with the latest trends and be able to discuss current movies with friends and family. Movies were discussed from a perspective of appreciating them as interesting, moving, and contributing to new things to think about.

They contrasted this with television, with some stating that the quality had deteriorated over the years and therefore they preferred to watch movies. Complaints were also raised about the increasing frequency of commercials on television. Another common comment was about the ability to hear dialogue in movies and television shows because a soundtrack often is superimposed with music or the actors do not enunciate. Ann M. said it sounds "as if they are mumbling, and I miss half of their sentences." Current technology allows for endless choices for variety of films for viewing at one's own convenience. This provided a sense of freedom to be able to select desired films rather than be limited to available programming.

Judi H. stated, "I really enjoy movies, in the evening or afternoon, and keeping up with newer ones." When asked about cultural event participation, Maxine replied "movies, it's nice to be able to go with friends, we enjoy a matinee." Bob M. shared that "I like to watch old movies, catch up on ones not seen, [either] on TV or from the library." Even the task of a movie rental was a nice opportunity to get out of the house and into the community and possibly visit with staff members or another patron at the library. Appreciating new options for viewing movies at home, Malcolm stated that he enjoys "artsy" movies, typically Janus and Netflix options.

Learning Activity 92: Movies, History, and Culture

1. Create a timeline of the last 100 years, with demarcations by decade.

2. List 5 top popular movies for each decade.

3. Select one of the classic movies from the 1930s, 1940s, or 1950s that you have never seen and view it.

4. Write a 1-page reaction paper on how the world has changed since that era and how the popular culture of that era may have influenced the individuals who are now seniors.

Creative Expression

Many participants identified creative endeavors, either newly learned or well-loved over past years. They included musical performance, painting and drawing, needlecrafts, woodworking, and creative writing, among others. Although some of the self-fulfilling activities were "for fun" or pleasure, many were specifically selected to relate to an interest, but also to facilitate some aspect of personal growth. Ken described attempting to master a musical instrument. Margie is a singer with a folk group in her church. Singing in church choirs was also enjoyed by Peggie, Geno, Judi, Jan,

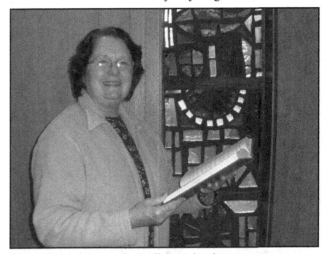
Figure 13-1. Judi sings in Senior Choir at church.

and others (Figure 13-1). Mary D. relaxes by playing the piano and plays for sing-a-longs at parties.

Signian identified her leisure interests as quilting, watercolors, colored pencil drawing, reading, swimming, gardening, dogs, travel, cooking, and walking. She did not describe any of them in particular, but it was known that she works diligently to develop skills for creative activities through workshops and classes. Jan also described a mix of interests and pursuits, stating that she does baking, sewing and other crafts in the context of church/social activities. Gloria stated that she enjoys needlepoint and crocheting, and that she knits clothing for new babies in her large family. A number of participants expressed that craft occupations were not for their personal use, but rather for gifts or donations to others.

Women tended to mention needle crafts most often, applying creativity in their color selections and designs. Nancy B. has a love of quilting. She has always enjoyed sewing, but in recent years became active with quilting. Along with making items at home, she works with others in a quilting group and a guild (Figure 13-2). "I work with people related to quilting on several levels for fundraising and exhibits. Now, I feel like I can do things again; I was so sick for so long." Mary V. described how "I like to crochet but I am having difficulty with arthritic bones. They say, 'use it or lose it' but it is too painful, so I don't."

June described her enjoyment of learning something new, "something you've never done before...I'm taking classes in painting and rug hooking, make it your own and be creative. Sometimes I do my own drawings on canvas. I go to thrift stores searching for good woolen clothes, and cut the strips for hooking original colors and textures."

Bob M. is very active with making wooden projects and restoring furniture (Figure 13-3). He has returned to a former interest of caning chairs, which requires immense skills for preparation, concentration, planning, and coordination. Because it is nearly a lost art, he finds great

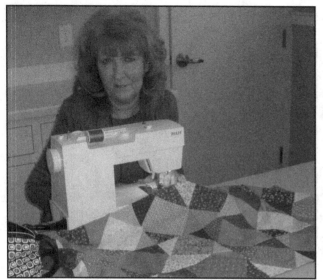

Figure 13-2. Nancy enjoys the creativity of quilting, as well as making a useful product for fundraisers.

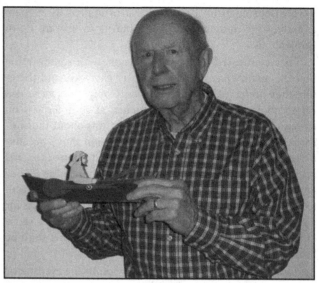

Figure 13-3. Bob M. enjoys woodworking in his retirement.

satisfaction in continuing on with this tradition of fine handwork. He also has a hobby of compiling old photographs into albums, which is much appreciated by his family. Recently, he discovered old photo negatives from his young adulthood and has been having them professionally developed. His children were fascinated as stories they had heard throughout their lives were now made real through these photographs.

Jack identified woodworking as an interest on many levels. He has a woodworking shop in his garage and described it as a social activity. For 11 years, he was the president of a woodworking guild and now acts as advisor to the president and is a member of the program committee. He loves making things from wood, especially using hand tools. He also does construction projects with his three sons, who are in that business. He helps with putting additions on homes, a new roof, a deck, or renovation projects. He states that "woodworking is relaxing, I like making useful things for friends and family."

Patricia described how she "loves writing poetry, memoirs, diaries, and autobiographical stories." She does this for her grandchildren. She is also writing cultural impressions of being an Australian who married an American, while living in India and then coming to America during World War II. It was inspiring to think of the valued memories that she was able to preserve and share for future enjoyment by family members. So many individuals think of such projects as a good idea but never get around to them.

Exercise and Sports

A personal fitness program was often identified as informal but important. Some participants would go to a gym on a regular basis, others walked or jogged a certain number of times a week. Most engaged in activities such as walking, swimming, or playing tennis with less of a scheduled plan, but many identified the need to remain active and moving in some way.

Maxine said that her "gentleman friend is 92, and he plays tennis three times a week. His mother died just before her 100th birthday and she was still volunteering. I like to watch sports on TV." Enjoying sports on television is a passive activity, yet because of the nature of the games, leads to mental stimulation and social interaction through discussion.

Until age 85, Bob M. was square dancing and bicycling, and continues to hike and sail. He remarked that, "I don't have any barriers except I have to let up on heavy lifting, but medium lifting is OK. Things seem to get heavier as I get older! I play one game of pool against myself to keep myself calmed down. I invented it: it is like golf except pool, I count how many balls in how many strokes." Malcolm, who has many intellectual interests, shares that he also enjoys professional sports, identifying football, hockey, boxing, and bullfights specifically, chuckling as he specifies that it is as a spectator. Jack utilizes a YMCA gym and finds that to be social activity as well. He enjoys biking with friends. He stays active in several ways, including playing sports, sailing, and doing yard work.

Learning Activity 93: Senior Sports and Exercise

Sports and exercise maintained a position as priority activities for the study participants.

1. Identify 10 sports activities that could be enjoyed by well elders.

   a.

   b.

c.

d.

e.

f.

g.

h.

i.

j.

2. For each activity, identify 3 ways in which it could be graded for simplicity as needed.

Men and Cars

Automobile maintenance and minor repairs were seen as almost "fun" for many of the men, who grew up in an era when most young men could fix their own cars. A few of the participants identified enjoying cars as an interest, appreciating either restoring an older model, or maintaining their current vehicle. Greg takes great pride in driving his Mercedes sports car, a gift to himself when he sold his business a few years ago. Ken restored a classic Corvette, which he drove to car "rallies" in good weather as a social activity, or to compete in mini-drag races (Figure 13-4).

Reading for Pleasure

Jan stated that she is a book club member, for both social and intellectually stimulating purposes, and enjoys the discussions. Maxine stated that she enjoys reading. She volunteers in a thrift store and many of the volunteers enjoy trading the latest bestsellers. Vi belongs to "two book clubs. You are forced to read books you wouldn't read otherwise, then you are able to discuss it with others." Phyllis said that she does "a lot of reading—mostly historical novels, and I have a Kindle, although I still like the feel of a book!" Dave H. described how "I read a lot. Historical or novels. I am interested in the history of my town, so I read a lot and I've...lived through it."

Marylyn commented how "some days are happily busy with a million things, and then there are days when I just sit and read all day. My eyes are still good, my ears not so much. I am sick of TV. I follow all trends, news, weather, stocks."

Learning Activity 94: Reading and Low Vision

Perform an online search for equipment and devices available for seniors who are visually impaired and wish to continue with their love of reading. Choose three devices or

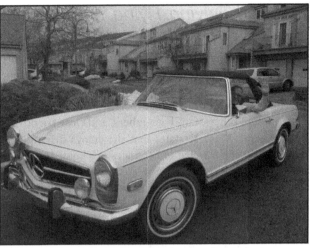
Figure 13-4. Greg's classic Mercedes.

applications to briefly describe below and provide the web references.

1.

2.

3.

Cooking and Gardening

Geno, in his early retirement, was enjoying having more time to cook, try new recipes, and learn about baking. "It's fun to enter contests at county fairs with my baking." Maxine stated that she enjoys eating out or cooking at home. "We belong to a group, once a week in the summer, we have a pot luck at the beach. In the winter, it is once a month in someone's home."

Mary said, "I garden as much as I can. It's not the same, but I do what I can do." Linval stated that he loves "to do gardening, plant flowers and make flower beds. Sometimes older people hire me to do that for their yards too." Phyllis described how "I had to stop outdoor gardening due to a back problem, but I still keep flowers in pots next to my patio."

Learning Activity 95: Adapted Gardening

Gardening remains a pleasurable occupation for many seniors.

1. What three considerations could the OT recommend if the person wished to participate in indoor or patio gardening?

2. How would you adapt an at-home gardening activity for a person who is confined to a wheelchair?

Traveling, Driving, Flying, and Touring

Travel for self-fulfillment can stem from the new freedom of being retired with no set schedule, from curiosity about other parts of the world, or as a way to spend time with family and friends. In most of the examples given, traveling was a co-occupation, experienced in the company of significant others, family members, and close friends.

In general, Mary V. states that she enjoys driving. She recalled how she traveled to her ancestor's home in Ireland after working on genealogy. She was excited that they were able to go to the actual ship area where her grandmother had traveled at age 19 to come to America to build a new life. "I hope I am from some of that stock." It was interesting to see how the research, designed with semi-structured and open-ended questions, led the participants to describe many parts of their lives—their memories, activities, and interests. Some topics brought back memories, but most were focusing on the here and now.

Maxine had been a travel agent and has traveled worldwide for many years. "We travel considerably, visiting friends, for pleasure, for example, an upcoming trip to Switzerland and we just got back from Hawaii for an Army reunion." Marilyn recalled how she and her husband traveled, "I have good memories of trips, and we traveled all over." She was proud of her exceptional ability to recall these memories that had deep meaning to her and she enjoyed reliving many adventures far from home.

Nettie exclaimed, "I can't believe it, but I fly in an airplane, a small one!! My friend knows a pilot and he takes us up!" She would never have dreamed years ago that she would be flying over local areas and seeing the sights from above, but now enjoys the thrill of it, awed at the opportunity. She also shared that she enjoys any kind of traveling, and often arranges for short weekend trips with friends.

In her earlier retirement years, Phyllis said that "it was a joy to travel, through the Elderhostel program in Arizona's Grand Canyon, the California Coast, the Shakespeare Festival in Ashland, Oregon, and the Canadian Rockies.... Also, it was an absolute thrill to go to Israel with a younger cousin and to England and France with an older son!"

Many of the participants were regular travelers for long distances. This was usually related to visiting with family who had moved from home or to return to the participants' native area. Women described how they had left the area in which they had grown up to be with their husband as opportunities for employment were available far from their home. Alice stated "I travel to see my grandkids—their parents are actors, they don't travel here together. I go to Washington, D.C., where my daughter is writing a musical. My own family [siblings] met in May, we decided to sell the farm. I just lost a sister, then my other sister took ill and her husband too. I stayed with my brother; we have to convert all the papers after she died. So, I'm involved in these long distance affairs [in the Midwest]." This highlighted that

some active seniors travelled not only for pleasure, but also for personal reasons.

Learning Activity 96: Adapting for Travel

1. What is the process (steps) for a woman at age 85 who is using a walker, for traveling by plane to visit a daughter in another state? List in priority sequence the steps from initial idea to arriving at the daughter's home.

2. Search airline websites and give one specific airline as an example of the accommodations available. What accommodations could the client in number 1 request from the airline?

3. What needed accommodations are *not* available? What might an OT, in a letter to an airline, report as areas of concern for older travelers?

Computers

New forms of entertainment may be found at various websites, such as YouTube, cable and network TV Websites, or computer game applications such as Words with Friends (a Scrabble-like game played through Facebook or e-mail). Generations can interact from afar through many of these sites.

Several of the participants were new or recent users of personal computers, while others had evolved with computer skills as technology developed. Malcolm said that "at this time, my principal activity is learning a computer language, JAVA, that is brand new to me. I'm doing this because my second son, who is not a programmer, must pass a JAVA-based course at Harvard Extension to complete his MS in information technology. He needs help and I will provide it."

Learning Activity 97: Computers for Older Adults

1. What interventions could an OT offer for a client who wishes to increase his or her skills with computer use, but:

   a. has some mild challenges with short-term memory?

   b. has limited endurance for sitting at a table?

   c. has visual perceptual problems?

Career Skills as Self-Fulfillment

Charlie explained that he transitioned from professional freelance writer for advertising and comedy for television to a more challenging type in his retirement. He currently writes crime fiction novels and self publishes on Amazon. He shared that he is "highly disciplined, focused, and creative," which contributes to his ongoing participation in his writing by choice.

Bob C. continues his former work role at home by managing assets for others, as well as their taxes. He describes himself as a planner and saver, and advises "having a stable allocation of assets so you can worry less in retirement." It was apparent that what would be considered difficult or tedious work to some individuals was viewed as an interesting and pleasurable pursuit by these participants. It was also impressive to note that no matter where they lived, the majority of the participants were aware of community resources and utilized them.

Other participants continued in their prior career occupations, finding them to be self-fulfilling. Although retired, Pearl maintains her identity as an English professor by continuing to teach part time. She continues to enjoy reading and participates in ongoing scholarship with former colleagues. Johanna recommended to others to "keep doing what you love" and she provided an amazing example in her own life. She continued practicing elder law, even while receiving chemo treatments in the hospital, up until 3 days before her death from ovarian cancer at age 73. Mildred also expressed that writing gives her the most fulfillment (she occasionally revises her chapters written for others), but that she also enjoys cooking, friendship, and family activities.

The activities described by participants often formed a part of another productive occupation. Cooking, gardening, and maintaining a car were self-fulfilling activities within the occupation of home manager, continued teaching and writing were part of paid worker roles, and voluntary musical and artistic performance might be part of a religious program or might help to raise funds for charity. Reading and traveling are also forms of lifelong learning. Good self-managers incorporate mental and physical exercise into an intentionally healthy lifestyle. In sharing their enjoyment of self-fulfilling activities with others, participants almost always described a social component. Many of the occupations described provided a valued end product, but the participants seemed to especially enjoy the process involved during the actual doing of the task.

LITERATURE REVIEW

Publications within and outside the OT body of literature describe and support the importance of self-fulfilling activities. This section attempts to pull together several related topics in relation to older adults: leisure, activities, interests, creative expression, social participation, and community engagement, among others. Some evidence supports the value of engagement in activities generally, while others study specific types of activities. John Dewey's classic 1899 perspective on occupation is interpreted by Cutchin (2013). Components include nature (occupation is a form of natural and social experiences), inquiry (a cycle of practicing and learning skills and habits), and aesthetics (occupations are creative and spiritual experiences) that contribute to a meaningful life. Over 100 years later, these premises stand true as descriptors for meaning and purpose in promoting wellness.

Developing New Interests in Retirement

The meaning of time and occupations in relation to role changes in retirement was studied by Chilvers, Corr, and Singlehurst (2010). The study identified tasks for daily performance as either required and necessary, or personal and enjoyable. Related to the latter, leisure types of occupations, the most commonly reported were TV, radio, and computer. Moderate was listed as hobbies, sports, and religious. Reading was identified as meaningful. As an interesting comparison to the PAS necessary and required skills, most frequent were sleep/rest, domestic chores, and eating and drinking; moderate were socializing and personal care; and minimal was considered shopping, appointments, travel, work, education, volunteering, and caregiving. They seemed to report time use in opposite proportions to what the PAS concluded as important to individuals.

To explore the occupations and issues of retirement, Pepin and Deutscher (2011) interviewed recently retired individuals. Five qualitative themes presented were as follows:

1. Time structure and meaningful occupations

2. Aging and performance capacity

3. Role changes

4. Emotional adjustment to retirement

5. Preparation for retirement

They synthesized their findings, portraying the importance of developing new interests, engaging in meaningful occupations, discovering a positive new identity, and accessing support regarding restructured use of time.

Another perspective in understanding occupations in later life was a study conducted with health science undergraduate students. Zecevic, Magalhaes, Madady, Halligan and Reeves (2010) wondered what their perspectives were on later life activities. The Australian participants viewed Western culture as healthy, successful, and positive when contributing to productive aging. The students viewed photographs of older adults engaged in activities and were asked to write reflections. Themes included the following: Importance of an active mind (puzzles, word games, attend a class), active occupations (travel, sport, work, play with grandchildren, pets, exercise classes, garden, cook, dance, play a musical instrument), and "being" (social activities, community programs, spiritual journeys). Happiness was seen as reflecting physical and mental health resulting from ability to "maintain self-control and efficacy as they age" (Zecevic et al., p. 17). Engagement required time and contributed to a sense of belonging. Participation continues even when frail, and on some level to the end of life, where importance was still connected to some form of continuous "doing."

A good example of this approach to retirement is a musical program for older people described by Habron, Butterly, Gordon, and Roebuck (2013). Participants worked with professional musicians to compose original compositions. Funded by "Arts in Health" initiatives in the United Kingdom, the participants were introduced to new and unfamiliar experiences. This resulted in opportunities for creativity, identity making, and validation of life experience with peers and the musicians. The group involvement also led to a sense of social engagement. On a personal level, they expressed a sense of well-being and a development of mastery related to the musical projects.

Religious participation falls within self-fulfilling occupations because it provides a meaningful spiritual dimension for religious elders, as well as a social connection with other believers. Loneliness can be a significant factor for older adults' quality of life. As family and friends may decrease in number over time, opportunities for social connections increase in importance. Rote, Hill, and Ellison (2013) discovered that religious attendance increased social integration and support and decreased loneliness.

Learning Activity 98: Self-Fulfilling Occupations in Retirement

1. Draw a timeline that extends by 10-year sections from your current age until age 100.

2. Underneath the line, list self-fulfilling activities that would be meaningful to you as aging progresses through each 10-year section.

3. Mark your expected retirement age. Which occupations continued throughout your lifespan?

4. Projecting into the future from age 70, how could you adapt as your skills change?

Facilitators and Barriers to Activity Participation

Public spaces can either facilitate or discourage the participation of older adults. "Older people hang out too" describes social behaviors of older adults studied in Tasmanian shopping malls (White, 2007, p. 115). The public spaces offered a sense of order, a self-contained environment, a controlled climate, and a certain element of predictability. The experience elicits the pleasure of being in a public space, "people watching," and just feeling connected to others by being present. Shopping malls offer possibilities

of spontaneous social encounters as well as planned time with known people. White (2007) continued to elucidate that "The vast majority of seniors are not in poor health" (p. 117) and that shopping malls and libraries offer occupations considered recreational, leisure, exercise, social, work, and consumer related. An "overly orderly" environment was seen as negative, but disorganized settings that are too disorienting or difficult to maneuver should also be avoided. Special environmental considerations for occupations of socializing or shopping in large public places included location, lighting, ramps, access to toilets, security cameras, seating, signs, and choice of music.

Factors leading to decreased activity participation were identified by Painter, Allison, Dhingra, Daugherty, Cogdill and Trujillo (2012). Fear of falling, depression, and anxiety were found to influence activity engagement. OTs were encouraged to screen for fear of falling because avoidance of mobility can become a self-fulfilling prophecy.

Low vision influenced occupational engagement according to McGrath and Rudman (2013). Factors were identified as age, emotional components (fear), behaviors (delay or refuse rehabilitation, stating will accept risks), accurate diagnosis, and environmental aspects (difficulty navigating unfamiliar places, struggling in social situations). These results represented a scoping review of literature in an effort to determine emphasis or gaps in the literature.

Related to sensory and auditory changes, Perlmutter, Bhorade, Gordon, Hollingsworth, and Baum (2010) describe how those changes often lead to increased depression and decreased participation. OTs may have an important role in recommending small, inexpensive changes at home to facilitate engagement in self-fulfilling activities or to increase ability to be more active in the community.

Cultural Expression

Awareness of cultural values is mentioned as important to participation, which may include age or gender sensitivity for some projects. Studying women in Crete, Tzanidaki and Reynolds (2011) interviewed practitioners of traditional indigenous crafts. Through weaving, lace making, and painting icons, the women promoted a respect for artistic tradition. They took pride in preserving and teaching skills, which contributed to their recognized roles and status in the community. This led to an affirmation and appreciation by others. A sense of personal history was expressed, as well as connecting to a continuity of their ancestors' lifespans. The activities, whether for leisure or for sale, promoted a sustained sense of physical well-being. The creative occupations enhanced self-expression, connection to others, and self-worth. In later life, the participants expressed how the crafts assisted with coping skills through loss and grief.

Wright-St. Clair (2012) explored occupations of importance to older adults in New Zealand. Through qualitative interviews of 15 participants, social, solitary, and shared activities were reviewed. All were believed to contribute to survival. Leisure was differentiated as active or passive (TV or radio). Solitary activities were considered handwork, hobbies, reading and writing, music, and art, with reports of these activities providing greater happiness than productive activities or social groups. Even as the quantity of activities decreased with aging, the associated happiness remained constant. Occupations had personal value and they incorporated routine tasks with unfamiliar ones. "Each person pointed to one pursuit as reflecting an essentialness of who they are" (Wright-St. Clair, 2012, p. 49). They reported the importance of having something pleasurable to look forward to each day to balance with all of their everyday required tasks.

Iggulden and Iggulden (2007) created a collection of "old fashioned" activities designed to describe creative/play/adventure/fun occupations that were popular decades ago. They capture the essence of curiosity, discovery, and "getting along with others" skills developed through projects like paper airplanes, tree houses, knot tying, poker, and building go-carts. With the increasing influence of technology, they hoped to portray the valuable skills and lessons available by identifying "boys" activities through stories and directions.

Learning Activity 99: Exploring Cultural Activities

1. Considering your cultural heritage, describe three common activities enjoyed by retired, active older adults in your family or cultural group.

   a.

   b.

   c.

2. Following your own descriptions, get together with others to create a poster or collage that represents a diversity of backgrounds.

3. Discuss: What do they have in common? How do they differ?

4. What values are reflected in each of the activity choices?

Creativity Through Activities

Observing 22 adults aged 22 to 55, Blanche (2007) explored the construct of expression of creativity through occupation. Although a younger age group, the findings were helpful in understanding experiences of leisure. Creativity extended beyond leisure and included meal preparation and planned daily attire. It transcended process and product-oriented frameworks to include using one's imagination, problem solving, or seeking variety and re-ordering of known routines. It was described as a means of losing oneself while in the process of an activity, which fed the spirit or led to some new aspect of self-discovery.

Meaningfulness

Meaningfulness of occupations is discussed by Ikiugu (2005). Occupations are seen as personal and idiosyncratic, with sense of meaning bound to personal identity. Meaning is seen as connecting past, present, and future. One's repertoire of occupations change over time and reflects enjoyment; usefulness in achieving important life tasks; value placed on participation by self, others, or God; accomplishment; and possible therapeutic value.

Kuo (2011) proposes the potential use of the task of creating meaningful occupations. Designing a plan for occupational choices includes possible courses of action that would contribute to health, well-being, and positive experiences. Social cultural factors are reviewed, highlighting the inseparability of the person, his or her environment, and the social world. When creating desirable experiences, attention would be paid to a sense of anticipation and hope for possibilities, and acknowledgment that results may be unpredictable.

An intergenerational program was designed to promote reminiscence through multimedia venues (Chonody & Wang, 2013). Through storytelling, focus groups, and social networking (websites and blogs), older adults were sharing their personal histories with their families and communities. Written stories and poems were collected and themes were determined to serve as a focus for group discussion. Through this activity, participants enjoyed learning about peers; family members appreciated the created materials. The authors believed that this group activity helped to dispel a bias that elder adults live in the past, as the participants revealed their full life course and related it to the present.

Williams and Murray (2013) identified conceptual themes related to engagement in occupations following a stroke. Participation created emotional responses, had an impact on identity, influenced roles with significant others, was related to community access, and contributed to the process of adaptation. The final conclusions related to the importance of environment, relationship to significant others through shared occupations, and emotional response.

Although not specifically related to older adults, some general reviews of personal meaning of leisure activities are presented. Macdonald (2003) relates experiences of healing from a motor vehicle accident through use of selected leisure activities. Crocheting, knitting, and quilting assisted with postural, mobility, coordination, and cognitive challenges. OT friends recommended solitaire, jigsaw puzzles, Scrabble, and macramé for visual perceptual skill development.

APPLICATIONS TO CONTINUUM OF CARE

Self-fulfilling activities have a central place in the lives of retirees, not only because they fill time or replace the worker role, but also because evidence supports their importance as a protective factor in prolonging health and well-being in older adulthood. Therefore, as they age, older people both prefer, and need to continue to engage in their best loved activities at every level of care.

Community and Aging in Place

The community dwelling seniors often continue on with self-fulfilling activities they have cultivated throughout their lives, and these might be hobbies, crafts, fine or performing arts, collections, sports or games, or other interests, either solitary or shared. OTs may encounter older adults who have acquired health conditions that interfere with their ability to engage in their activity priorities. For example, a widow with an acute back injury wishes to control her pain and increase her strength so that she might continue to participate in a bowling league to which many of her friends belong. Such self-fulfilling activities become the goal that OT and client will work to achieve.

For community dwelling older adults, abilities ranged considerably related to health status. Many seniors seek guidance for maintaining and promoting health through activity. Dr. Amen (2012) is a popular author and television personality who promotes activities to promote brain function, including the following:

- Learn a new language
- Play sudoku
- Play board games (trivia and Scrabble)
- Do online brain training games
- Create mnemonics to trigger a memory, such as rhyming a "first letter"
- Try healthy new recipes
- Break routines, especially bad habits
- Meditate
- Return to school, be curious, read, study
- Play a musical instrument
- Engage in a sport requiring brain power

The principle is to introduce new and different ways to approach familiar activities, as well as adding learning through new pursuits.

Primary Care

The best time to assist older adults in adapting their self-fulfilling activities and environments is when they first acquire a health condition. OTs have the best qualifications for doing this and will hopefully get the opportunity to do so in the near future as the wellness incentives of the Affordable Care Act are implemented.

Assisted Living and Retirement Communities

Most of these facilities pride themselves on the frequency and variety of interesting activities and recreational programs they offer residents. However, often the facility does not hire an OT practitioner to oversee their activity planning. OTs have an important role to play, especially in consulting or advising the staff of these facilities about the best way to structure activities to make them accessible to individuals with health conditions, disabilities, or limitations in functioning. OTs also encounter residents of these facilities as home care providers, following up after the onset of an illness or injury.

Rehabilitation Settings

Clients of rehabilitation settings are often high functioning and in the midst of healing from an acute illness or injury. The healing process may have affected their usual routine of outside the home activities. Many express that for now, they are at home with a lot of time and would like some guidance for leisure occupations. Some would need modifications to match current yet changing levels of ability. The OT could pursue past interests and "someday I'd like to try..." possibilities and arrange for trying sample projects. What is a new leisure passion to attempt?

Other clients would like assistance with learning or mastering skills for cognitively challenging hobbies or games. Examples could include collecting stamps or coins, board or card games, and word games. Many enjoy a sense of personal competition in completing crossword puzzles, Sudoku, or word search activities. The OT may make recommendations for "tips" for success, modifications (large print), or graded complexity. Clients may also be guided to apps and resources online for various resources for mental stimulation. The OT may teach about adapted technology and principles of joint protection and ergonomics to prevent poor positioning or joint strain.

Long-Term Care

Residents in extended care facilities rely on staff members such as OTs or recreation therapists to organize or provide leisure activities. While considering individual interests and abilities, much of such programming is based on the needs of populations, such as stroke survivors or residents with dementia.

There is a distinction between the role of OTs and our colleagues in therapeutic recreation with regard to self-fulfilling activities in long-term care. Recreation therapists often provide programs for small and large groups, promoting both active and passive participation, such as movie hours, special events, entertainment, and parties. While also attending to individual skills and interests, recreational goals are more focused on active engagement and social participation. In contrast, OTs may use leisure activities as occupation-based, purposeful, or preparatory interventions. They might be part of a longer term goal of development of a specific performance skill or self-care activity (e.g., a plastic canvas needlepoint activity to develop pincher grasp required for buttoning and zipping). The OT could also problem solve for adaptive techniques to promote successful participation for a beloved activity by creating a built up brush or means to stabilize the work surface. OT group interventions usually have different goals (e.g., modified sports activities that provide specific sensory input, following evidence of population needs, but with a client-centered focus).

Hatter and Nelson (1987) explored altruism as a motivating factor for long-term care residents. When told that a cookie decorating group activity was intended for presentation to local preschool children, participation increased. They deduced that purposeful activity and personal meaning contributed to life satisfaction. Altruistic activities were also described by Cipriani, Haley, Moravec, and Young (2010). Residents created floral arrangements and cards for local hospice patients. This led to a sense of connectedness as encompassing themes of reciprocity, reminiscing, sense of community, and well-being stemming from a creative and thoughtful activity.

For low functioning residents of an Alzheimer's special care unit, Wood, Womack, and Hooper (2009) used case study design to measure quality of life. They believed that insufficient attention was provided related to the residents' occupational needs, initiatives, and capacities. They believed that OTs could play an important role in goals to increase activity participation. Activity groups were introduced, including music, craft, games, exercises, and avocational interests. Observations included (during activity participation) attention to manifestations of interest, pleasure, sadness, anxiety, fear, and anger. They concluded that the residents would benefit from a careful balance of structured time vs. "down time." Smaller activity groups were recommended as an opportunity to increase social interaction beyond meals and larger activity groups.

Cultural heritage was a consideration when individuals were newly admitted to long-term geriatric care. Hersch et al. (2012) used culturally sensitive activities to aid in adjustment. Themes from the residents' lives were identified, including family, home, food, music, work, and leisure activities. Then, group protocols were designed to reflect those themes. Exercise, poetry, current events groups, and crafts were adapted to match special considerations of race or ethnicity.

The importance of staff member interest and engagement was interpreted by Leutwyler, Hubbard, Jeste, and Vinogradov (2013). Studying older adults with schizophrenia in long-term care environments, staff members recognized that they were barriers or facilitators to physical activity. They served as role models for physical and mental health and attended to institutional requirements and safety precautions. They sought to expand upon options for activities, especially those known to contribute to health. These included walks, Wii games, chores, Tai Chi, swim, dance, video games, volleyball, work, gardening, outings, and crossword puzzles. The staff carefully applied motivation techniques for every task. Incentives such as coffee, snacks, and prizes were used. Interventions were designed to match individualized needs in small steps with respect to whatever level of functioning a patient was exhibiting. They applied Bandura's (1989) social cognitive theory and Blumer's (1969) principles of symbolic interactionism, which proposes that personal understanding occurs within the context of relationships.

IMPLICATIONS FOR OCCUPATIONAL THERAPY PRACTICE

Crafts as Therapy

Because OT has a strong history in the use of crafts as therapy, many studies have supported their health benefits, including their graded use in building strength, endurance, sensory discrimination, perceptual accuracy, and other mental functions related to well-being. In using crafts, OT practitioners are applying an occupation-based approach only when the craft is chosen by the client as a self-fulfilling (or meaningful) activity. Traditionally, crafts have been used in OT mainly as a means to another, more health-related goal, such as increasing fine motor skills or eye-hand coordination, a process explained by Trombly as "occupation as means" (1995).

Monson (2011) suggests crafts as a healing medium. She reviews America's deep connections with art and craft pastimes. Traditional occupations such as drawing, crochet, and woodwork are as popular as ever, along with recent trends such as scrapbooking and jewelry making. Specialty stores featuring arts and craft supplies have been multiplying. Individually or shared with family members, crafting serves to relieve stress, promote a sense of creativity and accomplishment, and encourage social interaction. Projects

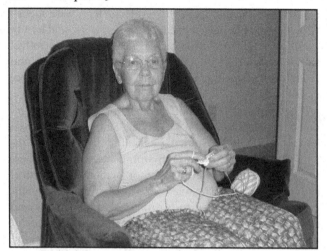

Figure 13-5. Alice loves to knit, a lifelong hobby for her.

may serve as a tool for expressing feelings or aid in distraction from difficult or painful emotions. Crafts are varied and can be selected to match almost any age or interest (Figure 13-5).

Use of crafts as a therapeutic modality is presented by Drake (1999). The OT role is compared to a teacher and learner. Client needs are analyzed and planning includes consideration of how activities may be used for treatment. Examples of use in the cognitive realm would relate to goals of increasing memory orientation, initiation and termination, and generalization of what was learned. The client is instructed in the principles of using a craft project as a purposeful method of matching therapy goals.

Therapeutic use of crafts is discussed by Johnson, Lobdell, Nesbitt, and Clare (1996), including principles of activity analysis and assessment of performance skills. Suggestions are provided for grading activities for performance complexity, attention to safety hazards, and adjustments for possible errors. The therapist is reminded to list all supplies, be cognizant of and cautious regarding a craft medium, and the importance of step by step instructions. Adaptations may include positioning or amount of repetition.

Leisure participation was studied by Stav, Hallenen, Lane, and Arbesman (2012) in relationship to health outcomes. Activities promoting health were listed as "playing games, completing crossword puzzles, gardening, outings, reading, visiting others, playing sports and participating in clubs" (Stav et al., p. 204). Participating in higher level cognitive activities, such as reading, museums, puzzles, and games, were seen as decreasing risk for dementia. In general, involvement in occupations was viewed as beneficial to widows and widowers to assist with coping and well-being.

Evaluation and Outcomes

Law, Baum, and Dunn (2001) promote continued development of outcomes measures to guide practice. Leisure performance, known to increase well-being and life satisfaction, is measured through categories of skills, roles, and motivational factors. Interests, skills, and pleasure are defined individually. Freedom to choose tasks was important, whether short- or long-term in nature. Most valued were occupations that were personally rewarding and offered a sense of immediate gratification.

Wood (2005) developed an observational tool to investigate activity participation, time use, and quality of life in individuals with advanced dementia in a long-term care settings. This was seen as a beginning contribution to relating individual to activity and environment through defined measures. The domains included ratings for engaged gaze, functional mobility, participation in conversation, and engagement in activity. The intention was to use the Activity in Context and Time (ACT) tool over time to determine patterns of behavior.

Therapeutic Use of Self

A person attracted to pursuing a career in OT presumably has a deep appreciation of the meaning and value of participating in activities. This might reflect a background interest in crafts and hobbies, sports, or games that may have made an impression about the personal and social value of occupations. Through therapeutic use of self, the practitioner may share expertise based on professional, education, experience, and reasoning to relate to a client. Along with those insights, personal experiences and traits may "bring to the table" another level of connecting with a client.

Occupation-Based Activities

Given the published evidence related to the importance of leisure pursuits in promoting quality of life, OTs may have important roles in community settings for health promotion. Working as a volunteer or consultant, OTs may lead a series of programs in a worship hall, senior center, or assisted living setting. Through instruction and demonstration, varied leisure skills could be taught, including the cognitive, emotional, social, and physical benefits.

Fidler and Velde (1999) expound on the use of activity analysis when planning for occupation-based therapy. This includes evaluation of form and structure (procedures, time, sequence), properties (materials, cultural consideration, one person or more, space/setting, and symbolic meaning), action (cognitive, social, sensory, motor, and emotional), and outcome (outcome expectations). These considerations were reviewed by Cynkin and Robinson (1990), who also included the following under the nature of an activity: historical context, individual relevance, relations to rituals, and idiosyncratic personal style.

Advice could also be provided to troubleshoot for challenge areas. For handwork, larger needles and yarn may be suggested to avoid prolonged tight grasp. The importance of rest periods and stretching could be discussed along with proper posture, pillow support as needed, and appropriate lighting. To aid in visual challenges, magnifiers may be used, along with color contrasts. For example, if a woman is knitting with navy blue yarn and is wearing navy blue slacks, figure ground discrimination is difficult. Placing a light-colored towel on the lap creates a visual contrast, or using a light pillow that also allows for support of the hands and project.

Leisure activities may be used by the OT for many health and wellness goals. Crafts promote self-expression and creativity. Sports such as bocce, bowling, tennis, or golf promote social interaction. Cards and "game night" events have activity demands of cooperation, competition, rule following, and communication—all important social skills to maintain. Leisure activities represent a continuity of a person's past to present and may reinforce personal identity despite altered abilities. Along with adapting activities to match skills, OTs may also assist in identifying and exploring new interests.

Purposeful Activities

When I received my undergraduate degree in OT, crafts were taught as an important therapeutic modality. Over a semester, we became expert in weaving, ceramics, printmaking, hand crafts, woodworking, metal work, leather crafting, and sewing (for adapted clothing). We created elaborate task analysis reports to describe how that modality could be used for rehabilitation of multiple conditions, along with possible modifications.

My first place of employment provided me with the challenge of opening their OT department. I needed to design and define all OT services. I was one-half employee for an adult day care center and one-half for the long-term care facility. For the latter, expectations were for ADL training, preparatory methods for ROM and strength, and many forms of purposeful activities. In the adult day care, individual rehabilitation and home visits were provided, but the greater role was developing and leading groups (exercise, health topics, reminiscing, and crafts). As the OT, I would often develop a group and then the leadership would be assumed by a recreation staff member, senior aide, or nurse.

Purposeful activities would often appear as "fun" or "keeping people occupied," but intentions for diversional activity were rare. One woman with dementia, Rose, would become agitated at mid-afternoon in the adult day care center. She would call out loudly and repeatedly, "Where's the jitney [bus to go home]?" This would upset the other clients, who would then also exhibit anxious behaviors. We discovered that Rose, although very visually impaired, could crochet, very simply (chain stitch only). It quieted her and focused her attention. Over months, Rose happily crocheted seemingly miles of chain stitch. Our staff enjoyed collaborating to dream up uses for those wound up balls. We invested in a frame to clamp to the table—a simple 2-foot board with 2 upright dowels at either end. One of the men enjoyed wrapping the created "yarn" around and around. When enough was wrapped, a staff member would carefully tie off one end and create a head, then the rest was braided. Another client, who was blind, enjoyed braiding to create eight legs for an octopus or segments for arms and legs and body for a doll. Another client created felt eyes and mouths, another fabricated small garments. The items were then sold at the center's craft table. Rose's need for calming activity triggered extensive and enjoyable group projects.

Purposeful activities play a vital role in individual rehabilitation for older adults. A hand therapist in private practice may use a variety of "tabletop" or manipulative types of activities to promote finger ROM, strength, coordination, and pinch and grasp. This could include puzzles, pegboards, or assorted craft projects, such as beadwork or needlepoint.

Through purposeful activities, the client may be using occupations seen as fun, familiar, and interesting, which assists in facilitating active participation. Increased practice and repetition are fostered when engaging in projects of personal significance. The OT seeks to discover specifics of needs for performance skills development, and selects activities to address therapeutic goals. Purposeful activities often increase levels of motivation, especially when related to leisure interests.

Occupational Therapy Group Interventions

Groups using self-fulfilling activities have been used successfully by OTs at every level, from community-to facility-based care. Pierce (2009) coined the term *co-occupation*, meaning shared activity. This is considered a joint performance, highly interactive, with varied roles, but a single goal. This does not necessarily imply the same shared time, space, or intent. For example, an older adult could be planning a birthday party to be held in her home, along with her family. The grandmother could take responsibility for preparing for guests and baking a cake, while her son offers to purchase and set up decorations and her daughter sends out invitations.

At the community level, a structured gardening program was offered for individuals with young onset dementia (Hewitt, Watts, Hussey, Power, & Williams, 2013). Clients participated in gardening group sessions based on principles of horticulture therapy. At the same time, family caregivers attended a group for support, socializing, and planning. This offered respite and a sense of "not in this alone" for the caregivers. The gardeners were assessed as having increased enjoyment, independent skills, feeling valued, decrease in anxiety, and increase in feeling a sense of achievement. Although cognitive decline continued, rating on a well-being scale (Bradford Well-Being Profile) increased.

In the long-term care facility, male residents seemed to isolate themselves and avoid attending recreational activities, whether small or large. As an OT, I identified a need for a men's group. Because generations of my family have been woodworkers, I had a background knowledge of simple woodworking using hand tools. A group of six men were identified, and the Men's Club was launched. At first it appeared awkward for them to get accustomed to me as a leader, but they became interested as I would assess their skills, divide up steps to match ability, and, using simple woodworking kits, grade the project to maximize success experiences. The group lasted for a few months, during which time they completed sanding, gluing and nailing, and finishing boxes and birdhouses. As the men attended, they became acquainted and slowly began meaningful conversations while working. To support that level of socializing, I began preparing for topics of discussion related to sports, politics, and history. By the end of the program, the men were speaking with one another outside of the group, and most were attending other opportunities in the facility, such as work activity center, residents' council meetings, and religious services. Bringing them together to share a common activity decreased isolation and increased willingness to explore other programs offered.

Case Example: Ira (by Dr. Estelle Breines, PhD, OTR/L)

As the president of Geri Rehab, Inc., a corporation I founded in 1977, my experiences with disabled and infirm elders is of long duration. This was enhanced by the opportunities I've had as an OT educator, writer, and researcher. My column in *Advance for Occupational Therapy Practitioners* was published regularly from 1994 to 2013. Now I find myself living through the many experiences that I formerly addressed through my patients and their families.

In August 2012, my husband Ira elected to have a hip replacement to relieve the arthritic pain he had been enduring for some time. Ira has been a gentleman farmer on a small farm in New Jersey for the 40 years we have lived here. Each morning he fed the cattle, peacocks, chickens, guinea hens, dogs, and cats before returning to the house with the eggs he found in the barn to cook breakfast. He ran the washing machine, made a shopping list for dinner, and rode to town to visit with his buddies at the bakery before he went shopping. Sometimes he went off to the grain store to pick up feed for the animals, then came back home to mow the grass. Considering all of the usual chores he encountered in a day, Ira was a very busy guy. I volunteered to feed the animals until October, by which time we thought he would be back on duty.

His surgery and recovery was uneventful, having the usual course of OT and PT following an anterior surgical approach that did not require the usual hip precautions. I elected to allow the professionals to do their part while I took the role of wife and driver. The surgical hose Ira had been wearing for 50 years remained his only obstacle, which he soon mastered using a pair of long-handled reachers. He progressed to the use of a cane, and managed the 13 steps up to our home.

All was going well until a hematoma broke through along the suture line, necessitating further surgery to clean out the wound. Now we were back to stage one of recovery. The wound defied closure, so a wound vac was inserted, which Ira wore for 6 weeks. My October commitment came and went, and I fed the animals through the winter months, while Ira's ambulation endurance began to increase. He resumed his cooking responsibilities and I took over as OT, making certain that Ira could manage the various activities he ordinarily engaged in.

Along about January, severe pain began and became excruciating. By the time his 80th birthday arrived in February, he was back using the walker. A series of visits to the orthopedic surgeon, the infectious disease doctor, the pain management specialist, and the neurologist resulted in a diagnosis of femoral neuritis and a referral to a neurosurgeon, who disagreed with the diagnosis. He referred us to a complex spine surgeon. Ira became further and further debilitated.

Throughout, our daughter, who is an internist at the Cleveland Clinic, was urging us to come to Cleveland for examination. Our frustration and Ira's pain clinched the notion. After arranging for help to care for the farm while we were gone, I fixed the back seat of the car so Ira's legs were elevated and we began our 7-hour trip, moving into a hotel in Beachwood for the duration. Our daughter's home was inaccessible, but close by.

Two hours into our visit with the orthopedic surgeon, we heard a diagnosis. Ira's hip was infected with a common but slow growing bacterium rarely found in the hip. The diagnosis was confirmed 10 days later by lab testing and surgery was performed, this time using a posterior approach, limiting his movement past 90 flexion of his right hip. The original prosthesis was replaced by a temporary spacer infused with antibiotics. Post-surgery, he had extreme edema of both legs. Neither compression hose nor his own socks would fit. I used retrograde massage and elastic wraps to reduce the edema. I was trained to deliver the 24-hour doses of antibiotic he would receive daily for the next 6 weeks.

Visiting nurses and therapists came to the hotel to provide care. A raised toilet seat was provided. I requested a tub bench so Ira could bathe on his own. He used his reachers and a leg lifter effectively. We purchased a pair of Velcro closure shoes online that could fit his swollen feet. Shorts with elastic waistbands were easy for him to wear, and worked well as pajamas too. Disposable underpants helped with the laundry until the wound healed.

At the end of 6 weeks, the antibiotics were discontinued. Two weeks later, his hip was aspirated to determine if the infection was gone. Surgery was scheduled to implant the permanent hip and begin his final recovery.

While initially I deferred to the therapists, I became more involved in Ira's rehabilitation as time went on. I found I could facilitate his involvement in healthful activities by partnering in them. Together we solved problems, and I did only as much as was needed, gradually restricting my assistance as his abilities increased.

The long periods of time between procedures made it important to fill that time purposefully. A trip to a museum required a call in advance to determine if there would be a wheelchair available, as long walks were too demanding because he was using a walker during most of his recovery. No weight bearing was permitted while he had the temporary spacer in place. The supermarket was possible if he used an electric cart. The walker sufficed when we went to cribbage club each week. We took a urinal with us when we travelled. Attending religious services necessitated a scouting trip to find the accessible yet locked doorway and park the car. Then I scampered around the building to enter at the front and go through the building to reach the appropriate door and let Ira in. His laptop computer consumed his interest for hours each day, sometimes with news and sometimes with Scrabble, which he enjoys. He set up a desk and took care of business matters, having arranged to receive a box of mail from home each week. He even helped me wind yarn, bringing to mind how he used to help his mother in the same way when he was a boy. Ira continued to make light meals and plan our menus, keeping our shopping list. On weekends, we visited our children and grandchildren, while they dropped by our place most evenings after work. Best was when some of our friends and neighbors traveling through would arrange to visit us, making our long stay tolerable.

Do I have recommendations for the reader? Develop respect for the importance of activity in maintaining health. Moreover, recognize that each individual has his or her own set of meaningful activities. Broaden your understanding of what makes life meaningful. It will be different for each person. Spend your own lifetime acquiring skills in as many activities as you can master. They will enrich your own life and will enhance your professional life as well. You never know when these skills will be called on. The more tools you acquire, the better you will become as a therapist. Make friends of all ages. They will teach you a great deal.

Summary

Older adults may have extensive experience with varied leisure activities or may have anticipated discovering new possibilities to explore creative outlets after retirement. OT practitioners offer assistance in defining areas of interest, exploring activity demands and available resources, and assisting with occupational performance. Adaptations may be needed if the client has skill challenges, including modifications for timing and frequency of activity performance. Self-fulfilling activities often pertain to interaction with other people, which promotes their health-enhancing values. The participants of the PAS shared personal stories about the many types of self-fulfilling activities that increased creative expression, community participation, and inner growth, all contributing to a sense of increased life satisfaction.

References

Amen, D. G. (2012). *Use your brain to change your age: Secrets to look, feel, and think younger every day.* New York: Crown Archetype.

American Occupational Therapy Association. (2014). The occupational therapy practice framework: Domain and process (3rd ed.), *American Journal of Occupational Therapy, 68,* S1-S48.

Bandura, A. (1989). Social cognitive theory. *Psychologist, 44,* 1175-1184.

Blanche, E. I. (2007). The expression of creativity through occupation. *Journal of Occupational Science, 14,* 21-29.

Blumer, H. (1969). *Symbolic interactionism.* Englewood Cliffs, NJ: Prentice Hall.

Chilvers, R., Corr, S., & Singlehurst, H. (2010). Investigation into the occupational lives of healthy older people through their use of time. *Australian Occupational Therapy Journal, 57,* 24-33.

Chonody, J., & Wang, D. (2013). Connecting older adults to the community through multimedia: An intergenerational reminiscence program. *Activities, Adaptation & Aging, 37,* 79-93.

Cipriani, J., Haley, R., Moravec, E., & Young, H. (2010). Experience and meaning of group altruistic activities among long-term care residents. *British Journal of Occupational Therapy, 73,* 269-276.

Cutchin, M. P. (2013). The art and science of occupation: Nature, inquiry, and the aesthetics of living. *Journal of Occupational Science, 20,* 286-297.

Cynkin, S., & Robinson, A. M. (1990). *Occupational therapy and activities health: Toward health through activities.* Boston, MA: Little, Brown & Company.

Drake, M. (1999). *Crafts in therapy and rehabilitation.* Thorofare, NJ: SLACK Incorporated.

Fidler, G. S., & Velde, B. P. (1999). *Activities: Reality and symbol.* Thorofare, NJ: SLACK Incorporated.

Habron, J., Butterly, F., Gordon, I., & Roebuck, A. (2013). Being well, being musical: Music composition as a resource and occupation for older people. *British Journal of Occupational Therapy, 76,* 308-316.

Hatter, J. K., & Nelson, D. L. (1987). Altruism and task participation in the elderly. *American Journal of Occupational Therapy, 41,* 379-381.

Hersch, G., Hutchinson, S., Davidson, H. Wilson, C., Maharaj, T., & Watson, K. (2012). Effect of an occupation-based cultural heritage intervention in long term geriatric carte: A two-group control study. *American Journal of Occupational Therapy, 66,* 224-232.

Hewitt, P., Watts, C., Hussey, J., Power, K., & Williams, T. (2013). Does a structured gardening program improve wellbeing in young-onset dementia? *British Journal of Occupational Therapy, 76,* 355-361.

Iggulden, C., & Iggulden, H. (2007). *The dangerous book for boys.* New York: Harper Collins Publications.

Ikiugu, M. N. (2005). Meaningfulness of occupations as an occupation-life-trajectory attractor. *Journal of Occupational Science, 12,* 102-105.

Johnson, C., Lobdell, K., Nesbitt, J., & Clare, M. (1996). *Therapeutic crafts: A practical approach.* Thorofare, NJ: SLACK Incorporated.

Kuo, A. (2011). A transactional view: Occupation as a means to create experiences that matter. *Journal of Occupational Science, 18,* 131-138.

Laslett, P. (1989). *A fresh map of life: The emergence of the Third Age.* Cambridge, MA: Harvard University Press.

Laslett, P. (1997). Interpreting the demographic changes. *Philosophical Transactions of the Royal Society B: Biological Sciences, 352*(1363): 1805-1809.

Law, M., Baum, C., & Dunn, W. (2001). *Measuring occupational performance: Supporting best practice in occupational therapy.* Thorofare, NJ: SLACK Incorporated.

Leutwyler, H., Hubbard, E. M., Jeste, D. V., & Vinogradov, S. (2013). "We're not just sitting on the periphery": A staff perspective of physical activity in older adults with schizophrenia. *The Gerontologist, 53,* 474-478.

Macdonald, K. (2003). Still climbing high. In D. R. Labovitz (Ed.), *Ordinary miracles: True stories about overcoming obstacles and surviving catastrophes* (pp. 260-264). Thorofare, NJ: SLACK Incorporated.

McGrath, C. E., & Rudman, D. C. (2013). Factors that influence the occupational engagement of older adults with low vision: A scoping review. *British Journal of Occupational Therapy, 76,* 234-241.

Monson, N. (2011). *Crafts to heal: Soothing your soul with sewing, painting and other pastimes.* Tuscon, AZ: Hats Off Books.

Painter, P. A., Allison, L., Dhingra, P., Daugherty, I. Cogdill, K., & Trujillo, L. (2012). Fear of falling and its relationship with anxiety, depression, and activity engagement among community-dwelling older adults. *American Journal of Occupational Therapy, 66,* 169-176.

Parham, D., & Fazio, L. S. (Eds.). (1997). *Play in occupational therapy for children.* St. Louis, MO: Mosby.

Pepin, G., & Deutscher, B. (2011). The lived experience of Australian retirees: I'm retired, what do I do now? *British Journal of Occupational Therapy, 74,* 419-426.

Perlmutter, M. S., Bhorade, A., Gordon, N., Hollingsworth, H. H., & Baum, M. C. (2010). Cognitive, visual, auditory and emotional factors that affect participation in older adults. *American Journal of Occupational Therapy, 64,* 570-579.

Pierce, D. (2009). Co-occupation: The challenge of defining concepts original to occupational science. *Journal of Occupational Science, 16,* 203-207.

Rote, S., Hill, T. D., & Ellison, C. (2013). Religious attendance and loneliness in later life. *The Gerontologist, 53,* 39-50.

Stav, W. B., Hallenen, T., Lane J., & Arbesman, M. (2012). Systematic review of occupational engagement and health outcomes among community dwelling older adults. *American Journal of Occupation Therapy, 66,* 301-310.

Trombly, C. (1995). Occupation: Purposefulness and meaningfulness as therapeutic mechanisms. *American Journal of Occupational Therapy, 49,* 960-972.

Tzanidaki, D., & Reynolds, F. (2011). Exploring the meanings of making traditional arts and crafts among older women in Crete, using interpretive phenomenological analysis. *British Journal of Occupational Therapy, 74,* 375-382.

White, R. (2007). Older people hang out too. *Journal of Occupational Science, 14,* 115-118.

Williams, S., & Murray, C. (2013). The experience of engaging an occupation following stroke: A qualitative meta-synthesis. *British Journal of Occupational Therapy, 76,* 370-378.

Wood, W. (2005). Toward developing new occupational science measures: An example from dementia care research. *Journal of Occupational Science, 12,* 121-129.

Wood, W., Womack, J., & Hooper, B. (2009). Dying of boredom: An exploratory case study of time use, apparent effect, and routine activity situations in two Alzheimer's special care units. *American Journal of Occupational Therapy, 67,* 351-350.

Wright-St Clair, V. (2012). Being occupied with what matters in advanced age. *Journal of Occupational Science, 19,* 44-53.

Zecevic, A., Magalhaes, L., Madady, M., Halligan, M., & Reeves, A. (2010). Happy and healthy only if occupied: Perceptions of health sciences students on occupation in later life. *Australian Occupational Therapy Journal, 57,* 17-73.

14

A Theory of
Conditional Independence

Karen C. Macdonald, PhD, OTR/L

"Under what circumstances, as established by careful OT assessment and intervention, is independence facilitated?"
(K. Macdonald)

Using qualitative methodology, the researcher may continue using the results of the PAS for an additional level of analysis leading to the development of a grounded theory. Scholars debate the differences between theory, conceptual or practice models, and frames of reference. For the purposes of this textbook, the PAS final analysis represents the application of themes as elements for further inquiry and includes some application possibilities for practice. The proposed theory derived from the PAS is entitled Conditional Independence, with principles related to any geriatric population. Conditional Independence is not a frame of reference because it does not relate to a particular diagnosis, condition, or population. A theory may stand alone as a structure for related constructs and concepts. Here, the theory is converted into an OT occupation-based model with categories representing facilitation of skills toward a final client goal of structured function.

EXPERT'S EXPERIENCE—
BY DR. ELIZABETH GRIFFIN
LANNIGAN, PhD, OTR/L, FAOTA

I have been an OT for 40 years, with a special interest in serving those individuals living with mental illness. I have been a clinician, educator, researcher, and consultant addressing the life experiences of these individuals. My own doctoral research utilized a qualitative research method to understand the experience of those living with severe mental illness as they participated in vocational rehabilitation programs to enter the workforce. While my research topic is a different focus compared to the research topic of this text, the use of the qualitative research method is central to understanding the life experiences of any individual, able-bodied or living with disabilities.

Cole MB, Macdonald KC.
Productive Aging: An Occupational Perspective (pp 231-242).
© 2015 Taylor & Francis Group.

To understand the "lived experience" of my research participants, I needed to be able to solicit personal descriptions through open-ended questioning. Collecting data through a specifically focused questionnaire would not have yielded the richness of participants' experience. By listening to the first-person voice, I was able to "hear" how individuals moved through the duration of their illness and recognize the value of entering a rehabilitation program devoted to individuals experiencing mental illness. The research participants acknowledged the difficulty of inability to be working members of society and of needing to be dependent on the agency's therapeutic services. My qualitative study yielded the following themes: (1) living with a mental illness, (2) descriptions of the benefits of participating in a vocational rehabilitation program, (3) discrepancy between life expectations and realities of missed life opportunities, and (4) their view that to be a worker is to be healthy. Collecting this personal experience data enabled me as a researcher to understand that these individuals had a view that they desired and could be "healthy" as workers, despite living with an illness.

Regardless of understanding the experience of living with a mental illness or being an older adult, the OT profession has relied extensively on qualitative research methodology. It is imperative that the profession utilizes the appropriate research methodology to suit the information needed to be collected and analyzed to reach professional knowledge. As a profession addressing the quality of daily living, OT has a long history of using both quantitative and qualitative methods. (Yes, we do need the numbers of statistical analysis for our professional knowledge base as well.) As the profession began to study *occupation* as the foundation of designing OT interventions for those with daily living limitations, the emergence of the qualitative method was crucial to understanding typical occupational performance of healthy individuals, as well as the impact of disabilities on the lives of many (Hinojosa & Anderson, 1991; Moll & Cook, 1997; Ruderman, Cook, & Polatajko, 1997; Siporin & Lysack, 2004; Tham & Keilhofner, 2003). These conceptual knowledge bases then support the OT profession to determine strategies to support healthy living and interventions to assist those in need of assistance. In this text, the daily lives of those active and productive older adults are explored to provide evidence of the characteristics of those elders who are thriving in life.

For OT students and clinicians who are beginning the task of conducting research, the qualitative research methodology must be considered for the type of knowledge to be developed. Although this chapter has outlined the rigors of conducting this qualitative research study for productive aging, it is possible to begin qualitative research on a smaller basis. Conducting open-ended interviews with a selected group of individuals enables the beginning researcher to "hear" and understand aspects of living from the individuals' perspective. The content of the interviews may be specifically focused on one aspect of life or may be broader, based on the research topic desired. Utilizing a mentor with experience in conducting qualitative research is especially helpful. Understanding qualitative research strategies for determining the accuracy of research findings through peer debriefing, triangulation, and member checking can be learned with the guidance of a mentor. Any research undertaking seems overwhelming, yet starting on a small project enables the beginner to develop competencies to produce significant research results. (Just like the support we give our clients as they approach the challenges of therapy!)

FINAL PHASES OF ANALYSIS

Generating Hypotheses

Four hypotheses were identified related to the span of OT interventions with older adults, including both medical and community models of service delivery:

1. With structured methods for assessment and direct intervention, including *client education*, OTs can promote optimized ability and quality of life for healthy older adults. OTs have expertise in teaching/learning and will use these techniques to promote self-management skills of older adults. This would pertain to instruction for self-management during therapy sessions, with anticipation of pursuing these strategies independently following discharge. Models will be developed to demonstrate effective service delivery in which OT practitioners develop programs for older adults to implement a self-directed program to maintain skills and prevent decline in physical, cognitive, social-emotional, and sensory areas of functioning.

2. Increasing roles for OT intervention with community dwelling older adults will have a significant influence in maintaining independence and the ability to remain living in the community. Structured intervention, as needed over time, would be provided through *consultation* to clients, family members, home care providers, and coordinators of home-based health care services. Evidence-based strategies will be used to maximize personal or assisted skills for performance of ADL and IADL tasks. Additional consideration will be made toward adapting needs and responding to life changes over time.

3. OTs will promote an understanding of the relationship of engagement in daily activity and social connectedness to sustained levels of health. *Community programs* for groups of older adults would offer skill development, interpersonal support, referrals to needed services, and ongoing instruction for compensatory techniques.

4. As models for service delivery evolve toward community-based services, OTs will have an increasing role in

advocacy and policy development to promote availability and reimbursement for their services that promote Conditional Independence for older adults.

Final Synthesis

In a boundary-setting effort to finalize topics for data analysis, we stepped back to consider whether we had covered all topics pertaining to Productive Aging. The interview results were self-eliminating for boundaries of discussion. We paused to respect another aspect of data analysis: what the participants did *not* discuss. The following areas were minimally raised and were obvious by their omission.

- Role of neighbors
- Sexuality
- Relocation and downsizing
- Details about current role of being a parent (their own adult children)

Because the study continually mushroomed for subjects of personally identified importance, limits were established on exploring additional topics. However, presuming these issues to be of significance, we wondered if these topics were so ingrained as "givens" that they were not raised by the participants. They were addressed as broad areas of interest or concern for older adults in the review of literature in previous chapters.

In reviewing all extensive analysis findings, final themes emerged about the qualities and abilities of the participants. What exactly contributed to their productivity? How do they do it? How can OTs apply the participants' skills as approaches for others as they grow older? Wherever the authors mentioned the project of writing this textbook, the listener would say something like, "When can I buy the book? I want to know how to age and be productive!"

In a final synthesis of objectively analyzing the participant's unique qualities, layers of brainstorming continued. The participants appeared to have in common traits such as being deliberate, aware, and end goal-oriented in their view of everyday activities. They had a sense of continuity from past, present, and future perspectives of plans, priorities, and purpose.

The participants had grown up in an era of traditional values and roles. They then experienced a lifetime of cultural, social, political, economic, and technological changes. They shared qualities of being motivated, having the self-ability to accept and adjust to change, and having a desire to be active and "doing." In their retirement years, they continued to be self-modulating, interested in others, and determined to remain able and active. In closing the collection and analysis of data, qualitative research continues to pose the questions: "So what? What does this all mean? How do we dissect and organize all of this information, and create final conclusions? What have we learned that will transfer to OT practice? Have we discovered the key to promoting and sustaining the well elderly stage of life?"

The participants' life long core belief systems appeared to directly influence their daily motivation and activities. Those included principles such as "can do," "go with the flow," respect for self and others, faith, and determination. Can these attitudes and beliefs in self-efficacy be taught to seniors who did not share these beliefs that supported skills? How could OTs facilitate these motivational strategies if not part of an individual's lifelong pattern? The participants had role models from their youth, and their parents' generation—inventors, innovators like Ford, Edison, Rockefeller, Carnegie, the Roosevelts, Amelia Earhart, Jim Thorpe—what influence did these have on the participant's development of a "can do" attitude? Did subsequent generations have comparable idols and heroes?

Questions continued to accumulate when considering the OT's potential roles. What else was unique about the participants? Some types of qualitative analysis reflect on identifying opposite constructs to aid in understanding a topic. The participants did *not* have characteristics of feeling the following: bored, nothing to do, fed up, "done it all," or worn out. Instead, they shared a sense of eager enthusiasm—What's next? Now what? Why not? They respected being satisfied with what they have and what they have accomplished and yet were continuing to strive even further. They consistently had a positive sense of anticipation and expectations and an eagerness toward future possibilities. They viewed themselves as capable and yet open to future learning and growth.

Their strong sense of self-direction and determination led us to wonder: "How will this current generation be different in seeking and responding to health care? Will professional relationships need to be structured differently? Will these capable productive agers accept help and advice? How may we promote compliance with recommendations by medical or community-based models of service delivery?"

As the months passed by in the preparation for the manuscript, we had the sensation of being challenged by the enormity of the project. We felt confident that we were discovering important aspects of defining and understanding productive aging. We experienced many hunches and surprises. One that we did not expect was the wisdom of hindsight. Only in the accumulated findings and synthesis of all materials did we begin to feel enlightened about the development of a new theory.

And Life Goes On...

In the course of the study, major changes occurred for a number of the participants.

Four participants died. Patricia passed at age 92, after a brief illness that followed a general decline over months. Ken experienced a fatal cardiac arrest at age 73. He had been extremely active and athletic, enjoying family, traveling, and recent retirement. Geno and Dave both experienced a stroke. Nettie had numerous surgeries for orthopedic and cancer-related conditions. Ray's cherished role as a caregiver to a lady friend changed when she experienced increased memory loss and a fall, which led to placement in a long-term care facility, followed shortly thereafter by her death. Judi had a number of family changes that led to her altering her social activities. Jim experienced a heart attack with a slow recovery. Signian became a widow. Pearl was diagnosed with Parkinson's.

In the 3 months since writing the above paragraph, and in the process of reviewing and revising, 2 more participants have passed away. Johanna lost her battle with ovarian cancer at age 73. She worked from her hospital bed to resolve open cases, making phone calls and signing documents, up until 3 days before her death. Suzie died at age 99, still living alone at home, cooking, cleaning, driving, and attending beloved social organization meetings. All her activities were slower, less frequent, but she was still an active participant enjoying her roles and routines. In discussing this, Marli and I marveled that none of these participants who passed away ever entered the Fourth Age. It appeared that participation in varied meaningful activities continued until their final day, *a final day of living*. Isn't this what we all would want for ourselves?

Because we knew our participants, we were aware of their life changes. We questioned ourselves further about the relationship between the original categories of attitude, ability, activity, and productive aging. We realized that the individuals who died had remained productive until their dying day. Those who experienced health or life changes needed recovery or reorganizing time, and then tenaciously moved again toward desired activities. We concluded that these individuals, no matter what the circumstances, could determine the means and methods for continuing to progress in life with purpose.

For active and productive agers, what might be OT's role in helping them maintain the ability to sustain self and activity? Although all OT intervention promotes performance skills and related task performance, what needs to be different for the emerging population who will become retirees during the 21st century?

PROPOSAL OF A GROUNDED THEORY

Based on the completed synthesis of the PAS, a final representative topic emerged, which we labeled Conditional Independence. For these older adults, many diverse components of occupations needed to be in place to enable engagement. To promote function, many habitual patterns were in place, representing decades of established routine. Other occupations required minimal to maximum adaptation to permit involvement. This reflected changes in health status,

time management considerations, finances, and social network. Over time, whether maintaining former or developing new activity interests, modifications became necessary to promote performance (Figure 14-1).

To explore constructs contributing to a new theory, we analyzed universal considerations for the task analysis of what are the desired goals; what are possible challenge areas; and what may be required to support performance through education, adaptation, or skill development? The older adults seemed to have innate problem-solving skills. This may reflect their unique generation's lifelong responses to coping with changes and challenges. They seemed to be natural trouble-shooters for problem solving, fixing things, and finding a new way to achieve a specified goal. Again, we wondered, how do they do this independently? How could we as OTs teach these abilities to other older adults who have never had that skill or are now challenged due to a health condition? Can we create a generic task analysis for promoting skills?

Conditional Independence is established when predetermined systems and structures are in place.

"I can _____ IF _____."

For example: "I can dress myself early in the morning if I lay out my clothes the night before," might apply to an individual who needs to avoid expending mental power first thing in the morning, reserving it for upcoming tasks. Established methods would be designed for performance areas of self-management, social connections, and self-fulfilling activities (leisure). When in place, the approach would ideally allow for higher levels of performance and result in supported function.

CONDITIONAL INDEPENDENCE

The theory of Conditional Independence is being defined as an abstract construct representing planned and purposeful efforts for self-directed ability. Although being proposed as a theory that would stand separate from practical application, the author wished to explore elements and relationships to OT intervention with older adults. Future deliberation is recommended for possible considerations of conceptual models or frames of reference.

Conditional Independence reflects a process of preparation and practice of skills for self-management, social connections, and self-fulfilling activities. By defining needs and goals, designing adaptive strategies for performance, and evaluating effectiveness, the older adult would gain skill during OT sessions. During those sessions, the client's capability when no longer within the simulated or structured environment of a treatment session would be determined. How can OTs promote skills for problem solving to foster maximum independent functioning in the home and community? The OT would facilitate planned skills for managing abilities within real life situations and

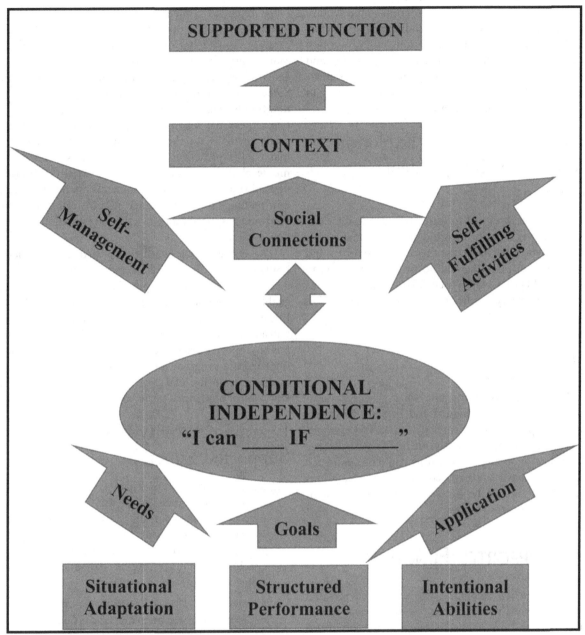

Figure 14-1. Theory of Conditional Independence. (Created by K. C. Macdonald, 2015.)

settings. By teaching principles of task analysis, compensatory techniques, and environmental modification, the OT would help the client to have the resources for ongoing life skill design for safety, survival, and participation in activities of choice.

The OT would assist with promoting personal insight for client needs, skills, and functional challenges. To determine an ideal plan for occupational performance, the OT would collaborate with the client to strategize individualized schedules and approaches for managing ADLs and IADLs. After design of sample techniques, and practice within the supportive milieu of a therapeutic relationship, the OT would guide the client toward transition-

ing application separate from the therapist's supervision and guidance. The client would progressively develop problem-solving and critical-thinking skills toward self-management. Ultimately, through this "self-help" program, the client would develop the capacity for consistently reasoning through challenging issues, recognizing needs for a planned approach, and creatively devising a suitable method to address the circumstances. This would require an ongoing mindfulness of personal skills and needs, as well as recognition of the influences of countless interpersonal or environmental variables.

The client would independently construct a unique system of approaches with long-term objectives of sustainable self-support. This custom designed program would require a perspective of enacted self-care, including activity performance, skill development, risk prevention, and promotion of wellness. With careful construction, repetition, and revision, the client would reinforce abilities toward creating habits and routines for supported function, resulting in sustained conditional independence.

Learning Activity 100: Exploring Conditions for Independent Functioning

This exercise is designed to raise your personal awareness of conditions for your own independent functioning. Imagine that you have moderate rheumatoid arthritis and are responsible for planning and hosting a birthday party for an 8-year-old girl. Create a list of 10 to 20 considerations for planning the party. Under the list, create a table as follows:

- Motor skills

- Process skills

- Social interaction skills

Next to each category, imagine what planned conditions would need to be designed and in place to enable successful completion of the party planning. For example, motor skills: if an individual had difficulty with fatigue and endurance, shopping and cleaning could be completed 2 days prior to the party. Finally, consider what adaptations or modifications would be necessary for independent or assisted performance of the task.

SUPPORTED FUNCTION

Supported function recognizes the set of behaviors and layers of established patterns required for optimal ability. It reflects successfully applied strategies for compensatory techniques, organized assistance of family or professional caregivers, and ongoing deliberate efforts for self-management. It implies continued attention to all that may be necessary to enable occupational performance. Over time, routines may become more "subcortical" or automatic in nature; however, if not adhered to, the structured set of skills could deteriorate.

Supported function represents the successful ongoing application of a desired program toward maximum abilities, both daily and over time. This would not represent a "single fix," but rather a systematic and comprehensive design for actual ability performance, considering the client's unique life circumstances, background, and current skill sets. Daily programming would be established for enhanced or optimal engagement in occupations.

To relate to contemporary thinking, the older client would be putting a positive spin on age- or health-related changes. A metaphor of a personal "makeover" would promote inspiration to integrate new skills and approaches with goals of personal transformation toward higher abilities. Some older adults welcome change and progress toward new trends, including rehabilitative equipment and modalities. Others may see the benefit of performance options but prefer to maintain their "hard wired" approaches. Some may try OT principles or assistive devices to restore a former level of ability but are unable to sustain their attempts beyond trial efforts. Finally, some clients refuse to attempt new methods for performance, and instead delegate many roles and responsibilities to others, resulting in increasing dependency.

The system for designing supported function does not imply external assistance provided completely by caregivers. Instead, it is a design of many types of support to enable the individual client to maintain optimal abilities through a personal plan. By establishing client potential and addressing pertinent topics for modified ability, the OT has an important role in assessing, fabricating, and helping implement a program for ongoing ability through applied adaptive strategies. The client then has a sense of regulation and control of planned performance.

Learning Activity 101: Exploring Supported Function

1. Recall an attempt to learn to use a new electronic device or appliance. What was the process that you used to motivate yourself to learn "how to"? What steps were required to support function and ongoing ability? Written instructions? Assistance, demonstration, or coaching from others? Reduced distractions? Trial and error? Take notes for reference?

2. Create a list of possible considerations that would be appropriate for an older adult. Focus on trying a new way (adapted technique) to perform the familiar activity of making a phone call, but now the individual has low vision and is trying to learn how to use a Smartphone. How would you approach the process of teaching new skills? How would you encourage the client, offer instruction, and promote ongoing independent application?

Supported function consists of a carefully structured system to enable ongoing performance. Over time, some of the support measures would be assessed for continued need or considerations for further modification. Many older adults, while considered well and high functioning, devise altered approaches as needed to maintain skills or prevent risk. For example, many seniors avoid driving at night after detecting challenges with distraction caused by oncoming headlights. For individuals seen by OTs in community settings, supported function is made possible by providing minimal planned assistance with tasks such as moderate to heavy IADLs (e.g., vacuuming, shopping, and yard care). The OT may be helpful in defining a spectrum of resources and referrals to provide for a balance of realistic performance of roles and responsibilities while maintaining a private residence.

PHASES OF PARTICIPATION

Phases of participation describe the process involved in any endeavor. Any activity typically has a process of before, doing, and follow-up. This represents the preparation, performance, and ongoing participation in an occupation. These three phases are respectively referred to with labels of *situational adaptation, structured performance,* and *intentional ability*. These constructs parallel with the AOTA (2014) OTPF III, which references steps of occupational pursuit such as seeking and acquisition, exploration, participation, performance, and adjustment.

The following sections break down these components of Conditional Independence with ongoing consideration of activity demands. These are approaches typically used by OT practitioners while offering direct intervention. We are proposing an expanded role for OTs—that of teaching these elements of conditional independence to older adults to promote their continue skill development toward self-management in varied roles and tasks. This would be appropriate during therapy sessions, and reinforced at the time of discharge from formal services. OT services could ideally be reintroduced in the event of future alteration in health or life demands affecting occupational performance.

SITUATIONAL ADAPTATION

This encompasses the beginning phase of any occupation—the "pre" or preparation phase, where needs are identified and exploration takes place for possible approaches. In this phase, a determination is made of the individual's background, interests, and goals, focusing on needs for adaptation. What occupation is presenting a performance challenge? Under what circumstances is this a challenge? Along with the initial assessment of the client's skills, attention is directed toward the evaluation of the nature of the task and the performance setting.

Situational adaptation is a phase of extensive deliberation required for preparation by the OT. What situations create the surrounding considerations to enable adapted performance (i.e., task-related equipment and supplies and the structural or social setting). The OT develops a second sense for expertise in task analysis. How can these skills be taught to an older adult who is being discharged with residual impairments or to clients who are group members of a senior center Living Skills group? Or to a healthy individual who seeks preventive measures for wellness through stress reduction techniques? OTs have opportunities to offer significant assistance in client education, teaching basics of self-directed adaptation for any situation, with attention to activity demands and performance environment.

Consideration of the client's personal needs, interests, and goals would be identified along with a description of known or anticipated challenge areas. For the latter, many current older adults have a proactive determination to modify their living environment while still at a higher level of functioning. For example, some may apply Aging in Place principles with modifications for ease of functioning in anticipation of its future importance.

The universe of occupation possibilities is endless, but OTs have the knowledge and skills to teach clients how to evaluate any activity and adapt it for enhanced successful completion. With this extensive scope of possibilities, a therapist could easily become overwhelmed. However, this holistic approach, considering the client's whole world of functioning, is the domain of OT. Methods are designed to plan, implement, and revise task performance to match varied details of individual engagement.

Situational adaptation represents the phase of planning a comprehensive program to identify task needs, examine the unique characteristics of any activity, determine possible approaches, and establish contingency plans. This phase of planning includes many details and often overlaps with assessment results of client functional status (Table 14-1).

To apply principles of situational adaptation, the dynamic nature of human living needs to be recognized. Even if a consistent activity plan is applied in a consistent manner, things change over time. Schedules of other involved caregivers may shift. Abilities may fluctuate by the day or over time. The planned program may be too complex or "a nuisance" for a client to implement or maintain. Some people resist or resent a conscious "to do" list for their daily living. Even if a program is well maintained, ongoing inspiration and support may be needed to adhere to the plan, expand possibilities for approaches, and creatively problem solve to recognize errors or omissions. Ongoing revisions need to match any fluctuations in ability.

Learning Activity 102: Teaching the Skill of Task Analysis to Older Adults

When teaching the skill of task analysis to older adults for their ongoing application toward future independent occupational performance, what are the unique characteristics of any given activity?

1. List your ideas for generic considerations for a task— what would an older adult need to consider about:

   a. Space:

TABLE 14-1
SITUATIONAL ADAPTATION EXAMPLES OF TASK ANALYSIS FOR ACTIVITY PLANNING AND PREPARATION
IDENTIFY CLIENT NEEDS:
Interests, values, motivation, access to location, skill levels, challenge areas
IDENTIFY CONTRIBUTING FACTORS FOR TASK PERFORMANCE:
Cost, space needed, supplies, time considerations, assistance needed, contraindications, amount of active or passive participation required, process from inception to completion, familiar versus new, purpose, positioning, pacing, learning or research involved, single or multiple sessions needed, safety or risk considerations, steps and sequence required for completion, typically an activity for one person's engagement or more, possibilities for multi-tasking
ANTICIPATE NEEDS:
• Evaluate performance capacity through rehearsal, trial and error, ability for decision making and problem solving, consideration of needed compensatory techniques and preventive strategies, including adaptive or assistive devices, work simplification, joint protection, energy conservation, and risk prevention.   • Appropriateness for functional capacity, balance with other daily, weekly, monthly demands.   • Ability to eliminate ineffective approaches, identify alternative options or solutions; considerations of variable abilities with establishment of a range of possible approaches.   • Ability to initiate and sustain participation and recognize parameters of an occupation, including boundaries of task completion.   • Ability to establish priorities, determine any assistance required by others.
Created by K. C. Macdonald, 2015.

b. Supplies:

c. Time:

d. Assistance needed:

e. Positioning:

f. Safety:

g. Sequence or steps:

2. What would you need to plan for the teaching of this skill to promote the older adult's understanding and follow-through when attempting task analysis independently, after discharge from OT?

Careful planning is needed to anticipate the needs for grading activities to prevent frustration or failure. Tasks may be modified for simplicity or complexity by adapting the time available, number of steps, materials available, positioning, and pacing for speed.

Understanding the client's perspective and comfort level regarding the situational adaption needs exploration. How does he or she react to change or applying a novel approach to familiar occupations? Does the client resent or resist a new way of performance? If needed, can personal standards be flexible for "good enough" results? If compromise is necessary to create trade-offs for skills, what is the emotional reaction and how is coping promoted? Does the client enjoy experimenting or trying new things? Will it be considered novel and fun or deeply frustrating to attempt an altered approach? The client's identity may reflect an attitude of "no matter what, I will find a way to accomplish this." Another individual may refuse options for approaches. Understanding the client's unique outlook as an involved instrument of change is important to the OT's efforts for collaboration in treatment planning and implementation.

Daily performance, whether for a well elder or an older adult with single or multiple health conditions, is a changing kaleidoscope that shifts despite all efforts to establish a predictable pattern for success. Most task participation is never a single step or event, but rather a complete set of connected small steps, often following a specific sequence. Adapting to varied situations is a conscious process, seldom "take it as it comes." Many older adults design and attend to patterns of activity that balance both structured and free time. This helps to focus on priorities and maximize capacity for completing favored or priority tasks. This incorporates attention to both highly structured and less structured hours of a day. By helping the client understand and appreciate the "anatomy of an activity," the OT promotes an awareness of methods to promote task participation and modification. Beyond the supported environment of the clinic or therapy session, the client would establish skills toward independently adapting occupations for his or her personal successful engagement. This would promote an increase related to ongoing participation in a variety of activities, all serving to promote health, well-being, and life satisfaction.

STRUCTURED PERFORMANCE

Structured performance is the continued anticipation of the doing of a desired occupation, but from the perspective of the client's identified skills, challenges, and goals. Some older adults attempt engagement in a beloved activity, experience challenge or difficulty, and then give it up. OTs may play a significant role in modifying tasks to enable participation. This would be the opposite of Nike's slogan, "Just do it." Instead, careful deliberation is devoted to establish means and methods for successful task completion. To determine the most effective and efficient "how to," conscious planning is directed toward understanding—in effect, "what you do, when you do it, and how you do it." Here, activity demands are specifically considered to match the person's unique set of performance skills. Specific goals for optimal activity and occupational competence are addressed through the formal and informal OT assessment procedures.

OT practitioners, through the use of occupations and activities, preparatory methods, education, and advocacy, promote self-directed and self-sustained engagement in desired real life roles and daily living tasks. We guide clients toward developing skills in "deconstructing doing," including planned design, participation, and completion of any selected activity. For structured performance, the therapist and client need to match skills to the demands of a task. This includes the mental planning of the process of a task, all materials needed, and modifications necessary to compensate for performance challenges. When learning a new task or applying a new adaptive strategy, an approach of "one task at a time, one step at a time" may be necessary until mastery is achieved.

Because older adults may have many demands related to ADLs and IADLs, multitasking may present challenges. Conscious attention to planning, and focused application of a structured routine appeared to promote the highest level of success, stability, and satisfaction for the PAS participants. Although some novel and spontaneous opportunities were also welcome and integrated, the more they arranged predictable patterns, the greater the variety in repertoire of occupations.

Most of the participants were experiencing relatively stable levels of ability, with many managing chronic health conditions. Because daily demands fluctuated, they had established methods to arrange for both predictable and unpredictable daily scenarios. For example, a request for childcare assistance with a grandchild may lead to rescheduling volunteer responsibilities. A follow-up to a physician visit may lead to a need to pick up a new medication, requiring an unexpected trip across town during rush hour. Daily living, usually within a known structure and schedule was, in reality, quite dynamic. Tactics for addressing daily needs were managed by careful identification of the goal and then pursuing approaches conducive to success.

If anything interfered with successful completion, they attempted alternative strategies. They would often identify and investigate possibilities and experiment with approaches. They had high skills for focusing on the "here and now," planning for future needs, and having the confidence, competence, and determination to complete a task. These well elders seemed to have a well-developed "savoir faire" and "stick-to-it-iveness." How might OTs promote these strengths for older adults with challenges or for the upcoming generations, as they retire and perhaps had fewer types of occupations, and less experience trouble-shooting?

The OT would complete the occupational profile and appropriate standardized and nonstandardized assessment techniques. The resulting information serves as a basis for determining and designing therapeutic approaches. Discussion with the client related to facilitators and barriers to occupational engagement help to establish personalized treatment goals. Through therapy sessions, the OT plays a role in teaching a client awareness for how to monitor performance capabilities. Consistent daily attention regarding any residual or potential symptoms that would affect performance should be part of a daily routine. For example, recommendations to observe for shortness of breath, edema, fatigue, or pain would be an aspect of structured performance. Consideration of any precautions or contraindications would also precede participation. For some clients, preparatory activities would be an integrated part of an activity. For example, stretching, doing relaxation techniques, applying of hot or cold packs may facilitate comfort and ease of performance.

Other topics to consider prior to Intentional Ability may include time management issues, scheduling, transportation, and family or professional assistance needed. The OT assists with raising the client's awareness of all aspects of the actual doing of any task in conjunction with the individual's unique skill sets. The client would then self-monitor for ongoing attention to whether activities are possible, realistic in scope, or need attention for possible modification.

Learning Activity 103: Applying Principles of Structured Performance

Tom, an 85-year-old client, recently had an annual physical, with his only complaint being stiffness after prolonged sitting. His primary care physician recommended yoga as an intervention and referred the client to an OT specializing in health and wellness programs for seniors. Consider an initial session, focusing on the principles of situational adaptation and structured performance:

1. How will Tom arrange for scheduling? Integrating into his daily or weekly routine? Are there any considerations for clothing and equipment? Is space available at home for follow-up application?

2. Tom has never been much of a joiner. How will the OT encourage his initial attendance?

3. What else might an OT consider as Tom begins involvement with an unfamiliar activity?

4. What would be possible approaches for therapeutic use of self by the OT?

Through structured participation, the OT teaches the client principles of self-monitoring for performance ability. This includes attention to skill levels and limits and methods for intrinsic motivation. This would be similar to a motto of "know thyself." The conscious step prior to activity engagement promotes ability to successfully attempt a desired activity, whether familiar, modified, or unfamiliar.

INTENTIONAL ABILITY

After considering the many aspects of preplanning through situational adaptation (task preparedness) and structured performance (determining how performance skills influence goals and ability), actual involvement in activity occurs and continues over time. The global goal of conditional independence and supported function would be the establishment of a program to promote autonomy for the client. *Intentional Ability* would be defined as the "follow-through" or ongoing participation in desired occupations, as structured and modified, to support and sustain health and quality of life. Application of modified approaches include the client's higher levels of task analysis, determination of skills and challenges encountered, and design of pertinent compensatory techniques to be applied over time. Techniques to promote follow-through would include design of systems for self-reminders, including checklists, calendars, schedules, and cuing from others. Over time, the client would self-monitor and evaluate the effectiveness of the program and determine needs for adaptation.

Following acute illness, injury, or chronic disability, the OT promotes a planned program for managing altered abilities to match occupational choices. The OT also designs systems for maximizing abilities through preventive approaches toward health and wellness. After discharge from services, the client needs to perpetuate these types of interventions independently.

The phase of intentional ability represents application of actual doing of occupations that have been analyzed and structured to enhance successful experiences. The client attempts participation in actual occupations, whether ADLs and IADLS, rest and sleep, education, work, play, leisure, or social participation. Through this, the therapist and client witness areas of success and difficulty. Ongoing intervention evaluates, in further detail areas of explicit challenge requiring skill development or compensatory techniques. The therapist works in collaboration with the client and other interdisciplinary team members to orchestrate pathways toward independence.

A repeated cycle develops: Plan … attempt … apply … revise … adapt …

Intentional implies deliberate, conscious, active application of successfully devised performance steps and patterns. Development of sustained new approaches become a habit or routine with repeated application and reinforcement. To incorporate new methods that enhance ability, the individual needs to incorporate personal insight and planned strategies to assimilate and accommodate the new patterns of performance. Given a realistic perspective on a finite amount of daily time, energy, and ability, the client needs to remember supporting systems for participation, promote the ongoing application of those systems, and continue with self-directed assessment of outcomes.

OTs would assist with designing built-in systems for when the client "goes solo" to independently maintain health promoting programs. Even for the most motivated individual, compliance is a challenge when follow-through is needed for indefinite periods of time. Human tendencies toward procrastination, avoidance, and backsliding may be discussed, with related strategies to enable return to goals. Some PAS participants stated that accountability measures helped them to sustain ongoing efforts. This included personal journals to record and rate abilities, or having a family member or peer serve as a sounding board to report successes or lapses.

On several layers, Intentional Ability was promoted through external supports. Many of the participants shared tips and techniques with peers about incentives to apply techniques toward maximum ability. They also reported that connectedness to family members promoted encouragement for pursuing healthful lifestyle and activity options. The participants often had an outlook of ability as "it depends." Performance depended on adaptation to whatever varying conditions existed. They often had to compromise standards of performance or establish trade-offs toward simpler activities. Regardless of barriers or challenges, they would find a way to "get out of the house," "do things," "have a positive outlook," and "be with people."

The OT's role includes assessment of all aspects of performance influencing engagement in occupation. When working directly with an individual client or group, pending discharge is an ever-present influence on treatment planning. The process includes anticipating the client's skills as he or she plateaus or has demonstrated cycles of altered ability. For productive aging, the OT would ideally help to design a thorough program for the client's ongoing implementation of a highly developed personal skill for designing means to match activity engagement to personal performance skills.

EXPERT'S EXPERIENCE— DR. ROSALIE MILLER, PHD, OTR, FAOTA

Dr. Rosalie Miller is Professor and Director of Doctoral Programs at Brenau University in Gainesville, Georgia. She is the author of *Perspectives in Theory* (1993). She participated in a telephone interview, discussing the need for theoretical frameworks in OT.

She stated that theory validates and guides practice. Since the beginning of the profession, questions have been raised about principles of OT intervention. She related that in 1938, in an editorial in the journal of *Occupational Therapy and Rehabilitation* (vol. 18, April, p. 127), psychologists and physicians were working with OTs. They questioned whether theory was applied to demonstrate how OT assisted in bringing about recovery. Dr. Miller reviewed some key leaders in OT over the following decades. In 1979, Florence Clark encouraged the development and use of theory in order to validate our professional level of service. She continued with a reflection that theories are often used without a great deal of thought … students learn basic theories, but it becomes a portion of their whole training … many clinicians don't consciously use a selected theory, but instead a conglomeration. In 1989, Diane Parham proposed that theory is a key element in problem setting and problem solving. It is a tool that allows therapists to "name it and frame it." Gary Kielhofner (2008) did much work at a time when there was growing complexity in the field. As a critical thinker, one would draw on the well-formed body of knowledge based on theory. Carolyn Baum stated that along with validating and guiding practice services to justify reimbursement, OTs need to conduct theory-based research to develop evidence for supporting OT practice.

Regarding advancement of the profession, Dr. Miller shared that, although we have had increases in research and theory development, it is still an issue. Because areas of specialization have evolved, many feel a need to explain common elements and connections among the variety of specializations. In general, they would help us to grow as a profession as we continue to define a distinctive and ever-evolving theoretical base. The application of a theoretical base to guide clinical decision-making distinguishes professionals from technicians. Academicians are dedicated to educating competent practitioners. Discussion about theory has continued to occur over decades. When Anne

Mosey presented her Slagle Lecture, she debated whether a single, monistic unifying theory would be ideal.

In commenting about progress in this area, Dr. Miller related a new theoretical development by Michael Iwama (2006). In the Kawa Model, he parallels human experience to the natural flow of a river, including reactions to barriers and obstacles. This reflects a cultural perspective stemming from Eastern traditions, adding new theoretical directions to consider.

Other areas of progress include theories from Fidler and Velde (1999), Mosey (1986), and Reilly (1962). Newer models of theories are broader, reflect person-environment occupation, and are more application-based for the whole of OT practice. In the end, the focus is always on occupation, which has been key in recent and developing theory.

For the future, as we move increasingly into community-based practice, we are bringing principles of OT into public health. For example Wilcock (2006) addresses issues of occupational justice. Dr. Miller stated that she currently works with a thesis group focusing on health promotion and fall prevention for older adults. Studies and practice in these emerging areas will continue to have an impact on the development of OT as a profession. New topics are always emerging for potential OT involvement: disasters, wars, occupational deprivation, and poor work conditions in factories in third-world countries.

When asked to make three recommendations for new OT graduates, Dr. Miller answered:

1. Be comfortable and familiar with occupation-based theories, as well as the most recent theories from medical and social sciences. Many theories have changed (e.g., motor control). Stay updated with theoretical changes and developments, continue to be a learner.

2. Really look at prevention and health promotion…don't wait until there is a fall and fracture and need for rehabilitation. There are lots of ways to promote older adults staying as healthy as they can for as long as they can.

3. We need to be doing evidence-based practice; not just reviewing recent research, but making sure it is sound and applicable. There is a triangle, with three related pieces:

   a. The client situation: carefully assess, understand, and listen.

   b. Review of related literature and research.

   c. The therapist's own experience, theoretical perspective, and knowledge guiding professional clinical reasoning.

SUMMARY

In bringing the PAS to a close, the large amount of data gathered and analyzed led to interesting implications for OT practice. Forty retired older adults, identified as active in several life roles, participated in semi-structured interviews that explored their history and current occupations. The main themes—self-management, social connections, and self-fulfilling activities—were explored from the participants' perspectives, a review of literature, and the application to OT practice. Considering both individual and group settings within the medical model and the community-based model of service delivery, the OT has many possibilities for direct intervention, client instruction, consultation, and advocacy. The theory that emerged from the data was labeled Conditional Independence, with elements of Situational Adaptation, Structured Performance, and Intentional Ability contributing to Supported Function.

Limitations to the study and findings include consideration of the parameters of qualitative research, in which the findings are representative of a unique group and are not intended to be generalizable to unrelated groups or settings. They do reflect the unique self-reported, subjective views of 40 community dwelling, well older adults at this time in their lives.

Recommendations for future research would include conducting similar semi-structured interviews with individuals representing other levels of ability, living environment, or varied culture or ethnicity. With a smaller number of participants, observations and/or follow-up interviews would be helpful to explore additional elements of ability. The theory of Conditional Independence would need to be analyzed further and determinations made for eventual translation into conceptual models of practice or frames of reference.

The findings support the view of OT practitioners that occupations are important, are varied between individuals, and contribute to the maintenance of life satisfaction and varied role performance. Social identity was seen as a facilitating factor for participation in daily tasks, both for self-care and occupations outside of the home. The findings reinforced viewpoints that OTs have significant roles in promoting health and enhanced function through invention, including remediation, modification, and prevention. The final chapter offers descriptions of realms of practice for specialization with older adults in a wide spectrum of settings, while anticipating the future of OT's expanding role in public health.

REFERENCES

American Occupational Therapy Association. (2014). Occupational therapy practice framework: Domain and process, 3rd edition. *American Journal of Occupational Therapy, 68,* S1-S48.

Fidler, G. S., & Velde, B. P. (1999). *Activities: Reality and symbol.* Thorofare, NJ: SLACK Incorporated.

Hinojosa, J., & Anderson, J. (1991). Mothers' perception of home treatment programs for their preschool children with cerebral palsy. *American Journal of Occupational Therapy, 45,* 273-279.

Iwama, M. (2006). *The Kawa Model: Culturally relevant occupational therapy.* New York: Elsevier.

Kielhofner, G. (2008). *Model of human occupation: Theory and application* (4th ed.). Baltimore, MD: Lippincott Williams & Wilkins.

Laliberte-Rudman, D. L.; Cook, J. V.; & Polatajko, H. (1997). Understanding the potential of occupation: A qualitative exploration of seniors' perspective on activity. *American Journal of Occupational Therapy, 51,* 662-670.

Miller, R., & Walker, K. F. (1993). *Perspectives on theory for the practice of occupational therapy.* Gaithersburg, MD: Aspen Publications.

Moll, S., & Cook, J. V. (1997). "Doing" in mental health: Therapists' beliefs about why it works. *American Journal of Occupational Therapy, 51,* 640-650.

Mosey, A. C. (1986). *Psychosocial components of occupational therapy.* New York: Raven Press.

Reilly, M. (1962). Eleanor Clarke Slagle Lecture: Occupational therapy can be one of the great ideas of 20th century medicine. *American Journal of Occupational Therapy, 16,* 1-9.

Siporin. S., & Lysack, C. (2004). Quality of life and supported employment: A case study of three women with developmental disabilities. *American Journal of Occupational Therapy, 58,* 455-465.

Tham, K., & Keilhofner, G (2003). Impact of social environment on occupational experience and performance among persons with unilateral neglect. *American Journal of Occupational Therapy, 57,* 403-412.

Wilcock, A. (2006). An occupational perspective of health (2nd ed.). Thorofare, NJ: SLACK Incorporated.

15

Future Opportunities for Occupational Therapy in Gerontology

Karen C. Macdonald, PhD, OTR/L

This final chapter reflects back on content from the PAS and literature reviews. It is a final synthesis of topics related to geriatric OT practice, with a focus on predicting future needs. Although the medical model is likely to continue to be a predominant area for employment, social and policy changes are occurring at a more rapid pace. These changes place expanding emphasis on health promotion and wellness programs. Therefore, attention to interventions through community-based services continue to increase. Regardless of setting, OTs will have ongoing responsibilities for defining their scope and range of services through evidence-based research. Demands for standardized assessment tools are likely to increase, along with means to demonstrate effectiveness in meeting long- and short-term treatment goals. Incorporated into all expectations will be methods for data management and recordkeeping through electronic recordkeeping systems.

MAKING PROGRESS

In the past 100 years, gerontology has evolved into an important specialty area. OTs have developed many recognized roles and functions in a spectrum of settings, from adult day care and home care to hospice services. Research and publications have blossomed, exploring assessment strategies, influences of various treatment methods, and client satisfaction with intervention. These expanding roles have also extended to involvement in community programs and education, consulting with organizations, and advocacy and lobbying offers to promote improved services for older adults.

New graduates will be entering the profession at a time of "pick up the baton and keep running." Public awareness of OT has increased. However, competition for shifting availability of funding resources influences our need to define OT's uniqueness and importance to a client's functional ability and quality of life. OT practitioners promote abilities for real life skills in relation to real life occupations and environments. The increasing demographics in older Americans will create a continued and perhaps increasing demand for our specialized services within an interdisciplinary team.

In approaching the centennial anniversary of OT's inception, leaders and literature continue to promote further areas of exploration and development. The participants in the PAS reflected two generations of individuals who have had increased attention and adherence to healthy lifestyle habits and diverse life roles. This leads to a changing set of likely clients with very different needs from those of past decades. Individuals are remaining at home for longer periods and fewer ever reside in a long-term care facility. When seen for rehabilitation, symptoms are often more advanced and represent multiple types of functional challenges. Traditional restorative intervention will continue to focus on promoting function and maximizing abilities in self-care, task performance, and social skills.

Cole MB, Macdonald KC.
Productive Aging: An Occupational Perspective (pp 243-252).
© 2015 Taylor & Francis Group.

As individuals have increased longevity, the likelihood of comorbidities and progression of chronic conditions increases. OT can be recommended for a client who has a combination of acute and chronic conditions. For example, a person with a long-standing diagnosis of diabetes may develop significant visual impairment or an individual with chronic obstructive pulmonary disease may experience a fall on ice and fracture a shoulder. The OT needs to examine all aspects of function and dysfunction in the context of past, present, and future participation and performance goals. These complex cases for clients with multiple challenges create a practice environment that is both demanding and exciting, as therapists strive to assess and address the unique needs of each client or group.

Perspectives on chronic illness as a general social concern are described by Edwards (2013), "Now more than 133 million Americans live with chronic illness, accounting for nearly three-quarters of all health care dollars and untold pain and disability." Historical viewpoints about illness have evolved from superstitions about "being punished," to "it's all in your head," to current neuroscience and genetic influences. Edwards (2013) praises recent decades of civil rights awareness movements, including gender equality, disability advocacy, independent living movement, and health care reforms. The OT profession and practice have been strongly shaped by each of these social paradigm shifts.

Along with individuals who have led healthier lifestyles, the current generation of older adults also reflects those who may have lived for decades with poor health habits. This has resulted in increasing health challenges due to obesity, alcohol and tobacco use, or a sedentary lifestyle.

Other areas of intervention are more related to prevention and wellness. Prevention principles may be introduced during middle-age and early senior years as developmental changes naturally occur (e.g., client education about joint protection, body mechanics, and positioning). Another principle of prevention is that of influencing the rate of decline of skills, or monitoring current ability. The progressive nature of many conditions, and aging itself, eventually leads to potential loss of mobility, sensory, cognitive, and social skills. Some intervention is designed to slow this decline through therapeutic interaction to retrain a current level of ability. Other interventions match declining skills through graded activities and modified performance training.

Learning Activity 104: Client Education

Clinical education is a key element of intervention regardless of the practice setting. When working with older adults, what would be considerations for teaching and learning? Design a 1- to 2-page handout as a group that identifies unique learning styles of seniors and also adapted teaching strategies beyond verbal dissemination of information.

Wellness and health promotion practices may also be introduced at younger ages, encouraging a life span program for optimum functioning. This may include promoting use of meaningful occupations, such as leisure and social activities, to create a basis for expanded exposure to "doing." A life history of varied interests or involvement was one of the key findings in the PAS; patterns of past experience with activity influenced health and life satisfaction in later years. Modifications creatively designed by OTs may be needed to promote continued engagement in their choices for meaningful and purposeful activities.

JOURNAL ENTRY (K. M.)

As the final month of our deadline presented "an end in sight," I just had to have faith that completion is possible. The research project finally ended...or did it? With the review of literature, we keep finding more new/different/exciting resources to incorporate. Great, but they add another dimension for comparing, contrasting, or adding to our findings.

What is the bottom line? My army of supporters keeps asking for updates and publication dates. "I want to buy that book! It will teach me how to live longer!" Do we have the answers? Maybe we do, and OTs can be helpful leaders in new forms of extending life and promoting quality of life through selected roles and structured occupations.

Our results? Skills for self-management included commonly recognized themes of attention to diet, exercise, and sleep, along with avoiding poor health habits of smoking and alcohol use and increasing attention to safety risks with aging. We discovered new layers of importance to self-management, including social identity, perpetuation of roles and routines, and function promoted by repeated performance of many ADL and IADLs that require sensory, motor, and cognitive skills. Social connections provided opportunities for countless skill maintaining/building areas: feeling a part of a group, participating in cultural interests or volunteer projects, and feeling supported by "like-minded people" created a sense of purpose and well-being. Self-fulfilling activities represented new or life long interests—hobbies, sports, games, and reading, all of which offered meaningful goals and pleasure, from completing a crossword puzzle to learning photography. If I had to boil it down to an "elevator speech," I would have to say our bottom line findings were as follows:

- Take care of your body (self-care).

- Always find ways to learn.

- Participate in work or volunteer activities.

- Discover your passions for meaningful activities.

- Join an organization or group.

These were their real secrets to productive aging. In combination, these activities prolonged independent skills, offered connections to others, and promoted a sense of continued growth, belonging, and participation.

CAREER OPTIONS

With a specialty in geriatrics, the OT may look forward to variety of career choices, with pathways that are truly unlimited. When working as a clinician, a rich and rewarding career is possible. Options exist for varying schedules and caseloads, from per diem to full time. Responsibilities may be endlessly creative and exciting for providing *direct treatment* to individuals and groups. Transitions to other settings on the continuum of care are also available. In addition, professional growth and advancement may also be achieved through advanced practice, administrative, academic, and leadership opportunities.

The following section describes possibilities for expanded roles, in addition to or as a "career ladder." In the clinical setting, a clinician's role may develop rather quickly from new graduate to clinical fieldwork *supervisor* and/or department supervisor. Department head and *administrative* promotions may occur over time (e.g., Director of Rehabilitation Services).

Learning Activity 105: Time Management for Administrative Responsibilities

Administrative and supervisory tasks define a large portion of responsibilities for the OT when working in geriatrics.

1. As a self-awareness exercise, create an activity to explore the topic of time management skills.

2. What are your strengths and challenges?

3. How can the OT best balance the demands of direct treatment with other required duties?

While remaining in the clinical arena, many other expanded roles are possible. Clinical *research* is encouraged, with possibilities ranging from single case studies to formal qualitative, descriptive, or quantitative studies, perhaps collaborating with a local university. *Teaching* opportunities exist, such as service training for staff development of varied disciplines. External to the clinic, OTs may engage in public speaking about various health topics. This author taught a community adult education class entitled "Understanding Your Aging Parent." Many OTs engage in writing activities. A variety of OT publications accept articles reporting research results, program descriptions, or essays supporting opinions on current issues. Many health care publishers promote work by OT authors featuring biographical, descriptive, and research-based materials.

Teaching is an avenue for experienced clinicians to expand their role and participate in the development of future practitioners. Part-time opportunities are often available for adjunct faculty members. Rich opportunities exist for the OT geriatric specialists to shift gears and enter the world of academia. As a full-time faculty member, the OT assumes a new assortment of responsibilities. These include teaching, advising, committee work, and, usually, participation in scheduling pursuits of research and publications. Within the academic arena, a different career ladder exists for advancement and promotion involving varied demonstrated competencies.

Consulting is a rewarding way for experienced OTs to offer highly developed skills. Consultants may perform a needs assessment for new services, recommend changes to existing programs, or assist in other specialized needs.

Learning Activity 106: Consultation in Your Community

1. Identify three unmet needs for elders in your community.

2. How could an OT develop a consulting position to serve one of those unmet needs? Consider all phases of initiating, implementing, and concluding the time limited project.

In addition to these layers of professional involvement, other areas of involvement and exposure exist. These include participation in local, state, national, and international *projects*. These may be paid positions but often are volunteer participation in committees, lobbying, or advocacy activities. An example would be serving as the president of a state OT association.

Learning Activity 107: Professional Advocacy

OTs may have a role on a national level, advocating for some issue related to health care services or the needs of an identified population.

1. Given your knowledge of current events, write a letter to a state representative about an issue related to occupational justice and senior issues.

2. Present a draft of the letter to others for review and editing.

3. Send the letter and report any results to OT peers.

Another perspective of career advancement would be through *continuing education*. Courses are mandated for licensure in most states. Separate from that, many OTs seek additional training, earning certificates or additional degrees in related specialized areas of interest.

Learning Activity 108: Private Practice Opportunities

Private practice opportunities exist in geriatric specialization as an OT.

1. Identify three possibilities in this arena.

2. Would these ideas be something that you would consider in the future? Why or why not?

3. What would be involved for each? List steps.

In *OT Practice*, a publication of the AOTA, a continuing education article highlights potential avenues from new practitioner to leadership positions. Ellison, Hanson, and Schmidt (2013) describe a need for development of future leaders. Career mapping involves goal setting, time frames, and strategies. Participating in a mentor relationship allows for growth through a partnership with an experienced practitioner. Leadership development often includes transitioning from a clinical role; educating oneself about departmental, facility, state, and federal rules and regulations; and a redefinition of relationships with former peers. Skills especially valued in managerial positions are critical thinking, problem solving, future planning, effective leadership, and fiscal responsibility. The variety of career options reflect the many possibilities for OTs to have a fulfilling career in gerontology. This flexibility allows for specialization in a single area of interest or explorations of many aspects of work with older adults.

The advanced practitioner may move toward independence and autonomy through *private practice*. This may include traditional, specialty, alternative, or newly designed programs and services. Background skills should include business management or networking as a means for referrals and personnel supervision.

For clinicians wishing to explore the possibility of opening a private practice, self-awareness of personal and professional skills and strengths is essential, as well as potential need for growth (Glennon, 2012; Harmon, 2014). Skills are necessary for technology, marketing and business management, administrative and supervisory responsibilities, and the ability to envision the full process of conceptualizing, initiating, and sustaining a small business (Glennon, 2012). Harmon (2014) recommends a full awareness of market trends, consumer needs of target client populations, sources for referral, and potential barriers. Harmon (2014) also suggests the need for understanding analyzing local competition, networking with others who also share entrepreneurial endeavors, and careful consideration of all financial responsibilities.

A final category of career flexibility is the *returning* or *transitioning* practitioner. This could represent a mother who has been a stay-at-home mom for a number of years wishing to reestablish her role as an OT practitioner or it could represent an individual who has specialized in another practice specialty such as mental health or substance abuse services and is looking to work with a different population. Re-entry and lateral moves are facilitated by review of recent literature, visits to local agencies, and participation in any local specialty interest section meetings. These practitioners are often encouraged to do a task analysis of their preceding roles in order to appreciate all of the related skills that they will be bringing to their subsequent place of employment.

Many aspects of the above may apply to OTAs. If the *OTA wishes to transition to an OT* level of practice, specially designed programs exist to complete a graduate degree and take the National Board for Certification in Occupational Therapy examination. These programs are often planned to meet the needs of working OTAs, such as weekend programs.

Learning Activity 109: Health Care Payment Systems

Identify reimbursement issues for elders.

1. What coverage is available for different levels of care?

2. Using online research, briefly investigate topics of private insurance, Medicare, Medicaid, and other third-party payers for senior citizens.

3. Discuss with others if available and review options for individuals who do not have any health care coverage.

Learning Activity 110: Documentation Procedures

Documentation systems and regulations vary by facility and state.

1. Investigate current models for documentation of services for extended care facilities in your region.

2. If applicable, during fieldwork experiences, request copies of their methods for record keeping.

3. Create a binder or electronic file for future reference.

EXPERT'S EXPERIENCE— DR. PAM STORY, OTD, OTR

Dr. Pam Story has had over 30 years of experience working in varied geriatric settings. Her career ladder has included roles as clinician, supervisor, and administrator. She is also currently an adjunct faculty member in OT programs related to gerontology. She reflected back on former practices and how OT roles have evolved and shared her perspectives on current and future needs for the OT profession.

In the early 1980s, Dr. Story worked in the Midwest in a geriatric nursing home. At that time, facilities formerly known as asylums and institutions were closing. The population in her setting had combined issues of mental illness and mental retardation. Many of them would not have been able to function in the community after many years in the structured care environment. Therefore, one residence area was allowed to remain and continue to "work the farm," participating in tasks to sustain the workings of the facility. The population changed to reflect new admissions, with diverse diagnoses such as cerebrovascular accident, Charcot-Marie-Tooth, muscular dystrophy, and cerebral palsy. Intervention included assessment, treatment, and documentation on a one-to-one basis. Additional roles included wheelchair fitting and modification as needed.

After that, she worked in a long-term care psychiatric facility with clients who were both acute and long term. Individual and group therapy was provided for a population including mental health, suicide attempts, dementia, and other geropsychiatric conditions. Referrals to OT also included fractures, nerve injuries, and traumatic brain injury.

After moving to the east coast, Dr. Story has worked in a long-term care/skilled nursing facility that also served a subacute population. In this setting, she treated assorted conditions such as aging individuals with schizophrenia and Down's syndrome. She has been promoted from practitioner to supervisor and administrator of rehabilitation. She replied to the following interview questions:

What would you define as current issues and challenges for occupational therapists?

Productivity expectations are high; we have to be able to give excellent outcomes to return subacute clients to their prior level of functioning. We need to clearly and thoroughly document what we are doing and define what our skills are and what we give. Now, there are so many other disciplines claiming "function" as their goal—we need to clearly define ourselves.

I believe the pendulum has swung to the "good old school" fashion of OT student. We need to prepare to be the best of what OT has always been. Considering that we need to learn medically based modalities, in practice, how can we make approaches into truly purposeful activities as opposed to strictly exercise and education?

We are dealing with much more complex patients, whether orthopedic or overall functional decline. We are seeing more for home care environmental adaptations. We see challenges with such a broad range of multiple comorbidities and family issues. Sometimes our attention is not as much directed at the client but more at the expectations of the extended family.

If you had a crystal ball, what would you predict about the future for geriatric OT?

The best case scenario would be for students to be truly expert in task analysis. That means to be grounded in our original truly occupation-based principles, blended with a medical model for understanding the human body. We need to be well versed in the medical model and pull it into our overall treatment for both assessment and treatment. We need to pull in the extended family and develop their involvement. We need to be much more integrated for physical, mental, and psychological approaches.

For the environment, this needs to be not just the actual physical environment; we have to consider where they came from and what they are going to and, if feasible, offer resources to point them toward [making] it happen, such as resources for finding contractors.

We need to understand more about "money follows the person" programs. Other disciplines are working quickly and effectively to claim reimbursement or funding for goals of function. We need to better define occupation and its relation to function. We are lacking one overarching definition of occupation, and I keep looking for it. I find more about this in international OT literature.

The challenge for students is going to be knowing about the facilities they are going to; many facilities are not equipped for true function. Occupational therapists need more involvement in the design of long-term care facilities' environments. I would like to see us go beyond a "gym" OT department and get back to purposeful activities such as a kiln, weaving, and woodworking.

What do you think is the meaning of OT in today's society and health care system?

Occupational therapists are the only habilitative and rehabilitative professionals who are trained and experienced in dealing with the whole: person, environment, situations, and lifespan. That is both our strength and stumbling block. We focus on integrating, others focus on dis-integrating.

Do you have any special recommendations for new graduates?

There are several areas of geriatric practice that I would not suggest until a clinician is more experienced. I would suggest working for a few years and have diverse experiences with a mentor, otherwise you shortchange yourself and your clients. This relates to roles such as health care, consulting, private practice, and traveling therapist.

What are three things you wish you had learned to prepare you for geriatric specialization?

I didn't learn much about "geriatrics"…we learned about conditions. I wish I had a better foundation in what would be considered "normal" aging and what is "extraordinary aging," like all the centagenarians we are seeing today. More about the role of family and community, and their role in influencing function for a client. Task analysis related to the whole scope of performance, beyond the medical model.

In summarizing, Dr. Story reflected a full circle in her experience. Therapy was fully holistic and then replaced by a long trend for fully medical models of intervention. Now, the larger picture is pulling back and returning to and advancing occupation as opposed to strictly function. She expressed a positive acknowledgment of occupational therapists' steady contributions for geriatric rehabilitation. She encourages her students to continue to grow in recognizing the core uniqueness of clients and respecting the importance of promoting ability in meaningful occupations.

EXPERT'S OPINION—
MICKEY REED, MS, MSED, OTR/L

Mickey Reed discussed the future role of OT in geriatrics. She is the Program Director of the Occupational Therapy Assistant Program at Housatonic Community College in Bridgeport, Connecticut. In considering both medical and community models, she promotes that the practitioner needs to know "that when your focus is to 'help somebody,' you've already lost your original path, but if you come in with the idea that my liberation is tied up with your liberation, then you've got a much better chance of freeing the person from whatever the difficulty is." This gets away from a therapist's perspective of "I've got it together and you don't and I'm the one to help you." The therapist often experiences personal or professional growth as a result of the therapeutic relationship with a client.

Ms. Reed confirmed an awareness that the Baby Boomers will represent a new generation of clients. They will be taking more control of their health or ability concerns, have more access and skillful use of technology, and expect health care providers to be respectful of their autonomy. They have so much more of a voice, having had access to education and many avenues for being an informed consumer. They will be aware of many options as they have witnessed the medical system changing.

She concluded that OTs need to rethink professional distancing and boundaries, and that will provide a richer perspective. In the therapeutic relationship, the client and therapist are both growing and achieving goals. Therapists need to feel a solid confidence in expressing their needs and expectations and find a way to meet them or be open to others' discovery of ways to meet them.

EXPANDING ROLES AND SETTINGS
FOR OCCUPATIONAL THERAPISTS

OTs have been encouraged to expand their roles in settings such as mental health, environmental consultation, and health and wellness programs. Beyond individual one-to-one services and groups, goals of increased presence in organizations and community agencies have been promoted. In viewing an increasing movement toward community-based services, OTs will continue to be com-

petent for designing programs to match home or local settings.

Based on the findings from the PAS, the authors discovered many possible roles for OTs to participate in prevention and health promotion. As "successful seniors" strive to maintain or increase abilities, OTs have expertise to assess and address skills for self-management, caregiving, volunteering, social connections, paid work, and self-fulfilling activities. These occupations were identified as influencing health and increasing life satisfaction and quality of life. For each of the activity categories, OTs have unique skills for task analysis, compensatory techniques, graded activity, and supported learning. These task areas occur in a social context of family and friends and within a setting of home or community structures. The OT may have a significant role in matching ability to relationships to others and to their physical environment.

Given these preferred occupational pursuits, the practitioner could potentially identify many possible activities for intervention. Some ideas include the following:

- Lead groups for older women in senior centers focusing on adapted grooming and dressing skills.

- Offer cooking classes for widows and widowers.

- Evaluate elder drivers.

- Teach caregiving skills in adult education.

- Teach programs in a public library for introduction to computer use for seniors.

- Work with volunteer department heads to successfully identify work opportunities matched to an individual's abilities and interests.

- Contract with a corporation to consult regarding pre-retirement planning for employees; participate in evaluations for safety hazards and promoting protective ergonomics.

- Consult with architects and subcontractors regarding principles of universal design.

- Co-lead community groups to teach resources for immigrants dealing with chronic health conditions.

- Participate in travel and educational service programs for active seniors, with roles as coordinator for scheduling and planning of group activities.

- Serve as a public speaker to local service organizations about providing leisure-cultural activities for seniors.

This list depicts possibilities for paid or unpaid roles for the OT. When an OT designs a new niche in a volunteer position, it frequently demonstrates fulfillment of a need and often develops into a paid position as a consultant or clinician.

Witnessing the expanding proportion of older adults in our society, OTs may continue to offer important services to promote independence and social participation. Types of intervention are likely to continue to develop to best promote ability and function in those who are healthy, experiencing acute illness or injury, or living with a chronic condition. Because this population is likely to have comorbidities, OTs will continue to demonstrate expertise in understanding the unique individual client's goals and establish programs to promote meaningful participation in preferred occupations.

EMERGING AREAS OF PRACTICE

OT has evolved as a dynamic profession, reflecting development in its own evidence-based practice and changes in health care and society. As a profession, it has acknowledged the changing nature of knowledge and practice, and the need to work in collaboration with other disciplines, who also continue to evolve.

Advances have been made in recent decades with expanding practice in medical and community-based model settings. Group programming has been encouraged as a means of addressing many conditions for increasingly varied populations of older adults. Increasing attention has been given to research, and the need for standardized assessments and expertise to tailor treatment planning to specific client-centered needs. Educational programs have stressed the development of critical thinking and clinical reasoning skills. Beyond direct intervention, local, regional, and national initiatives have promoted efforts to expand OT's scope of practice to additional consultation and advocacy roles.

For three areas in particular, OT has been in the forefront of developing areas of intervention. The profession continues to explore needs in these areas for additional research, and for establishment of treatment programs.

Health and Wellness

These programs are preventive in nature and address holistic issues for life satisfaction and maintaining well-being. An OT's individual or group intervention may include the following:

- Fall prevention
- Safety training for home, yard, and community
- Consumer protection
- Exercise programs
- Support groups
- Stress reduction
- Referrals to community opportunities for volunteer roles
- Driving considerations
- Coping with age-related changes

- Adjusting to new roles and life transitions (retiree/widow)

Technology

OT roles in technology have matched advances in all forms of electronic devices. Historically, OTs have assisted with adapted switches for assistive technology and use of software programs to promote specific skills.

With the advent of the personal computer, tablet, and Smartphone, older adults have had increasing participation in developing computer literacy. OTs could increase involvement in skill training for use of electronic devices from beginner to expert levels. Teaching strategies would be designed to match learner need, ranging from logging in to sophisticated online research. As technology shifts quickly in format and methods for use, OTs could help with transitions to promote user independence.

Primary Care

A recent area for proposed growth is the OT role in primary care. The OT would work directly with a physician to determine degrees of functional challenges caused by an identified condition. The therapist would assess how a condition is affecting ADL and IADL status, and the influence of the client's performance environment and social network. The OT's holistic consideration of physical, cognitive, sensory, and emotional factors and how they relate to occupation provides information to strengthen treatment planning for interdisciplinary team members, including nurses and social workers.

Learning Activity 111: Interdisciplinary Teamwork

In many settings, interdisciplinary teamwork is the norm.

1. What have you noticed in clinical observation related to how different disciplines work together or separately in various settings?

2. Reimbursing agencies will not recognize duplicate services. Consider the topic of professional boundaries and how four different health care providers, in addition to OTs, will meet the needs of productive agers.

EXPERT'S EXPERIENCE— DR. JODY BORTONE, EdD, OT/L

Dr. Jody Bortone participated in an in-person interview. She is the Associate Dean in the College of Health Professions, and Chair and Director of the graduate program in Occupational Therapy at Sacred Heart University in Fairfield, Connecticut. When asked about future roles in OT and preparing the students for emerging areas of practice, she focused on the topic of primary care. She remarked that at the recent AOTA National Conference in Baltimore, Maryland, increased attention was given to this area.

"Primary care is going to be a critical emerging area of practice for our profession, especially considering the increasing populations of elderly who have diverse needs. It will encompass home care, leadership, advocacy, and consulting all rolled into one.

"Preparation is going to increase, as programs and the profession are just beginning to prepare for these roles. It's going to require that the profession make connections with primary care physicians to create these roles, because they don't exist. Currently the jobs and payment systems don't exist. If we wait for reimbursement to exist first, we will be closed out of these roles. We need to create these positions before there is identified reimbursement.

"Primary care goes beyond health and wellness. For OTs, it is working with people with several major medical conditions, who are taking a plethora of medications...we won't find them in rehabilitation or well elder centers, we will be seeing them as the Aging in Place, which too often translates to Isolating in Place.

"In terms of needs for students, they will need to be prepared for the challenges of new kinds of leadership, assertiveness, and advocacy...they will need to go out and create jobs for themselves. They will be explaining 'This is OT' if the vision isn't there. We need to help students to create a vision of what OT could be in primary care, inspire a passion, and then work on the skills. However, we need to consider whether this is really an appropriate role for a new graduate...it will require personal and professional maturity. Now, with a graduate program, we do get second-career students who have this personal maturity to feel comfortable approaching physicians to get a foot in the door to create these new roles.

"This is all innovative and just novel and right now. The profession is assessing the needs of older adults in home care, varied settings, and primary care. Working with a physician, the OT would offer immediate assessment and recommendations for managing habits and routines to support health and function. This is beyond ADLs and transfers and extends to broader occupations and life roles. The OT will have important roles for helping to develop and maintain skills needed for everyday living."

ANTICIPATING FUTURE ROLES

Health care systems of service delivery and reimbursement policies fluctuate in unpredictable ways. OTs need to be sensitive to needs for new research, the avenues for increasing our roles to match consumer need, and dem-

onstrate effective outcomes. What are OT roles in the future for working with older adults? They may include the following:

- Bariatrics
- Substance abuse
- Veteran needs
- Survivors of trauma
- Disaster assistance
- Promoting universal design
- Suicide prevention
- Designing living spaces for seniors
- Assisting with program design for individuals with dementia
- Establishing wellness services
- Homelessness

Learning Activity 112: Past, Present, and Future

1. Past: Consider the year that you were born. What were three public health issues of that era? Did OTs have roles for intervention?

2. Present: List three current public health issues at a population level. Do OTs have a current role in addressing them? How could that be expanded? If OT is not yet involved in this issue, what are some possibilities?

3. Future: Imagine three public health issues for the future OT practitioner. What would need to change to enable expertise and involvement in those areas?

OTs have the skills to identify an issue of occupational challenge, define strategies for adaptation and compensation or skill development, and structure function for maximizing independence. New graduates are encouraged to embrace the responsibilities of continuing to promote the benefits of OT as a key profession to assist with enabling ability and assuring quality of life.

Learning Activity: Career Timeline

Create a timeline representing your projected career as an OT practitioner from graduation to retirement. For each decade, list the type of practice setting, specialty, and level of responsibility that would be a goal for you. Compare with other group members.

SUMMARY

Throughout the project of the PAS, related research and writing, the authors discovered that anyone who heard about the project was very excited about the topic. Participants enthusiastically "signed on" and commented throughout about their belief that the topic and what they contributed was very important. The authors' social networks and acquaintances often asked, "Why didn't you interview me? I would have a lot to say!" Students were interested in learning the real life perspectives of older adults.

The participants were also firm in their statements that students needs to know this information for two reasons. First, so that students could empathize and understand the realities of daily living of healthy older adults. Second, because most of their comments reflected decades-long healthy habits; they want students to begin to develop positive lifestyles for themselves, and also promote them for their middle-aged clients.

The classic "common sense" secrets to successful aging were supported in our findings, including attention to a healthy diet, exercise, positive attitude, rest, and avoidance of negative health habits. Additional findings in the PAS included the importance of other aspects of occupational engagement, including self-management, caregiving, paid work, social connections, volunteering, home management, and self-fulfilling activities. Those findings were supported by interdisciplinary review of literature.

Final synthesis of all findings contributed to the development of an emergent theory. Based on the process of qualitative inquiry and analysis, it was labeled *Conditional Independence*. The OT practitioner assesses the client's needs, goals, and challenge areas and then creates an adaptable system to match facilitated performance to variable abilities. This includes instruction methods specifically geared toward promoting client skills for problem solving and adaptive strategies. This ability to modify or manage life skills and chosen occupations would lead to continued independence in many areas of functioning.

REVIEW OF OUTCOMES

Throughout this process of research, review and writing, we kept in mind the richness of the OTPF III (AOTA, 2014) and the AOTA's (2007) Centennial Vision. As a self-check, a review of *Types of Outcomes from the OT Process* was performed.

- *Occupational Performance:* The PAS identified key areas of occupational performance as important to retired older adults. The participants specified self-management, social connections, and self-fulfilling activities as a means to improve and enhance life satisfaction and quality of life.

- *Health and Wellness:* The participants took pride in long-established positive lifestyle choices. Many were especially interested in sharing their stories in hopes

that others would be inspired to initiate their successful strategies for full and fulfilling lives.

- *Participation:* A strong finding was the meaning and power of varied types of participation as an influential life factor. Whether individual pursuits (crossword puzzles) or involving social contact (volunteering), repeated examples were offered regarding the importance of activity and involvement.

- *Prevention:* Preventing illness or injury is an important "other side of the coin" to promoting health. OTs have a professional legacy of both areas of intervention through safety awareness, compensatory techniques, health/ergonomics, education, and intervening for indications of mental or physical decline. The participants valued professional input and reported many examples of personal problem solving. They had perspectives of "nip it in the bud" and welcomed medical advances for preventive measures (e.g., shingles vaccination).

- *Quality of Life:* The review of literature substantiates the views of the participants and OT principles about the importance of the interaction of activity participation, structural context, and interpersonal relations. In combination, these defined individuals' identity, sense of purpose, use of time, and life satisfaction. Whether traditionalists or Baby Boomers, the participants shared a perspective of future orientation. They anticipated future events of personal significance, leading to a sense of purpose and increased participation in planning of upcoming occasions. OTs could assist with promoting quality of life by assisting with assessment and intervention for participation in upcoming activities through structured performance.

- *Role Competence:* The consolidated evidence from the PAS and the review of literature supported the importance of all performance patterns. Roles established over a lifetime were supported and adjusted to match health or ability changes. Post-retirement roles, habits, and routines were established, which often included new social connections and patterns of performance. Preserving and promoting a sense of sustaining self-identity is an important underlying goal in geriatric OT. The PAS participants represented an array of role diversity. They each had differing roles encompassing a variety of assorted settings: self and home care, family, friends, and community. OTs could assist with the identification, exploration, and pursuit of additional meaningful roles.

- *Occupational Justice:* Much of the literature reviewed included summary section recommendations for OTs to participate in development of public policy. This would include issues such as advocating for expanded services for seniors, improving funding for supportive programs, and lobbying for legislative issues that promote health and wellness for older adults. The OT may

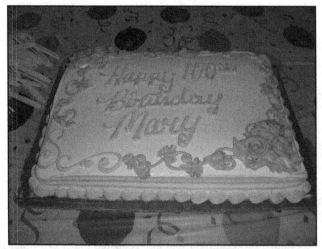

Figure 15-1. The authors look forward to celebrating the American Occupational Therapy Association's 100th birthday in 2017.

partner with a former client to offer testimony about the need for universal design for a proposed new senior center.

The outcomes relate to potential roles and functions of the OT and OTA. Through the process of evaluation and intervention, needs are explored, goals identified, and therapeutic strategies are designed in collaboration with the client. Because clients experience occupation in the context of their larger world, including family, community, and nation, outcomes may be narrowly focused or expansive. Throughout their education and professional careers, OT practitioners are encouraged to consider the needs of individuals, groups, organizations, and populations. As OTs continue to expand into community-based services, more clients will be exposed to the value of structured occupation for promoting health and wellness for older adults.

In conclusion, we hope OT practitioners will enable all our clients to reach 100 years in good health and living productively. Happy birthday, AOTA: 1917-2017 (Figure 15-1)!

References

American Occupational Therapy Association. (2007). AOTA's Centennial Vision and executive summary. *American Journal of Occupational Therapy, 61*, 613-614. Retrieved from http://dx.doi.org/10.5014/ajot.61.613.

American Occupational Therapy Association. (2014). The occupational therapy practice framework: Domain and process (3rd ed.), *American Journal of Occupational Therapy, 68*, S1-S48.

Edwards, L. (2013). *In the kingdom of the sick: A social history of chronic illness in America.* New York: Walker & Company.

Ellison, J. S., Hanson, P. C., & Schmidt, J. L. (2013). Journey of leadership, steps for a meaningful career. *OT Practice, 18*, CE1-CE7.

Glennon, T.J. (2012). Starting a private practice: The first steps. *OT Practice, 17*, 12-15.

Harmon, S. (2014). Entrepreneurial options: Steps to consider in starting a private practice. *OT Practice, 19*, 8-11.

Appendix I

Methodology for the
Qualitative Productive Aging Study

Karen C. Macdonald, PhD, OTR/L

This appendix describes the complete process of creating a textbook of this type. Original research was designed and completed using qualitative methodology. As authors, we wished to describe in complete detail the many steps involved. The AOTA (2007) Centennial Vision encourages a client-centered focus and promotes evidence and occupation-based practice and recommends research conducted by OTs. We decided to base this textbook on those considerations. The following is a description of the process involved from research design to analysis, to application to literature and clinical practice, and to final synthesis into emergent theory. We hope this may encourage readers to appreciate the depth of this method of inquiry and perhaps to consider attempting qualitative methodology in relation to their own topic of interest. Details about the publishing process are also included as a guide for readers who may be our OT authors of the future.

Marli Cole was contacted by the editors at SLACK Incorporated in 2011 to explore the possibility of a need for a current textbook on the topic of productive aging. The intent was not to update existing literature that explores gerontological conditions and related intervention exclusively. This text would include some of that content, but also broaden the scope, including group populations and community models of service delivery. Initial ideas included recognizing the issues and needs for modern day senior citizens who are living longer, with varied lifestyles, beliefs, and approaches to health care.

Marli contacted me to be coauthor. We submitted a preliminary proposal and table of contents that was reviewed by SLACK Incorporated's editors. They offered helpful comments, critique, and suggestions, and supported the current need for a book of this type. A contract was signed with a 2-year deadline for final manuscript submission. As we continued with preliminary thoughts and ideas, we were asked to submit suggestions for a cover design to be used for marketing. As creative OTs, we enjoyed the process of debating color use, representational graphics, and spatial considerations for the elements of the book cover. To represent active seniors, we created silhouettes of them engaged in a range of meaningful occupations. We chose red, white, and blue to denote traditional American values and culture. The publisher's experts adapted several versions until we were all pleased with the results.

RESEARCH DESIGN

From the beginning, we decided to create and conduct an original study, wishing to explore the actual subjective perspectives of individuals currently experiencing productive aging as retirees. How do they do it? What are their secrets? As we discussed the most appropriate means of inquiry, we decided on qualitative methodology. The rationale for this was based on a wish to study a group with in-depth interview questions and to explore their unique personal perspectives using a naturalistic format, studying the individuals "as is" (i.e., with no introduction of variables or comparisons), as would be the basis of other types of research.

Heaton (2004) reviews how all qualitative inquiry seeks to see through the eyes of participants, describes their social

Cole MB, Macdonald KC.
Productive Aging: An Occupational Perspective (pp 253-261).
© 2015 Taylor & Francis Group.

setting, and describes their creative behavior and events in their current historical and social context. Although qualitative methodology may also include observation of behavior over time, we limited our study to interviews. A sample introduction was written as a means to begin to "frame" the boundaries of our topic, which we knew to be huge in its holistic considerations. In determining the relevance of a topic and development of a research question, Marshall and Rossman (1995) proposed considering the larger need for the study, and the researcher's skills and practical ability to design and complete the project. Qualitative studies are time- and thought-consuming in their many intensive steps. The researcher should be able to justify the usefulness of the research and demonstrate compliance in the conceptual framework of the project's design. This includes clear formulation of the problem and its significance, focus, and limitations. Many skills—scholarly, technological, and interpersonal—are required.

In January 2012, the research design process continued. We selected a semi-structured interview format, meaning using a limited number of open-ended questions. We began to narrow our inquiry into research questions: What are the "secrets to success" for retired seniors who are representative of productive or successful aging? Who are these people what skill/resources do they have? By retired, we meant people who were no longer employed in their career jobs, even though some chose to continue working for pay.

A great deal of thought and planning went into the design of the interviews. Considerations were discussed, such as inclusion and exclusion criteria, how to document for identifying information and demographics, and sample questions.

Initial planning also included careful planning for gaining entrée, including initiating contact with individuals, description of the nature of the project, informed consent issues, and documentation systems for data collection. Dworkin et al. (1981) suggested careful attention to respecting "The use of persons as a means…" (p. 247) with avoidance of "…manipulation, deception, exploitation and coercion" (p. 247). Along with standard professional awareness of ethical and moral concerns, provisions should be made to respect and protect the autonomy of participants. Data analysis is an ongoing process of construction and deconstruction (Altheide & Johnson, 1994). The researcher considers relationships with the participants' culture, place in history, and personal meanings for behavior, habits, and rituals. Because the researcher's own perspective influences interpretation, care needs to be taken to objectify personal biases or viewpoints.

Ethical considerations are essential in the design of behavioral research (Cozby, 2001). These are varied and include protection from deception, harm, or stress and defining privacy and confidentiality expectations. The researcher is expected to demonstrate professionalism by honoring commitments, complying with any rules or laws regarding human subjects, and minimizing invasiveness into the participants' lives.

Patten (1998) proposes that researchers identify their own theoretical predisposition and make explicit their own paradigms. Zou et al. (2013) provide details of the full process of a qualitative study. Findings may be validated via interpretation by additional experienced researchers, inclusion of a participatory design, and a large, diverse sample size.

Before the research began, we also needed to plan for initial data analysis (which would begin as soon as data collection was started) and make decisions about protecting our own objectivity (purposely put a "hold" on review of literature until we had the bulk of our own data collected). Although we started with some early theoretical frameworks, such as modern gerontology and developmental and historical perspectives, the health care literature was saved for later aspects of triangulation during data analysis. Mitchell (1993) explains that a researcher is never truly autonomous or self-directed. Even the choice of topic is somehow directed by personal interest and experience. Resulting design and findings are, in many ways, inseparable from personal viewpoints and background influences.

We began files on our own personal immersion on the topic, including jotting down thoughts, ideas, and questions that would come to mind about the project or related to our own extensive personal and professional experiences working with seniors. This included a list of "words" that might be representative of a concept to investigate at a later date, in an interview, or in literature search, such as "resourcefulness." "Hunches" were identified, as we jotted down things that we might expect to discover in the course of our research and perhaps to explore if not raised by participants (e.g., relationships with neighbors). Additionally, we collected any relevant literature or information for future consideration, gathering community pamphlets, newspaper articles, and quotes from personal communication separate from the interviews. We attended public forums and lectures when the topic seemed relevant to our inquiry.

We created a draft of the interview and conducted preliminary fieldwork with one individual to assess the effectiveness of our form and questions, gauge the time needed for the interview, and determine anything to add or subtract from our form. Feedback from that participant helped to clarify some of the elements of the interview.

Before scheduling interviews, a cover letter was created. This included a formal invitation to participate, description of the project, statement of confidentiality, "no harm" clause, commitment of participant, and request for signature for publication and photograph use. Contact information for the researchers was provided. A space for completion of their signature and date was provided to establish their consent.

To identify and select potential participants, we conducted purposive sampling—meaning participants were

TABLE AI-1
INTERVIEW QUESTIONS USED FOR PRODUCTIVE AGING STUDY
CURRENT PRODUCTIVE OCCUPATIONS: PLEASE CIRCLE ALL THAT APPLY Self-manager, home manager, paid worker, volunteer, caregiver, lifelong learner
BACKGROUND INFORMATION • Age, productive occupations, work history • Living arrangement, family information • Leisure interests • Describe a typical day
QUESTIONS • We've already identified you as a successful ager. How do you do it? What are your secrets? • Tell me about the occupations/activities you are currently engaged in. • What are your social identities? What roles do you play in family, work, community, and social groups? • What are your challenges and barriers to being productive? • How do your home and outside environments affect your ability to participate? • What recommendations do you have for others about aging productively? • How would you define productive aging in your own words?
Created by M. B. Cole & K. C. Macdonald, 2015.

purposely selected—because we knew they met our initial criteria for inclusion. Inclusionary criteria consisted of retired, community dwelling individuals known by the authors to be active seniors who self-identified three of six productive roles/occupations:

- Self-manager
- Home manager
- Caregiver
- Volunteer
- Paid worker
- Student/lifelong learner

Participants were neither included nor excluded because of the presence of any health condition. We then realized that the initial group of individuals contacted was rather homogeneous for age and background. We experiences a "snowball" effect of people who had heard about our study and were eagerly volunteering to participate. All participants were known, at least somewhat, by one of the authors. We initially anticipated in-depth interviews for five to eight individuals. As we added for diversity, including gender, marital status, socioeconomic status, and geography, the total number of participants reached 40! Although this level of diversity is not required for qualitative analysis, we were eager to explore as many perspectives as possible. Although

more people kept volunteering, we stopped at 40, anticipating the extensiveness of the analysis. After an 8-month period, from January through August 2012, redundancy of findings was also occurring. This represented "saturation" of findings, indicating a need to conclude the interviewing process, known as "exiting the field" (Table AI-1).

After beginning the interviews, we revised the long form, adding specific entries for background information such as roles and describing a typical day. This was followed by the specific open-ended questions that allowed for prompting and cuing to gather further detail. We eventually saw a need for a short form because a few individuals were limited in time or ability to manage the full interview. We created and used a short form for them when needed.

DATA COLLECTION

Beginning in January 2012, over an 8-month period, each author independently scheduled and conducted 20 interviews, for a total of 40 participants. The majority were conducted in person, usually at the participant's home. Some were completed online or by telephone at the participant's request or due to location.

As the results of the interviews were becoming available, we developed a uniform technique for data collection: hard copies of consent and interview forms were used, and were taken notes by hand (not recorded). Throughout, we needed to evaluate how we were doing, adapt procedures, and continually remind ourselves of the primary focus and purpose of the study. This became a repeated issue because the findings were so extensive, leading to many other areas that would be tempting to explore in detail.

We noticed a trend in which extensive information was provided during the introductory section of identifying information, especially when asked to describe a typical day. Therefore, a great deal of material was provided before the actual semi-structured interview was initiated. As the interview proceeded, we were prepared to offer prompts or cues as needed if short answers had been provided. For example, "Could you tell me more about _____?"

Each interview took approximately 45 to 90 minutes. Photographs with "in action" poses were taken. Some participants had anticipated and prepared formal or informal notes to make sure they expressed what they wished to about the topic. As we began initial data analysis, we would mention early findings and response trends of earlier participants, and ask a subsequent participant's opinion.

Throughout the process, many participants appeared eager to be involved, stated that there is a strong need for a book of this type; they continued to ask for updates about progress and when they might be able to buy a copy. Some other participants seemed to view their participation as a private single event and did not ever raise it in conversation again when in contact with the authors for other occasions.

The qualitative interview is intended to be conversational, flexible, and purposeful (Mason, 2002). Active engagement is established by the interviewer. As the exploration of the topic continues, many abstract topics may arise, such as ideas, values, beliefs, and attitudes. Because responses are dynamic and contextual, the researcher explores specifics vs. generalities. Determination must be made about the "face value" of replies as opposed to representational or other significance. Because qualitative research is semi-structured by nature, participants may bring up a tangential or related topic. This may open up additional avenues for exploration/investigation.

Mitchell and Jolley (2007) address issues of construct validity, especially regarding what may be observed or inferred. Psychological constructs are described as characteristics of an individual that can be directly observed, including traits, intentions, and abilities. Assigned interpretations need to be carefully reviewed for accuracy. As the process proceeds, the researcher and participant develop an interdependency (Higgher, 2001). Together, they are illuminating a topic and constructing a meaning in the process of seeking a fuller understanding of a topic. Responses rarely reflect opinions at that moment in time and could fluctuate with changing circumstances.

DATA ANALYSIS

In qualitative methodology, data analysis begins as soon as interviews are completed and continues throughout all interviews and afterward. Findings become categorized in progressive attempts at sorting data into meaningful themes. This was especially challenging due to the large number of participants and the rich material each individual provided. Fielding and Fielding (1986) propose that interviews are considered higher in "validity" because it represents the participants' views, not the observers' interpretation. The researcher carries a basic assumption that the informants are reliable in their reporting verification.

The researcher needs to be warned of contrived consistency of findings between participants stemming from highlighting certain topic areas and avoiding others. In reality, the researchers are inferring similarities until further investigation.

The authors would meet weekly and read the results of an interview aloud while the other took notes, highlighting themes. We marked outstanding direct quotes so that they could be interspersed within the narrative of the book as the text developed. Together, we identified outstanding themes, trends, and similarities. As time went by, we noticed some "expected" content to be missing, or gaps in findings that were obvious by their omission.

Techniques of constant comparative analysis were used throughout. This refers to a system of early coding by sorting initial data into categories and themes. We began to use the OTPF Domain as a holistic conceptual model for organizing some data, especially related to ADLs and IADLs. Early literature review was related to developmental, adaptive, and aging theories, including the Third Age.

Concept mapping was used, creating diagrams and outlines on large flip chart sheets of paper. Color coding was used for themes as they became apparent. By creating bubbles to represent concept areas, three preliminary overlapping themes emerged:

1. Ability

2. Activity

3. Attitude

We had great difficulty "dividing" and assigning many topics to a category because the meaning was contextual to the participant. For example, a passion for tennis could be referred to as an ability that is maintained by ongoing gym attendance when off court; the activity of tennis could have meaning as a leisure or exercise or social networking goals; or an attitude as related to methods for how to self-motivate for participation even when experiencing a bad day.

At times we returned to our initial hunches, preconceived notions, and possible biases based on our own personal and professional experiences with older adults. To maintain a sensitive level of objectivity, qualitative methodology refers to *trustworthiness* (similar to reliability) and *triangulation* (parallel to validity in quantitative designs). Myrdal (1970) states that biases in social science research always exist, even with every effort for "...keeping to the facts" (p. 17). The researcher makes choices in the research intent, development, and interpretation. These choices are inevitably influenced by apparent and nonapparent influences, including personal, professional, cultural, and political influences. The suggestion is to identify and make explicit influences of research design, analysis, and presentation of findings.

Creating meaning from qualitative data initially focuses on recognition of the single participant viewpoints. Barber (2006) stresses that understanding of the participant needs to consider forces that contributed to their perspectives. However, an individual's personal meaning cannot be separated out from relationships to their personal background, society, and their fiscal world. Therefore, an argument may be made that no individual acts alone from personally unique motives. Attention to this perspective reminds the researcher that inferences drawn as findings common between participants reflect the forces of multiple realities and priorities.

Trustworthiness occurred as we checked back at the end of interviews and, as they proceeded, asked a new participant to comment on our emerging findings. Triangulation took place through ongoing literature review to support or contrast with our findings, as well as forms of peer debriefing. An example of the latter was contacted for two sessions at a local Toastmasters International meeting. The group was asked to identify a "successful senior" in writing and list the attributes that contribute to their skills for a happy and healthy life. The group members confirmed the exact topics that we had been identifying as themes.

We continued to review, summarize more comprehensively, and use funneling as we went further into analysis and synthesis. *Funneling* refers to the management of data by means of inductive reasoning. Vast amounts of general information, in small discrete pieces of data, are clustered for shared elements. This leads to a narrowing down as content areas become grouped and labeled due to similar characteristics.

In qualitative research design, Lincoln and Guba (1985) explain the parallel to quantitative research's concepts of reliability and validity. Instead, in naturalistic inquiry, terms such as credibility, generalizability, transferability, dependability, triangulation, and conformability are used, along with confirmability. In a naturalistic paradigm, multiple realities are considered and constructed in a holistic manner (Higgs, in Byrne-Armstrong et al., 2001). Findings lead to hypotheses, which due to their descriptive nature are not designed to define a cause and effect. Instead, through the interactions' relationship with the researcher, findings are identified true to that particular setting and temporal context.

As themes developed and changed with further results of interviews, we saw a need to revise the original table of contents, which was approved by the publisher. The authors determined systems for dividing the content into chapters and determined individual responsibilities (Table AI-2).

The authors engaged in the very lengthy process of transcribing answers to interview questions. We devised a template system for categorizing their quotes into content areas for easier access when selecting quotes for specific chapters.

The final interview was completed in August 2012. Follow-up letters were sent to each participant thanking them for their participation and informing them of the early findings.

MEANWHILE

This section is included to demonstrate the vast amount of opportunities available to OTs. Both authors enjoy participation in lecturing, teaching, research, and writing. We received a Call for Papers from the Gerontological Society of America and submitted a proposal for a Poster Session based on our findings. In preparation for that San Diego event in November 2012, we need to complete a higher level of analysis and begin with the development of initial findings. The conference was an excellent opportunity to share our interests with an international and interdisciplinary audience. Many commented that the findings were pragmatic and very current to today's aging population.

Revised representative themes were:

- Self-management
- Social connections

The 4x8-ft poster was designed, including review of literature, method, initial conclusions, and application to practice. Other preparation included handouts and business cards.

Overlapping with this, the American Occupational Therapy Association had a Call for Papers, and we were fortunate to receive notice of acceptance. We continued to develop our findings into representational themes, appropriate to an OT audience for April 2013. By then, an additional theme of self-fulfilling activities had emerged, representing many meaningful occupations that had been embedded in the first two themes. The final three themes were as follows:

- Self-management
- Social connections
- Self-fulfilling activities

In addition, we presented a poster session for the World Federation of Occupational Therapy conference in Yokohama, Japan; in June 2014 (Figure AI-1).

As months passed, we allowed for some preparation time and for some "time off" to permit some needed reflection

TABLE AI-2	
PARTICIPANT DEMOGRAPHICS	
INCLUSIONARY CRITERIA	**AGES: RANGED FROM 54 TO 98**

• Retired
• Community dwelling
• Known by author to be an "active senior"
• Self-identified three of six roles:
  1. Self-manager   40
  2. Home manager   38
  3. Caregiver   13
  4. Volunteer   28
  5. Paid Worker   13
  6. Student   18
	• 50 to 55 1
	• 56 to 60 1
	• 61 to 65 4
	• 66 to 70 9
	• 71 to 75 5
	• 76 to 80 7
	• 81 to 85 3
	• 86 to 90 7
	• 91 to 95 2
	• 96 to 100 1

MARITAL STATUS	**EDUCATION**
• Married 15 • Widowed 14* • Divorced 5* • Single 6* *Of the above 25 unmarried individuals, 9 currently considered themselves in a committed long-term relationship.	• 1 High school not completed • 9 High school diploma • 6 Associate's degree • 10 Bachelor's degree • 11 Master's degree • 3 Doctorate
AREA OF RESIDENCE	**ETHNICITY**
• 26 suburban • 7 urban • 7 rural • 28 Connecticut • 12 out of state (New York, New Jersey, New Hampshire, Georgia, Florida, Washington)	• 37 Caucasian • 1 African American • 1 Latino • 1 Asian
SPIRITUAL	**GENDER MALE 13 FEMALE 27**
• 19 Protestant • 10 Catholic • 5 Jewish • 6 Other* *Identified self as "spiritual but not religious," Buddhist, agnostic.	Sexual Orientation—Some diversity was known to researchers for three individuals but was not mentioned in the course of the interview. Socioeconomic Status—Middle to upper middle class

and renewal after the intense year of research and analysis. We then felt that some time away from the study led to a clearer view of "the whole," as well as the sum of the parts.

In February 2013, data analysis continued, with a final "wrap up" contact with the participants, which represented "exiting the field." We felt a need for a final step triangulation and member checking of trustworthiness, and therefore devised a cover letter that explained our progress to date. This included research findings and sharing the experience of the GSA conference. On a separate page, we asked for feedback related to nearly completed findings. The format was sections for open-ended comments: agree/disagree/other comments. We included a self-addressed, stamped envelope and asked for return by March 1. We were amazed at the immediate responses. This reinforced our discoveries of the shared traits of these responsible, interested, committed, and "take action" men and women. They also included many personal comments of encouragement and belief that this book would be beneficial to both students and seniors who wish to understand approaches for productive living. These results were also transcribed and coded for themes. At this point, we were discovering a redundancy in findings, which signified what is known as *saturation*, which signals the conclusion of data gathering.

Figure AI-1. Gerontology Society of America poster session.

DATA SYNTHESIS

As we completed data analysis by the end of April 2013, we began serious planning for the writing of the manuscript, with a first draft due at the end of November 2013. *Data synthesis* refers to the consolidation of all analysis and transforming it to an emergent or grounded theory. In qualitative methodology, the findings may end with the data collection and posing of hypotheses for further inquiry for theory development, but we believed that our findings were solid evidence for new theory development.

Many final loose ends were completed in preparation for the writing of the text phase of our project. We began to communicate via Skype. We needed to determine ways to protect confidentiality through pseudonyms. We decided to use a few full case studies to get a complete perspective of select individuals. We decided to contact selected colleagues to offer their professional insights through "Expert's Experience" Sections. We continued to revise chapter responsibilities. We anticipated writing the body of the book and then, when reflecting upon the completed results of interviews, conducting the literature search, and reflecting on our personal and professional experiences, a new theory to summarize the entire text was developed.

Qualitative research is exciting and allows the researcher to explore the "real" world of the participant's views and experiences. The process is lengthy and requires intense planning and prolonged involvement with interviews and analysis. Because it is so client-centered in exploring unique personal perspectives of individuals, it is an excellent method for OTs to consider to investigate many aspects of human performance.

FINAL PARTICIPANT FEEDBACK

The responses from final contact with participants are summarized below and represent the "exiting of the field" with participants. For the reader, this will serve as an introduction to how our participants expressed themselves. Most made reference to concurring with our findings and added some reinforcing comments. Many stated that the summarized results were thorough and relevant. Assorted examples of comments agreed with stated results.

Comments on self-management:

- Self-management is a must for productive aging. Continued pursuits are important whether through learning, activities, or volunteering. (Signian)

- With a new diagnosis (of a progressive condition) it challenges my ability to manage the various compartments of my life. It will continue to change my self-reliance as my skills change and I become more dependent. (Pearl)

- It is all about a perspective of reasonableness, hopefulness, and rewarding oneself with self-appreciation. Motivation has to be fed. (Mildred)

- To have a successful retirement, you need a roadmap for success. (Signian)

- Flexibility is most important. (June)

Comments related to social connections:

- It is a must to plan for retirement and to maintain or develop social contacts. (Ken)

- The relevance of different roles would increase or decrease depending on the individual. (Bob C.)

- I find it important to remember internalized messages from my youth—minimize your own needs (challenges) and serve others. (Mildred)

Comments related to self-fulfilling activities:

- Lifelong learning is especially important and also leads to increased social contacts. (Johanna)

- Activities give me purpose, help me to maintain interests, and keep my mind sharp. (Jim)

- Self-fulfillment comes from leading a satisfied lifestyle at a comfortable pace. (Kenny)

- Continue to be curious, know how to manage money, be involved with the computer and classes. Keep your interests and activities. (Peggie & Jack)

Under "further comments," participants wrote the following additional thoughts:

- It all boils down to selfhood. I define that as being aware of taking care of oneself...house, cooking that is done for health, and exercise. It is important to "give back" by volunteering. People need to keep and find friendships, varied. (Betty U.)

- We need information on selecting and monitoring health care agents, attorneys, and service people. "Family" is not always best. (Gloria)

- Emphasize under self-fulfilling, group exercise, concerts, movie outings with others, board games, cards, dancing, community education classes. Under social connections, include church groups, choir, church committees, and political activities. (Peggie and Jack)

- One needs to transform and modify former roles into scaled down but similar things. Grandparenting is a special joy. (Pearl)

- For self-management, it is a planned lifestyle. This is not automatic, it is developmental and trial and error. (Vi)

- For self-fulfillment it is a collaboration, especially with family involvement and support. (Valnere)

- For social networks, "family, family, family" starts networks. (Valnere)

- Self-management is fine, but it is OK to get help. There are so many city, state, and federal agencies. Or you can barter with others for goods and services with an honor code. (Geno)

- Everything is a developmental process, whether it is skills and abilities or activities. (Vi)

- Simple—follow diet, have interests, and walk—live fully and creatively. (Bob M.)

- Balance everything for a healthy and wholesome life. (Dave)

- Maintain your contacts near and far. Volunteer or whatever to keep structure in your life. Be mindful of your body—how you eat and exercise. (Mary)

- As your network of friends decreases, it becomes more important to have family ties. (Vi)

Participants suggested the following areas they believed need inclusion or further emphasis:

- Include more on health routines. (Jim M.)

- Increase information on role of family as supportive. (Vi)

- More needed on diet and exercise. People need to broaden their health consciousness and observe for balance—what is repetition or omission. (Bob C.)

- Add more about various and common pitfalls to aging and agencies that could provide aid. (Nan)

- On self-fulfillment, the only benefit is personal to relax and relieve tension. It is not benefiting my fellow human beings. As my mother said, getting old stinks! The only benefit is beating the alternative. (Jim M.)

- Include the importance of music and travel. (Judi)

- Frugality! (Ray)

- Involvement with job, friends and family. Continuing with activities such as yoga, etc., keeps my mind in the positive direction. I need to be successful. (Johanna)

These comments represented their ongoing interest in the Productive Aging study and commitment to verifying the emerging findings. They served as a helpful summary of priority perspectives as the data gathering with participants concluded, and they reinforced many findings and suggested additional topics for consideration. These final results helped in designing the structure and content of the chapters of Section II and contributed to the foundation of emergent theory as the process of qualitative research continued.

JOURNAL ENTRY (K. M.)

When I decided on a qualitative design for my doctoral dissertation to fulfill the requirements for a Ph.D. in OT at New York University in 1987, qualitative research was not well known/accepted/used. Although not a foreign approach, those using qualitative methodology felt a need to justify the choice. Quantitative or experimental designs were deemed more "scientific" with respected norms for reliability and validity. Qualitative research was newer on the scene, and seemed ideal to me for social sciences. I loved everything about it! Really exploring a topic, from the perspectives of people who were actually living the described experiences. Intentionally not manipulating or modifying behaviors in any way, but analyzing their real world. Now, 35 years later, extensive research that occurred for this textbook showed a mushrooming of respect, acceptance, and uses of qualitative/naturalistic/ethnographic designs. Findings have been useful in building the body of knowledge about performance, myriad activities, and environmental and interpersonal relationships. Piece by piece, foundations to understand the meaning of health value participation in occupations has been building.

SUMMARY

This chapter reviewed the process of designing, developing, and implementing an original research project that we labeled the Productive Aging Study. A qualitative design was used, with 40 retired older adults participating in semi-structured interviews. Details of the process are shared for the reader's understanding of the many layers of analysis and interpretation involved in qualitative methodology. Data analysis includes the researcher's coding of data and comparison with related literature. Results were shared with the participants for their additional feedback and input for the three themes: self-management, social connections, and self-fulfilling activities.

The remaining chapters in Section II describe findings in the three main theme areas. The results of these findings are then synthesized in Chapter 14, as the basis for a proposed grounded theory.

Learning Activity 113

Discuss the need for evidence-based research in geriatric OT practice.

1. Describe the pros and cons of qualitative vs. quantitative research methods related to an older adult population.

2. Distinguish how issues of "reliability" and "validity" are addressed in both experimental and naturalistic designs of research.

3. Would you have an interest in participating in clinical research as a practicing clinician? Why or why not?

4. After reading this chapter, can you identify any way in which you would have designed the research project differently?

5. Conduct an interview (10 to 15 minutes long) with a "productive" older adult who is retired, and ask about his or her "secrets of success." Write a one-page summary with three paragraphs. One is a description of the individual and the setting. Two is a summary of findings. Three is a statement of how this type of experience felt to you.

6. Find examples to aid in understanding the difference between deductive and inductive reasoning.

7. Through role play, practice the technique of "gaining entrée," which represents a researcher's initial contacts with a potential participant. This would include explaining who you are, your goals and methods, as well as expectations of their participation.

8. Explain the difference between random and purposive sampling. Why is the latter indicated in qualitative inquiry?

9. Discuss issues of confidentiality in respect to the participants. How could this be defined to them? How would you insure that their privacy is respected as defined by the parameters of a study?

REFERENCES

Altheide, D. L., & Johnson, J. M. (1994). Criteria for assessing interpretive validity in qualitative research. In N. K. Denzin & Y. S. Lincoln (Eds.) *Handbook of qualitative research*. Thousand Oaks, CA: Sage Publications.

American Occupational Therapy Association (AOTA). (2007). AOTA's Centennial Vision and executive summary. *American Journal of Occupational Therapy, 61*, 613-614.

Barber, M. D. (2006). Occupational science and the first-person perspective. *Journal of Occupational Science, 13*, 94-96.

Cozby, P. C. (2001). *Methods in behavioral research* (7th ed.). Mountain View, CA: Mayfield Publishing Co.

Dworkin, G. (1982). Must subjects be objects? In T. L. Beauchamp, R. R. Faden, R. J. Wallace, & L. Walters (Eds.). *Ethical issues in social science research* (p. 246). Baltimore, MD: Johns Hopkins University Press.

Fielding, N. G., & Fielding, J. L. (1986). *Linking data*. Beverly Hills, CA: Sage Publications.

Heaton, J. (2004). *Reworking qualitative data*. Thousand Oaks, CA: Sage Publications.

Higgs, J. (2001). Charting standpoints in qualitative research. In H. Byrne-Armstrong, J. Higgs, & D. Horsfall (Eds.). *Critical moments in qualitative research* (pp. 44-67). Woburn, MA: Butterworth-Heinemann.

Lincoln, Y. S., & Guba, E. G. (1985). *Naturalistic inquiry*. Newbury Park, CA: Sage Publications.

Marshall, C., & Rossman, G. B. (1995). *Designing qualitative research* (2nd ed.). Thousand Oaks, CA: Sage Publications.

Mason, J. (2002). In T. May (Ed.). *Qualitative research in action*. Thousand Oaks, CA: Sage Publications.

Mitchell, M. C., & Jolley, J. M. (2007). *Research design explained* (6th ed.). Belmont, CA: Thomson Higher Education.

Mitchell, R. G. (1993). *Secrecy and fieldwork*. Newbury Park, CA: Sage Publications.

Myrdal, G. (1970). *Objectivity in social research*. London, UK: Gerald Duckworth & Co, Ltd.

Patton, M. Q. (1980). *Qualitative evaluation methods*. Beverly Hills, CA: Sage Publications.

Zou, H., Li, Z., Nolan, M., Wang, H., & Hu, L. (2013). Self-management among Chinese people with schizophrenia and their caregivers: A qualitative study. *Archives of Psychiatric Nursing, 27*, 42-53.

Appendix II

Participant Thumbnail Sketches

The following list represents brief identifying facts about participants in the Productive Aging Study, whose photographs and perspectives appear throughout this book. The information included was voluntarily provided to the authors at the time of the first interview. Some examples given in the text portray them as older, since the writing has occurred over almost three years. The age range is 54 to 98 years, with an average of 76 years.

Bob M.—86, high school diploma (HS), veteran, married, 3 children (c), 3 grandchildren (gc), 1 great-grandchild (ggc).
> Private house, suburban Connecticut (CT).
> Widowed 2008, remarried 2010.
> Retired ice cream executive, food oil manager.
> Scottish, German Protestant.

Ann—73, Bachelor of Science (BS) in education, Master of Arts in reading education, 4 c, 5 gc, 1 ggc due.
> Private house, suburb CT.
> Widowed 2006, remarried 2010.
> Retired Kindergarten teacher.
> French, Roman Catholic.

Nancy—63, HS, married, 1 c, 1 gc.
> Private house, CT.
> Retired hairdresser.
> Scottish, Protestant.

Geno—70, Associate of Science (AS), legal assistant, 3 c, 4 gc.
> Private house, urban CT.
> Divorced, remarried 1993.
> Retired mechanical designer.
> Italian, Catholic.

Mary V.—69, licensed practical nurses school, 3 c, 3 gc.
> Private house, suburban CT. Son and his family live with her.
> Widowed 2006.
> Nurse, geriatrics. Current part time work, private duty.
> Raised Catholic, now Protestant.

Maxine—83, HS, 2 c, 4 gc, 4 ggc.
> Condo with significant other (SO), suburban CT.
> Married and widowed. Married and divorced.
> Retired, office worker, travel agent.
> Grew up in West Virginia, German, Protestant.

Linval—66, HS, 6 c, 15 gc, 1 ggc.
> Condo, urban CT.
> Married, lives with spouse.
> Stock clerk, maintenance to head custodian, church custodian, just retired. Continues with part time work and handy man jobs.
> Jamaican, Christian.

Cole MB, Macdonald KC.
Productive Aging: An Occupational Perspective (pp 263-265).
© 2015 Taylor & Francis Group.

Judi—69, HS and some college, 3 c, 4 gc.
   Private house, suburban CT. Lives alone.
   Divorced.
   Retired, homemaker, assistant teacher, office work.
   Current part time baby sitting or house sitting.
   Irish/Scottish/English, Protestant.

Vi—83, Master of social work, 4 c, 10 gc.
   Private house, suburban CT. Lives alone.
   Widow.
   Retired social worker (3 years) and homemaker.
   Japanese, Protestant.

Jim—76, BS in marketing, 1 c.
   Private house, urban CT.
   Married.
   Retired businessman, now part time in grocery stores.
   Irish, Catholic.

Ray—86, HS dropout, veteran, then junior college (JC). 1 c, 2 gc.
   Townhouse, urban CT.
   Divorced. Spends all but night with SO.
   Retired, quality assurance.
   Protestant.

Marylyn—93, BS and Master of Science (MS) in teaching, 6th year. 3 c, 3 gc, 8 ggc.
   Private house, suburban CT.
   Widow. Daughter lives with her.
   Retired special education teacher.
   Grew up in the Midwest, Protestant.

Alice—86, HS, 2 years of business school, 3 c, 2 gc.
   Condo, suburban CT.
   Widow, lives alone.
   Retired school secretary.
   Grew up in the Midwest, Protestant.

Phyllis—83, JC, 2 c, 2 gc.
   Condo, suburban CT.
   Widow. Lives alone.
   Retired at 67, executive secretary. "I always worked."
   Jewish.

Ellen—54, BS in occupational therapy (OT), MS in Gerontology. No children.
   Senior housing, private unit, Denver, Colorado (CO).
   Divorced, lives with SO.
   Retired occupational therapist.
   Jewish.

Nan—60, MS in health promotion/disease prevention, no c.
   Senior housing, private unit, Denver, CO.
   Single, lives with SO.
   Retired therapeutic recreation director.
   German.

Suzy—98, 9th grade, 1 c, 3 gc, 3 ggc.
   Private house, urban CT
   Widow, lives alone.
   Retired "domestic engineer."
   Italian, Catholic.

Nettie—73. Nursing school, AS in gerontology, 3 c, 7 gc.
   Private house, suburban CT
   Widow for 2nd time. Lives alone.
   Retired registered nurse (RN) but works part time in agencies.
   Italian, Catholic.

Dave—87, Bachelor of engineering, veteran, 2 c, 5 gc, 4 gg.
   Condo, suburban CT.
   Married.
   Retired but works many hours consulting.
   Protestant.

Johanna—71, juris doctor attorney, elder law practice, 3 c, 5 gc.
   House, suburban CT.
   Widowed 2 years, and lived alone.
   Working full time, in treatment for ovarian cancer.
   Catholic.
   Died Nov 2013.

Malcolm—77, BS in marine engineering, Master of Business Administration (MBA), MS in electrical/computers, 1 c, 2 gc.
   House, suburban New Jersey, c and gc, ages 12 & 13, live with him.
   Retired naval officer, retired engineer/Information technologist.
   Widowed 20 years, significant other of 12 years.
   Retired, does not mention religion.

Signian—67, MS in OT, 2 c, 4 gc.
   House, suburban CT.
   Widowed 6 months, lives alone.
   Retired but teaches part time.
   Not religious, oldest of 6 siblings.

Patricia—91, Bachelor of Arts (BA) in languages, Melbourne University, 4 c, 8+ gc.
> Retirement community apartment, rural New Hampshire.
> Widowed, Episcopalian, Australian.
> Died December 2012, stroke.

Jan—70, BS in OT, widowed 13 years, 2 c, 4 gc.
> House, suburban CT, lives alone.
> Retired.
> Episcopalian.

Ken—68, Doctor of Philosophy (PhD) in zoology, marine biologist (retired professor), 2 c, 4 gc.
> House, suburban CT, lives with spouse.
> Not religious.
> Died of heart attack, March 2013.

June—71, 1 year of college, divorced many years, 3 c, gc??
> Retired executive recruiter.
> Apartment New York City (NYC), lives alone.
> Jewish, Hungarian ancestry.

Greg—69, general educational development, haircutter license age 17.
> Condo, suburban CT.
> Lives with partner of many years.
> Retired business owner (has twin sister).
> Not religious, not a gay activist, Italian.

Valnere—68, BS in OT, MBA, widowed, 1 c now deceased.
> House, suburban. CT.
> Lives alone, oldest of 4 siblings.
> Retired, Australian ancestry.
> Episcopalian but married a Catholic.

Betty—89, BA in art history, widowed, divorced, 2 c, 2 gc.
> Apartment NYC, lives alone.
> Retired, active volunteer.
> "Collapsed Jew."

Gloria—79, never married.
> Retired teacher.
> House, suburban CT, has lived with sister for 45 years.
> Catholic, Italian ancestry.

Charlie—77, BS in English, married, 1 c, 3 gc.
> House, suburban CT, lives with spouse.
> Retired freelance writer (TV comedy).
> Non-religious.

Pearl—80, PhD in English, 2 c, 4 gc.
> House, suburban CT, married, lives with spouse.
> Retired professor, teaches part time.
> Catholic, Cajun ancestry.

Mildred—86, BS in OT, divorced, 3 c, 1 gc.
> Congregate housing, rural CT, lives alone.
> Retired.
> Jewish.

Peggie—77, RN, BS in nursing, 5 c, 11 gc, 2 ggc.
> House, Seattle, Washington, married, lives with spouse.
> Retired but works part time, nurse practitioner.
> Catholic, Croatian ancestry.

Jack—79, BS degree, 5 c, 11 gc, 2 ggc.
> House, Seattle, Washington.
> Retired ship builder, human resource manager.
> Catholic.

Sue H.—65, HS (United Kingdom [UK]), married, 2 c, 2 gc.
> House, suburban CT, lives with spouse, son, and mother-in-law.
> Works church administrator 6 hrs/day.
> Episcopalian, "Englishwoman" (born in UK, married an American).

Gerry—90, HS, widowed, 3 c, 3 gc, 10 ggc.
> Condo, suburban CT, lives alone.
> Retired secretary.
> Episcopalian, Irish.

Bob C.—62, MBA, never married, girlfriend of 25 years.
> Apartment NYC, lives alone.
> Retired financial analyst/manager.
> Not religious.

Margie—64, BS in early childhood education, 4 c, 7 gc.
> House suburban, Georgia, married, lives with spouse.
> Retired, full-time caregiver of 2 gc.
> Episcopalian, Hispanic, oldest of 8 (born in Puerto Rico).

Bob T.—73, military graduate, retired Navy pilot, never married.
> Condo, Florida.
> Retired international pilot (TWA 35 years).
> Protestant, Midwestern roots, political conservative activist.

Mary D.—75, PhD in OT, never married, 4 siblings.
> House, suburban New York (now New Jersey), lives alone.
> Retired Catholic nun, retired university professor (teaches part time).
> Catholic, Irish, Italian.

Index

Printed in the United States
by Baker & Taylor Publisher Services